Back Pain Remedies For Dummies®

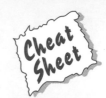

Cheat Sheet

P9-DDF-754

Checking Up on Your Doctor

Finding the right practitioner can be the key to solving your back pain problem. Before a physician or specialist treats you, do a little checking up on your own to be sure that the healthcare professional is right for you and your back pain problem. Take the following questions into the doctor's office with you to help ensure that you find the right doctor:

- ✔ What is your degree and where did you do your training?
- ✔ Are you board-certified in your specialty?
- ✔ To what medical and professional societies do you belong?
- ✔ How long have you practiced in this area?
- ✔ Do you have special training in treating back pain problems?
- ✔ Are you comfortable treating back pain problems using a conservative (non-surgical) approach?
- ✔ What percentage of the patients you see have back pain problems?

Checking Up on Your Medical Testing

If your doctor recommends that you have a medical test for your back problem, you should get answers to the following check-up questions first:

- ✔ What is the name of the test, and what do you expect to learn from it?
- ✔ Why is the test performed, and why am I being advised to have it?
- ✔ What can I expect before, during, and after the test?
- ✔ What does it mean if the test is positive or negative?
- ✔ How is the test related to developing a treatment plan for me?

Checking Up on Your Treatment

Be an active partner with your doctor in the treatment of your back problem. The following checklist helps you get the answers you need:

- ✔ Why are you recommending this treatment for me?
- ✔ What benefit should I expect, and how long will it take to determine if the treatment is working?
- ✔ Are there any possible problems that can occur with this treatment? What should I do if these occur?
- ✔ Is there any problem doing this treatment along with the other treatments I am pursuing?

...For Dummies: Bestselling Book Series for Beginners

Back Pain Remedies For Dummies®

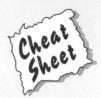
Cheat Sheet

Warning Signs That Indicate You Should See Your Doctor

Initially, you can self-manage most episodes of back pain. The following warning signs, however, may indicate more serious problems that your doctor needs to check:

- ✔ Problems with your bowel (loss of feeling), bladder (trouble with urination), sexual function (inability to get an erection for men), or numbness in your groin area
- ✔ Weakness in one or both of your legs and/or feet
- ✔ Back pain that awakens you at night that is throbbing and aching
- ✔ A serious trauma to your spine, such as a car accident or fall
- ✔ Excruciating back pain or new symptoms
- ✔ Problems with your medications, or using alcohol or other substances to manage your back pain problem

Managing a Back Attack

Try the following regime to get your back pain attack under control:

- ✔ Go to bed, but not for long: Limited bed rest (one to three days) can help calm down back pain.
- ✔ Use ice and heat: Applying ice and heat to your back can help control the symptoms and make you more comfortable.
- ✔ Use anti-inflammatory medication: Unless you have a medical reason for not taking over-the-counter anti-inflammatory medications, Advil, Aleve, Motrin, Nuprin, and other medications work very well for pain.
- ✔ Start moving around even during the bed rest phase: Limited bed rest is helpful, but you should gradually increase your activity as soon as you can. Walking is one of the best and safest exercises.
- ✔ Return to normal activity: After limited bed rest, gradually increase your activities each day until you return to your normal levels.
- ✔ Seek professional help: If you experience any of the warning signs mentioned in the preceding section get professional help. (We discuss warning signs in Chapters 5 and 21.)

If this self-management approach to your back pain doesn't provide significant relief after about one week, then you should see a doctor if you have not already done so.

Wiley, the Wiley Publishing logo, For Dummies, the Dummies Man logo, the For Dummies Bestselling Book Series logo and all related trade dress are trademarks or registered trademarks of Wiley Publishing, Inc. All other trademarks are property of their respective owners.

...For Dummies: Bestselling Book Series for Beginners

Praise for *Back Pain Remedies For Dummies*

"If you suffer from back pain like I do, it's no laughing matter. Anyone with back pain should read this book now. It will put you on the road to recovery and get you smiling again."

— Sid Caesar

"This is a tremendous book. After reading this book, you will go from being a 'Dummy' with back pain to just being a 'Dummy.' I highly recommend it . . ."

— Don Rickles

"Dr. Sinel has broad experience with a wide range of musculoskeletal pain disorders. His work is a must read for anyone suffering from one of these disorders."

— John E. Sarno, M.D, Professor, Clinical Rehabilitation Medicine, New York University School of Medicine

"This book may be more helpful than a dozen 'back specialists' — it won't keep you waiting!"

— Theodore B. Goldstein, M.D., F.A.C.S.

"In a clear and concise manner, *Back Pain Remedies For Dummies* distills the essential information needed to understand back pain basics and treatment alternatives. It provides up-to-date mind-body techniques to effectively combat most back pain. If you suffer from back pain, this book can help. Read it, use it, and get better."

— John L. Reeves II, Ph.D., past president of The American Pain Society

"Anyone who has ever sought treatment for chronic back pain knows that it can be a bewildering maze of diagnostic tests, medical jargon, and confusing treatment options. Well, no more. *Back Pain Remedies For Dummies* is like having an old friend — who also happens to be an expert in the field — to point you in the right direction. It is the simplest, most easy-to-understand back pain book on the market today, bar-none."

— Allan F. Chino, Ph.D., ABPP, and Corinne D. Davis, M.D., Las Vegas, Nevada

"Finally, a book to help patients communicate with their doctors. The authors have done an excellent job of summarizing a complicated problem so that those with back pain can make well-informed choices regarding their treatment."

— Virgil T. Wittmer, Ph.D., Clinical Psychologist, Director of Pain Rehabilitation, Brooks Rehabilitation

"The most common cause of back pain is poor resting posture — so fellow Dummies, let's get smart about the way we sit, recline, and sleep to not only end the EPIDEMIC of back pain, but also live a more healthy, active lifestyle. Read this book — you'll look and feel years younger!"

> — Dairl M. Johnson, Ex-back pain sufferer and President of Relax the Back Corporation

"*Back Pain Remedies For Dummies* cuts a clear path through the jungle of back problems and treatments. For anyone with back pain, or anyone who knows anyone with back pain, this book will set you straight on what to do."

> — Fred N. Lerner, D.C., Ph.D., F.A.C.O., Beverly Hills, California

"*Back Pain Remedies For Dummies* will equip you with the knowledge and skills to take an active role in treating and relieving your pain. Drs. Sinel and Deardorff's integrated approach will put you in control of the recovery process. Spanning the fields of medicine, rehabilitation, health psychology, and complementary medicine, this book is an invaluable resource for patients and practitioners alike."

> — Louis F. Damis, Ph.D., ABPP, Clinical Health Psychologist, Florida Hospital's Center for Rehabilitation and Sports Medicine

"The authors have provided a concise, user-friendly overview of what everyone should know to prevent and treat back discomfort."

> — Stephen H. Hochschuler, M.D., Spine Surgeon, Chairman of the Texas Back Institute

"Dr. Sinel and Dr. Deardorff have created a user-friendly reference for all those suffering from lower back pain. Clear and precise explanations, coupled with sound clinical and common sense advice make *Back Pain Remedies For Dummies* an outstanding reference."

> — Andrew J. Cole, M.D., Medical Director, The Spine Center at Overlake Medical Center, Bellevue, WA

"*Back Pain Remedies For Dummies* is an easy-to-read guidebook that educates readers on the importance of back pain prevention and intervention. The emphasis on helping readers choose practitioners among the wide range of choices available in today's healing disciplines, as well as providing clinical and insurance information, makes this book a must read for anyone interested in maintaining a healthy back."

> — Thomas F. Zenty, III, Senior Vice President, Clinical Care Services and Chief Operating Officer Cedars-Sinai Medical Center

"If you have a back problem and are considering spine surgery, read this book first."

> — J. Patrick Johnson, M.D., Neurosurgeon and Co-Director, UCLA Spine Center, Los Angeles

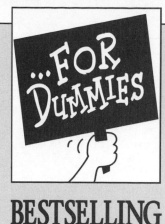 TM

References for the Rest of Us!®

BESTSELLING BOOK SERIES

Do you find that traditional reference books are overloaded with technical details and advice you'll never use? Do you postpone important life decisions because you just don't want to deal with them? Then our *For Dummies*® business and general reference book series is for you.

For Dummies business and general reference books are written for those frustrated and hard-working souls who know they aren't dumb, but find that the myriad of personal and business issues and the accompanying horror stories make them feel helpless. *For Dummies* books use a lighthearted approach, a down-to-earth style, and even cartoons and humorous icons to dispel fears and build confidence. Lighthearted but not lightweight, these books are perfect survival guides to solve your everyday personal and business problems.

Already, millions of satisfied readers agree. They have made For Dummies the #1 introductory level computer book series and a best-selling business book series. They have written asking for more. So, if you're looking for the best and easiest way to learn about business and other general reference topics, look to For Dummies to give you a helping hand.

Wiley Publishing, Inc.

5/09

BACK PAIN REMEDIES FOR DUMMIES®

by Michael S. Sinel, M.D. and
William W. Deardorff, Ph.D.

WILEY

Wiley Publishing, Inc.

Back Pain Remedies For Dummies®

Published by
Wiley Publishing, Inc.
909 Third Avenue
New York, NY 10022
www.wiley.com

Copyright © 1999 by Wiley Publishing, Inc., Indianapolis, Indiana

Published by Wiley Publishing, Inc., Indianapolis, Indiana

Published simultaneously in Canada

For general information on our other products and services or to obtain technical support, please contact our Customer Care Department within the U.S. at 800-762-2974, outside the U.S. at 317-572-3993, or fax 317-572-4002.

Wiley also publishes its books in a variety of electronic formats. Some content that appears in print may not be available in electronic books.

Library of Congress Cataloging-in-Publication Data:

Library of Congress Control Number: 99-62838

ISBN: 0-7645-5132-9

Manufactured in the United States of America

10

3B/RV/QW/QT/IN

About the Authors

Michael Sinel, M.D. is a nationally renowned back pain expert. He received his medical degree from State University of New York Downstate and then completed a residency in physical medicine and rehabilitation at New York Hospital-Cornell University Medical Center. After serving as Director of Outpatient Physical Medicine at Cedar Sinai Medical Center, he became board-certified in both physical medicine and rehabilitation and pain management.

Dr. Sinel is a co-founder of California Orthopedics and Rehabilitation (COR), a prestigious multi-specialty medical group in Beverly Hills, California. He is also an assistant clinical professor at UCLA Medical Center and attending physician with the UCLA Comprehensive Spine Center. He lectures regularly to various medical and lay audiences and is actively involved in clinical research of spinal disorders.

As a specialist in non-surgical approaches to spinal problems and pain management, Dr. Sinel has made numerous national radio and television appearances and has been quoted in The New York Times, Los Angeles Times, and Reader's Digest.

William W. Deardorff, Ph.D., ABPP received his doctorate in clinical psychology with a special emphasis in health from Washington State University after completing an internship at the University of Washington Medical School. He then completed a post-doctoral fellowship in behavioral medicine at Kaiser Permanente Medical Center in Los Angeles.

Dr. Deardorff is board-certified in clinical health psychology and specializes in the evaluation and treatment of psychological issues related to medical problems. He is a Fellow of the American Psychological Association and Past-President of the American Academy of Clinical Health Psychology. Dr. Deardorff is in practice with California Orthopedic and Rehabilitation group in Beverly Hills, California. As an assistant clinical professor at the UCLA School of Medicine, he is active in teaching and research.

Dr. Deardorff has published extensively in the area of health psychology. His previous patient guidebook, Preparing for Surgery: A Mind-Body Approach to Enhance Healing and Recovery won the Small Press Book Award in Health in 1998. He has made numerous national radio and television appearances, and has been quoted in a variety of general publications.

Dedication

Michael Sinel: To my wife, for her never-ending love and commitment. To all those who suffer from back pain, and all those who help.

William Deardorff: To my wife Janine ("not Jeanine") for her support, patience and putting up with my never-ending "projects." To my sons Paul ("Mr. P") and James ("Squeaks") for their constant encouragement in the form of the regular retort, "How many pages to go, Daddy?"

Acknowledgments

Michael Sinel: I want to thank my wife and my parents for their support and encouragement. I want to thank my first mentor, John Sarno, M.D., who taught me the strength of the mind-body connection, and my present and forever mentor and friend, Ted Goldstein, M.D., who remains the premier "spine doctor" in my eyes. Finally, I would like to thank my patients who will always be my true teachers.

William Deardorff: Aside from my family, I want to thank my close friends for their consistent support throughout the past year: Jeff and Kimberly Steinbach, Brian and Nicoli Tucker, Rick and Joanne Wilson, Ron and Gerri Day, and "Uncle" Dr. Allan F. Chino. I would also like to extend special thanks to Dr. Theodore ("Teddy") Goldstein for his friendship, support, and professional practice style.

I want to thank Brian Kramer, our project editor, for keeping me on track and on time, as well as immersing me in the ... For Dummies style. Also, thanks to Tami Booth, our executive editor, for being an excellent problem-solver and for taking the time to be sure that this book gets to the people that need it the most, the back pain sufferer.

From both authors: We would like to extend our sincerest gratitude to the many experts who made invaluable contributions to this book, insuring that the information presented is "cutting edge". First, special acknowledgments are given to the following who made major contributions to specific chapters: to Theodore Goldstein, M.D., for his contribution to the surgery chapter, to Jay Triano, D.C., Ph.D., for his contribution to the chiropractic chapter, and to Larry Payne, Ph.D. for his contribution to the yoga chapter.

We would also like to thank the following for their contributions to various parts of the book (listed in alphabetical order): Aaron Filler, M.D.; Mary Jo Ford, M.D.; Stephen Hochschuler, M.D.; Patrick Johnson, M.D.; Fred Lerner, DC, Ph.D.; Joshua Prager, M.D.; John Reeves, II, Ph.D.; Risa Sheppard; Stephen Sideroff, Ph.D.; Steven Waldman, M.D.

Lastly, we would like to thank our technical reviewers Anthony Cole, M.D. and John Reeves, II, Ph.D. for ensuring the accuracy of our information and strengthening the presentation of the material overall.

Publisher's Acknowledgments

We're proud of this book; please send us your comments through our online registration form located at www.dummies.com/register.

Some of the people who helped bring this book to market include the following:

Acquisitions and Editorial

Project Editor: Brian Kramer

Executive Editor: Tammerly Booth

Copy Editors: Christine Meloy Beck, Tamara Castleman, Kathleen Dobie, Patricia Yuu Pan, Susan Diane Smith

Technical Editors: Andrew J. Cole, M.D.; John L. Reeves, Ph.D.

Editorial Manager: Leah P. Cameron

Editorial Assistants: Beth Parlon, Alison Walthall

Special Help
    Donna Love; Larry Payne, Ph.D.; Douglas Barenburg, D.C.; Laura Johnston

Production

Project Coordinator: Regina Snyder

Layout and Graphics: Linda M. Boyer, Laura Carpenter, Angela F. Hunckler, David McKelvey, Anna Rohrer, Brent Savage, Janet Seib, Michael A. Sullivan, Brian Torwelle

Illustrator: Kathryn Born

Photos: Custom Medical Stock Photo (page 81); P. Saluotos/Custom Medical Stock Photo (page 84); M. Moreland/Custom Medical Stock Photo (page 189)

Proofreaders: Kelli Botta, Laura L. Bowman, Betty Kish, Nancy Price, Marianne Santy, Rebecca Senninger

Indexer: Steve Rath

Publishing and Editorial for Consumer Dummies
    Diane Graves Steele, Vice President and Publisher, Consumer Dummies
    Joyce Pepple, Acquisitions Director, Consumer Dummies
    Kristin A. Cocks, Product Development Director, Consumer Dummies
    Michael Spring, Vice President and Publisher, Travel
    Brice Gosnell, Publishing Director, Travel
    Suzanne Jannetta, Editorial Director, Travel

Publishing for Technology Dummies
    Richard Swadley, Vice President and Executive Group Publisher
    Andy Cummings, Vice President and Publisher

Composition Services
    Gerry Fahey, Vice President of Production Services
    Debbie Stailey, Director of Composition Services

Contents at a Glance

Cartoons at a Glance

By Rich Tennant

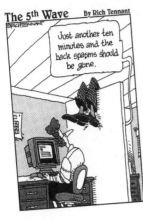

page 7

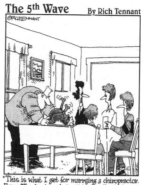

page 133

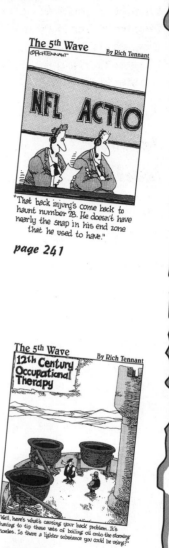

page 241

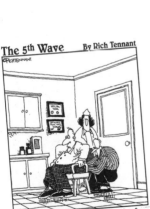

page 65

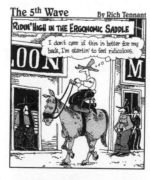

page 283

page 193

Cartoon Information:
Fax: 978-546-7747
E-Mail: richtennant@the5thwave.com
World Wide Web: www.the5thwave.com

Table of Contents

Part V: Resuming Normal Activity and Preventing Future Injury: Work, Play, and Sex......................................241

Chapter 16: Getting Back to Work 243

Chapter 17: Safely Returning to Your Favorite Sports: The Weekend Warrior 255

Introduction

● ●

"*O*h, my aching back!" If you've ever uttered these words, then this book is for you. Back pain is a very common problem. In fact, almost everyone has or will experience back pain at some point in time.

We know how miserable back pain can be — many of our patients struggle with chronic back pain, while others come to us searching for an end to pain that began after an auto accident or some other trauma. Several things can cause back pain; this book offers multiple remedies to manage — and conquer — this frustrating condition.

We also know that any pain is frightening. You may be afraid to move for fear you'll injure yourself further. You may worry that you'll never regain normal functioning. And you may be shaken when your doctor starts suggesting tests with high-tech, hard-to-pronounce names. This book works to put you in charge of the pain and to remove the intimidation factor from common medical procedures.

About This Book

In our practice, we use a *whole-person, multidisciplinary approach*. When treating the whole person, we look at all the factors that contribute to a back pain condition. With a multidisciplinary approach, we often combine treatments from different disciplines (for instance, medical approaches, exercise, chiropractic, acupuncture, bodywork, and so on) to help our patients overcome back pain problems. We believe that back pain is completely manageable and that surgery is avoidable in the vast majority of cases.

Throughout the book, we look at both the physical and emotional causes and ramifications of back pain. We also look at ways you can manage and relieve your pain, including everything from aerobics, nerve blocks, and medication to yoga and guided imagery. We also cover common treatments and diagnoses, and we look at ways in which pain affects your life at home and at work.

Back Pain Remedies For Dummies is organized in an easy-access manner. We start with the most basic information (such as an overview of back pain and back anatomy) and move through to more specific topics like conventional and complementary approaches, as well as rehabilitation. The book is chock-full of tips and anecdotes from our practice (many derived from our patients) who have overcome the challenges of back pain. You'll find detailed explanations of common conditions, tests, and treatments — all described in plain English. (If we ever lapse into medical jargon, our editors make sure that we explain exactly what we mean in layman's terms.)

Finally, this book is a tool that empowers you to get the best possible treatment — and results. We give you lists of questions to ask your doctor, and we prepare you for interaction with the medical community. No more will you find yourself nodding your head while your doctor talks, only to scramble to figure out just what he or she meant after the appointment. When you're talking about your body, you deserve to be in control.

Foolish Assumptions

As we wrote this book, we did make a few assumptions about you, the reader:

- ✔ You or someone you care about suffer from occasional, chronic, or recurring back pain.

- ✔ You want to educate yourself about back pain conditions and common treatments.

- ✔ You are frequently frustrated by the information — or lack of it — that you receive from the medical community.

- ✔ You want to take charge of your own treatment, and you want to make intelligent decisions about any tests or surgeries your doctor suggests.

- ✔ You are interested in exploring some of the emotional aspects of living with back pain.

- ✔ You want to feel better.

- ✔ You like chocolate ice cream. (You don't actually have to like chocolate ice cream, but we try to add a little humor here and there.)

What You're Not to Read

You don't have to read this book from cover to cover. Feel free to skip around and read what interests or applies to you and your situation. The book is *modular,* so you can start in the middle of Chapter 13 and then go to the beginning of Chapter 1 without losing any important information, and no matter how much you skip around, the book will still make sense. We've loaded the book with cross references to other chapters, so you know right where to jump for more information or a further explanation of a given term or treatment.

Of course, if you're one of those people who must start at the beginning and go to the end, we won't stop you. The book does have a logical progression, so you can read from front to back. Just remember that even though back pain can be scary, we didn't write this book like a Stephen King thriller. Use what you need; skip the rest.

How This Book Is Organized

Remember back in high school when you had to provide your teachers with an outline of a chapter or a report? This book is organized in much the same way. We start out by dividing the text into parts. Each part covers a general area of back pain and treatment. The parts are further divided into chapters. Each chapter deals with a specific issue that pertains to the entire part. Chapters are broken down by headings that separate the main ideas we cover, and sometimes, we even use subheads. Our English teachers would be so proud!

Part I: Getting Back to Back Basics

Most importantly, this part explains how common back pain really is. After reading this part, you'll be relieved to discover that you don't need to be embarrassed by your back pain — millions of people are facing the same challenges. We also spend a bit of time looking at spine anatomy and the causes of back pain. This part ends with a chapter that tells you when you need to see a professional, and what kind of professional can help you the most.

Part II: Conventional Treatment Options

We hate to hit you over the head with the obvious, but this part looks at traditional treatment options. When you first have a flare-up, you may want to try some home remedies, so we talk about which of those may work in your situation, and when you need to trade in the home remedies for a visit to your doctor's office.

Our goal is to help you make the best decision possible about the course of treatment you choose. Physicians have several options for treating back pain, so in the next couple of chapters, we explain common tests and common medical treatments. We also spend a chapter exploring the surgery option (and we tell you how to find a good surgeon if you go that route). By the end of this part, you should have all the tools you need to make intelligent decisions about your course of treatment.

Part III: Complementary Approaches: Are They for You?

If you have a mother or a financial advisor, then you know that putting all your eggs in one basket is almost never a good idea. So in this part, we explore treatment options that you can use in conjunction with standard medical treatments, including the following (to name a few):

- ✔ Acupuncture
- ✔ Bodywork
- ✔ Magnet therapy
- ✔ Biofeedback
- ✔ Massage
- ✔ Yoga

We spend some time discussing the mind-body connection, and how you can use it to help manage your pain. No back pain book would be complete without a chapter on chiropractics, and we're nothing if not thorough. Well, we're also responsible, and to that end, we tell you how to recognize the charlatans out there of all types who offer quick cures that result in worsened pain.

Part IV: Rehabilitation

This part gets into the hands-on stuff. We tell you what kinds of exercises and treatments your doctor is likely to recommend, and we walk through each of them with you. This part is also full of tips and tricks that you can do on your own to manage your pain and speed recovery. We help you design an exercise program tailored to your condition. And, finally, we offer you a chapter's worth of products that can work to make you and your back more comfortable.

Part V: Resuming Normal Activity and Preventing Future Injury: Work, Play, and Sex

Bet you can't guess what this part covers. Seriously, though, as you are painfully aware, a bad back can affect your overall quality of life. Once you finally get the pain and the condition under control, returning to normal activities can be a daunting thought at best. And after a siege of back pain, you certainly want to prevent any future injuries. By following the tips in these chapters, you can safely return to work and engage in extracurricular activities — all without fear of reinjury.

Part VI: The Part of Tens

All books in the ...*For Dummies* series contain a Part of Tens part. These chapters offer tidbits of information in easy bites. We cover ten (or so — ...*For Dummies* books aren't big on rules) of the following:

- ✔ Common questions about back pain
- ✔ Steps to a healthy back
- ✔ Reasons to see a doctor for back pain
- ✔ Tips for working successfully with your doctor
- ✔ Hot topics in back pain

If nothing else, you won't run out of conversation starters at your next cocktail party.

We also end the book with two appendixes. The first is a glossary that gives you an at-a-glance definition of common terms in the world of back pain treatment. The second is a list of resources. You can contact the organizations here for further information and support or visit some helpful Web sites.

Icons Used in This Book

As you thumb through the book, you'll notice that many paragraphs are set off by little icons. We put them there to draw your attention to information that is especially important, or that you may find particularly interesting. We use the following icons:

This icon alerts you to those instances when you should see your doctor right away.

We occasionally add some information that is pretty technical in nature. If you really want to delve into the topic, you'll enjoy the information we present here. Otherwise, feel free to skip right over these paragraphs.

You're not alone if your back pain causes you anxiety. We understand, so paragraphs marked with this icon offer you healing, motivational, or stress-relieving ideas.

These are things that we simply don't want you to forget.

We give our patients all kinds of tips for dealing with and managing their pain and their interaction with the medical community. We're happy to share them with you, too, in the paragraphs marked with this icon.

This icon's not a picture of a bomb for nothing. These paragraphs warn you of things you shouldn't do and symptoms you shouldn't ignore. Think of this information as giant stop signs on the back pain highway.

Where to Go from Here

You've already made a commitment to helping yourself by getting this book. Just as you need to choose the treatment options and remedies that are best for you, you should choose where to start reading. Take a gander at the Table of Contents. When you find a topic that interests you, start reading your way to pain-free living.

Part I
Getting Back to Back Basics

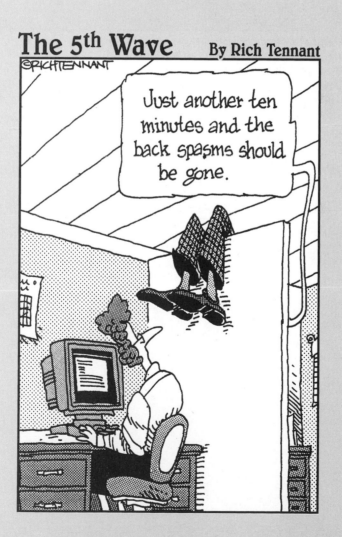

In this part . . .

You are not suffering alone.

Back pain can be embarrassing and make you feel isolated from friends, coworkers — even your family. In this part, you discover just how common back pain is — actually, almost everyone suffers from at least one bout of back pain during his or her life. We also give you an overview of spine anatomy, which is essential to understanding your pain, and then we go on to discuss the things that can cause back pain.

Chapter 1

Ouch! The Problem of Back Pain

. . . .

In This Chapter

▶ Digging into the who, what, when, where, and why of back pain

▶ Getting successful treatment

▶ Combining traditional and non-traditional treatments

. . . .

*U*nless you find the topic of back pain as exciting as the latest Tom Clancy novel, we're guessing that you or someone you care about is experiencing back pain. Finding appropriate treatment that actually works can be frustrating, to say the least. And everybody seems to have an opinion about what you should do: Your mother-in-law swears by her chiropractor, your son thinks you should try yoga, your boss touts physical therapy, and your best friend raves about the results of his surgery.

In addition to getting more advice than you want, you may also notice that people treat you differently. For instance, how many times have you heard the following statements (or made them yourself):

✔ Don't lift those boxes without bending your knees; you'll hurt your lower back.

✔ You can't play golf — that twisting motion is bad for your back pain. You'll throw your back out for sure.

✔ You have a bad back. Don't even think about trying to sit in a movie theater for two hours. In fact, you should rest while we go out.

Even though back pain is an incredibly common condition, the preceding examples illustrate just how much confusion surrounds the problem of back pain, both for patients and healthcare professionals. If you have spent any time searching for a "remedy" to your back pain, then you are familiar with the bewildering number of opinions and treatment options out there. Two things cause this state of confusion:

- In the majority of cases, the exact source of the pain remains unknown.

- Healthcare providers show considerable disagreement as to specific diagnoses and appropriate treatment plans.

These two problems mean that you are likely to get a wide variety of diagnoses and treatment recommendations as you search for answers to your back pain. In fact, the more you search, the more bewildered you may feel.

With all this conflicting information, you may not be sure which route to follow. Chapter 1 to the rescue! We start by giving you a solid definition of back pain and go on to discuss treating back pain. Read on to get a leg up on the whole issue of back pain as it applies to you.

Defining Back Pain

A section that asks, "What is back pain?" may seem crazy. Your answer may very well be, "Why, pain in the back, of course!" However, (as you may have already experienced) a general back pain problem or a spinal condition can include many different symptoms.

You may notice that we use the terms *back pain* and *spinal condition* somewhat interchangeably, although sometimes the terms mean something different. For instance, a spinal condition may cause pain down your legs but no pain in your back.

As you experience back pain or a spinal condition, you may experience a variety of symptoms, including:

- Pain that has a throbbing, aching, shooting, stabbing, dull, or sharp quality

- Pain down one or both legs with very little pain in the lower back

- Numbness or weakness in the legs

- Pain in the lower back and legs that only occurs in certain positions

- Sleep problems, decreased energy, depression, and anxiety

- Pain that seems to move to different parts of the body, including the back

- Pain that stress and emotional issues cause or make worse

The preceding examples represent just a few of the many ways that a back pain problem can present itself. In order to get good treatment and ensure that treatment doesn't actually make your problem worse, you must have a good understanding of the different types of back pain problems (see Chapter 3 for details). Having this knowledge helps you gain control over your particular back pain or spinal problem.

Who experiences back pain?

Back pain is a very common condition that many doctors and researchers consider a normal part of life, similar to having an occasional cold or flu. As a back pain sufferer, you are not alone:

- Back pain affects more than 80 percent of the population at some time during their lifetime.
- Back pain is second only to the common cold as a reason for visits to the doctor and it is second only to childbirth as a reason for hospitalization.
- Approximately 50 percent of the working population reports back problems every year.
- The total medical cost of back pain exceeds 20 billion dollars a year in the United States.

What causes back pain?

As we detail in Chapter 3, back pain has a great many known medical causes. If you venture outside the realm of traditional Western medicine, then the list of possible reasons for back pain becomes even longer. For the purposes of the discussion in this section, we only present a few examples of the more common causes of back pain.

One point — one that most practitioners often ignore — is absolutely critical: When you're investigating the various possible reasons for your back pain, remember that all pain has physical *and* emotional components. If you ignore either physical or emotional influences, you're less likely to find a remedy. We discuss the components of pain in Chapter 3.

Probably the most important thing to keep in mind regarding the causes of back pain is that in the majority of back pain problems, doctors never determine an exact reason for the pain. Even so, you shouldn't be discouraged, because the majority of back pain problems resolve completely even when the exact cause is unknown.

One of the most common causes of back pain includes problems with the muscles and ligaments. Similar to other tissues in your body, the muscles and ligaments of your back can be injured, irritated, or weakened, which then causes pain.

Another cause of back pain (often in conjunction with pain down one or both legs) is a disc problem. Two common disc problems are a *disc bulge* or a *disc herniation.* As we discuss in Chapter 2, the *disc* is a "cushion" that lies in between each of the bones of your back (the *vertebra*). Problems can occur when part of the disc either *bulges* (pushes out) or *herniates* (breaks through) out of its usual space and either presses or comes close to nerves that go down your legs. (This pressing and irritation of the nerve is why a back problem can cause pain down your legs.) Irritation can result even if the disc is not actually compressing the nerve but only comes in close proximity.

We would be remiss if we did not mention that *disc bulge* and *disc herniation* are no longer the "cool" medical terms to describe disc problems. In the ever-changing area of medical terminology, the new labels are disc protrusion and extrusion. A *disc protrusion* is roughly equivalent to a bulge, and *disc extrusion* approximates the definition of a herniation. (You find some other, very slight technical differences between the old and new terms, but nothing that would ever come up in light conversation.) Even though the terms protrusion and extrusion are now more technically correct, we generally use the terms bulge and herniation throughout the book. Also, the labels of bulging and herniation are still the most commonly used terms by health professionals, both in practice and in back pain books.

Another common reason for back pain (which we believe doctors often miss), is stress. In this case, back pain either starts, maintains, or becomes worse by emotionally stressful experiences. Stress (conscious or unconscious) can cause your back muscles to tighten, which then causes pain. Stress can also amplify the amount of pain coming from some other back problem, such as a herniated disc. Consequently, paying attention to emotional and physical aspects of back pain is very important.

Treating Back Pain

As you try to manage your back pain problem and investigate various treatment approaches, you can help yourself by being assured and hopeful that you can remedy your problem. Back pain does get better, and successful treatment is possible. You can find the best treatment for your back problem when you have some understanding of who treats back pain, how he or she treats it, and why using a multidisciplinary approach is important.

My back pain can get better, right?

Although back problems are very common, the good news is that they generally resolve on their own. In fact, the usual outcome of low-back pain symptoms is very favorable, often with or without treatment.

Determining which treatments are successful and which are not is often challenging because of back pain's natural tendency to improve — in many cases, the pain goes away on its own whether or not you receive treatment. However, even with the human body's natural pattern towards improvement, many back pain sufferers experience pain that lingers, worsens, or seems to come and go. Chances are good that, as a reader of this book, your back pain problem falls into the category of not getting better on its own. Some of the more common back pain situations include

- ✔ Flare-ups of back pain that seem to come and go over several years
- ✔ Chronic back pain problems that go on for more than three months
- ✔ Pain for which the recommendation is surgery
- ✔ Back or leg pain that continues even after having a spine surgery (called a _failed low-back surgery syndrome_)

The preceding types of pain don't resolve themselves quickly and can become increasingly frustrating for you and those close to you. Getting accurate information about whatever type of back pain problem you suffer from is your most important resource for getting better.

Often, the appropriate timing and integration of treatment options — traditional or nontraditional — is the key for you to successfully overcome your back pain problem. For example, you may improve with physical therapy treatments (such as electrical stimulation, ice, and heat) in combination with an exercise program and acupuncture if you receive all these treatments in a specific, overlapping time frame.

The importance of treatment integration extends to the broader category of surgical interventions, which in and of themselves may or may not be effective depending on a number of factors. Spine surgery is appropriate in certain cases. However, you may have a much better outcome when you add additional treatments such as psychological preparation for surgery (undergoing relaxation training, gathering information about your surgery, and having a healthy attitude towards the operation) and postoperative rehabilitation (exercise, psychological techniques, and alternative medicine approaches) to your treatment program. (See Chapter 8 for more on psychological preparation for surgery and Chapters 12 and 14 for more on postoperative rehabilitation.)

Who can treat my back pain?

A variety of practitioners treat back pain problems by using medical and non-medical approaches. Although you'll find many specialties involved in back pain evaluation and treatment, the following specialties are common. These specialties are in alphabetical order and are not meant to imply that you should proceed in this order when seeking back pain treatment. Actually, we recommend starting your treatment with a general type of practitioner (family physician, chiropractor, or osteopath) and then moving on to specialists (physiatrist, orthopedist, neurosurgeon, and so on) as necessary. (We discuss each of the following specialties in greater detail in Chapter 4.)

✔ **Anesthesiology:** The area of medical practice that focuses on decreasing or abolishing a person's sensation of pain. An anesthesiologist can obtain specialized training in treating pain problems. The treatment approach may include such things as medications, spinal injections, or general anesthesia (inducing a state that allows for surgical intervention). For more information about anesthesiological pain treatments see Chapters 7 and 23.

✔ **Chiropractic:** This system of evaluation and treatment is based upon the belief that abnormal function of the nervous system causes disease. Chiropractors restore normal function by treating and manipulating different body parts, especially the spine. Beyond manipulation, most chiropractors provide a variety of other treatments such as massage, physical therapy, nutritional counseling, and vitamin therapy.

✔ **Internal medicine, family practice, and general practice:** Doctors in these groups may have slightly different training, but they all generally function as your family, or *primary care,* doctor and are often the first ones you consult for a back pain problem. Because many cases of back pain get better without treatment or with minimal treatment, your family doctor is fully equipped to handle the problem initially. Primary care doctors have general training in all areas of medicine. If you need a more specialized approach, your family doctor can refer you to an appropriate specialist.

✔ **Neurology:** This branch of medicine deals with the nervous system. Neurologists often use non-surgical treatment approaches to diagnose and treat back pain.

✔ **Neurosurgery:** This medical specialty focuses on the surgical treatment of nervous system problems. A neurosurgeon generally uses a surgical treatment approach and may be involved in such things as removing tumors from the brain or repairing damaged nerves after a severe injury. Neurosurgeons who specialize in spine problems use a surgery treatment approach (see Chapter 8 for more information about spine surgery).

✔ **Orthopedic surgery:** This area of medicine focuses on the surgical treatment of skeletal problems. For example, general orthopedic surgeons may perform hip and knee replacement surgery, repair severely fractured bones, or do other types of joint surgery. Some orthopedic surgeons specialize in the treatment and surgery of spinal problems.

✔ **Osteopathy:** This system of medicine uses traditional physical, medicinal, and surgical methods of diagnosis and treatment while also emphasizing *body mechanics* (for example, your posture while being still or moving — see Chapter 13) and manipulative techniques (such as moving or adjusting your joints — see Chapter 10).

✔ **Pain psychology:** A specialized branch of clinical psychology that uses psychological methods to diagnose and treat pain problems. Examples may include helping you identify thoughts or emotions that make your back pain worse, teaching you relaxation exercises, and helping you change your attitude towards the pain. (For more details about pain psychology treatment see Chapters 8, 12, and 23.)

✔ **Physiatry:** Although the word *physiatry* resembles *psychiatry,* the two specialties are very different. A psychiatrist (note the spelling) is a medical doctor who treats various types of emotional and mental problems. In contrast, a physiatrist is a rehabilitation physician. Physiatrists specialize in nonsurgical approaches to muscle and skeletal problems. Physiatrists often are involved in rehabilitation programs after you suffer a stroke or an injury to your muscles or joints, or after you undergo surgery. Some physiatrists specialize in the treatment of spinal problems and back pain.

How is my back pain treated?

Your physician or specialist may recommend that you try a variety of more traditional treatments like the following:

✔ **Physical therapy:** Your doctor may prescribe physical therapy treatment for your back pain problem, which a physical therapist completes. Examples of the treatment include special exercises, manual therapy or manipulation, deep-tissue massage, heat and cold treatments, water therapy, and treatments that use electrical stimulation, among others.

✔ **Medications:** Doctors use a variety of medications in treating back pain, including, analgesics (painkillers), anti-inflammatories, muscle relaxants, among others. The physician most involved in treating your back pain problem usually prescribes these medications. Sometimes, a specialist (such as an orthopedic surgeon) may prefer that your family doctor manage your medications because of his or her familiarity with your entire medical history. (We discuss medications in detail in Chapter 7.)

✔ **Braces and corsets:** Braces and corsets restrict motion, provide support, may decrease pain, and correct posture in the lower back area. General back supports are available without a prescription at many health and drugstores. Your family doctor or specialist physician can also prescribe other types of braces. Your doctor or physical therapist should always guide your use of a back brace (for more info see Chapters 7 and 23).

✔ **Exercise:** Exercise is probably one of the most important treatments for back pain. Your doctor may recommend different types of exercise programs for back pain, including lumbar stabilization, cardiovascular conditioning, and others. We discuss these more fully in Chapter 14.

✔ **Spinal epidural steroid and nerve blocks:** These treatments involve injecting certain medicines (usually steroids or anesthetics) into a particular area of the spinal canal to help with back pain and nerve irritation. We discuss this treatment further in Chapters 7 and 23.

✔ **Trigger-point injection therapy:** This treatment involves injecting a small amount of anesthetic painkiller (or other medicine) into *trigger points,* the areas of a muscle that seem to trigger pain in a given region of the body.

✔ **Pain management:** Pain management combines a variety of approaches — psychological avenues, medicines, exercise, and working with family members — to address your pain problem. The doctor most involved in your back pain treatment usually recommends the treatment combinations, but you may decide to add treatments yourself. We discuss pain management more in Chapters 3 and 12.

✔ **Stress management and posture:** Stress management such as relaxation training, yoga, and thought analysis can help with back pain problems (see Chapters 11 and 12 for more information). Also, addressing your posture in your work or home environment can also be an important part of your treatment (see Chapter 13).

Diagnostic and treatment approaches that are not normally associated with mainstream medicine are termed *nontraditional, alternative,* or *complementary* medicine approaches. We believe that complementary treatment approaches definitely have a place for back pain problems. We use the term *complementary* to describe these approaches because this term best describes how we believe you should incorporate them into a back pain treatment program. These treatments should always be a *complement* to medical management rather than an *alternative* to medical management. Incorporating mainstream medical management and complementary approaches is the only safe way to combine these different treatment philosophies. We discuss the specifics of safely pursuing complementary medicine treatments in Chapter 9. Examples of more common complementary treatments include the following:

✔ **Acupuncture:** An ancient Chinese medicine approach in which small needles that pierce the skin are placed at specific body locations (*acupoints*) to cause healing and other benefits, such as pain relief. We discuss the details in Chapter 9.

✔ **Bodywork:** Therapies such as massage, deep-tissue manipulation, movement awareness, and energy balancing can improve the body's structure and function as well as reduce pain (see Chapter 9).

- ✔ **Chiropractic:** This treatment influences the body's nervous system and ability to heal through adjustments of the spine, muscles, and joints, as well as other treatment approaches (see Chapter 10).

- ✔ **Herbal therapies:** Herbal therapies use herbs to address a wide variety of medical problems, including pain (see Chapter 9 for more details).

- ✔ **Magnet therapy:** This therapy involves the application of a magnetic field (produced by a magnet or electrical device) to a body part. Magnets have long been thought to have healing properties, and recently, magnets have been used to relieve back pain (see Chapters 9 and 23 for more information).

- ✔ **Mind-body approaches:** A number of different approaches can promote the body's own ability to heal itself and increase the mind's power over the body. We discuss a number of these treatments in Chapter 12.

- ✔ **Yoga:** A system of health that uses physical postures, breathing exercises, and meditation to relieve suffering and enhance overall well-being. We discuss yoga approaches for back pain in Chapter 11.

How do I choose a multidisciplinary approach?

A *multidisciplinary approach* is the idea of combining a variety of treatment approaches to address a back pain problem. Research shows that back pain problems (especially those that are not improving) best respond to using a number of different approaches, delivered in a coordinated fashion. If you are not responding to a single approach (such as an exercise program or medicines), you may want to consider a multidisciplinary approach.

You can get multidisciplinary treatment for your back problem in a number of ways. For instance, you can participate in a structured *pain program* in which the treatment components (such as physical therapy, medicines, nerve blocks, and so on) are preset and you receive pretty much the same treatment as anyone else on the program. These programs generally have a medical director who oversees and coordinates the treatment. The programs are not very common, tend to be very expensive, and are often based within a hospital setting.

Other multidisciplinary treatment approaches are less formal and less structured than pain programs. The informal multidisciplinary approach can take on many forms and the types of treatments that can be combined differ from person to person. In some cases, your doctor helps you construct an individually tailored multidisciplinary program. In this situation, your doctor works with you in determining the best treatments to combine, as well as assisting you in the coordination of these treatments.

Unfortunately, many doctors do not think in terms of a multidisciplinary approach and you may have to design and coordinate your own program. You can still have a good outcome — you just have to work a little harder. The information in this book will give you an idea of the various treatments that are available as well as the ones that may address your particular back pain problem.

A multidisciplinary approach for back pain may involve the following:

- **Medical management:** A multidisciplinary treatment program may be overseen by your doctor, osteopath, or chiropractor who is responsible for prescribing the treatment components. (In some cases, you may put together your own multidisciplinary program.) If a physician is overseeing the treatment, he or she is responsible for prescribing any medications, manual medical techniques, invasive procedures, or physical therapy exercises.

- **Physical therapy:** Many multidisciplinary treatment approaches include an aggressive rehabilitation program, focusing on muscular *reconditioning* (strengthening) especially around your lower back area. A physical therapist may also utilize physical therapy *modalities,* techniques to relieve pain such as hot and cold packs, ultrasound, and massage.

- **Complementary approaches:** Complementary medicinal approaches are often part of a treatment program and may include such things as magnet therapy, yoga, and acupuncture (see Chapters 9, 11, and 12 for more details).

- **Stress and pain management:** A pain psychologist can teach you home techniques for relaxation and help you gain insights into the role that stress plays in your back pain (see Chapters 3 and 9).

- **Body mechanics and ergonomics:** This treatment may include such things as teaching you proper posture and making sure that your work area is safe for your back (see Chapter 13).

Although your back pain may improve when working with a single practitioner, sometimes an individual specialist cannot adequately treat a difficult back pain problem and associated complications. In a multidisciplinary treatment, you complete all appropriate treatments simultaneously in a coordinated fashion, which offers more powerful results than going through one treatment at a time.

Chapter 2

Introducing the Parts of Your Spine

. . . .

In This Chapter

▶ Recognizing your spine's strong structure

▶ Increasing your spinal awareness

▶ Understanding how the parts of the spine work together

. . . .

You know where your spine is, but you may have no idea what it actually looks like. This chapter acquaints you with your spine and helps you understand the various terms your doctor may use when discussing your back pain.

Too often, doctors speak to you as though you're a walking medical dictionary. The information in this chapter prepares you to "talk the talk" when it comes to your spine. Your head may start spinning when your doctor tells you that you have "lumbar-sacral sprain-strain injury," but rest assured that this complex phrase simply means that you have sore muscles in your lower back and with the proper treatment (such as time to heal and mild exercise) you can be back to your normal life.

Familiarity with the language of spinal anatomy helps you

✔ Ask better questions

✔ Get better answers

✔ Obtain better treatment

As you begin to explore the parts of the spine, don't fall prey to *medical student syndrome* (thinking you have every disease whose symptoms you read about in a medical book). In this syndrome, having a little knowledge can actually make things worse. We have had patients study the parts of their spines, only to worry that each area they studied — no matter how small — was weak or malfunctioning.

As we progress through this chapter, remember five important things:

- **Extensive muscles and ligaments support your spine, creating a very strong structure:** Your spine is very flexible, allowing you to bend forward and backwards while supporting your head (which weighs 12 to 16 pounds) and your torso (90 to 125 pounds). At the same time, your lower spine has a lifting capacity of up to 300 pounds per square inch! For a pile of bones strung together with ligaments and muscles, that's truly an amazing feat.

- **Doctors identify no specific structural problem in the majority of back pain cases:** The structure of your spine is usually in good shape and your pain isn't due to anything that is life-threatening or requires surgery. Your pain should respond to healing time and appropriate treatment, such as exercise.

- **Surgery is rarely necessary in order to become pain free:** As we explain in Chapter 8, surgery is almost always your personal choice.

- **Effective treatment is possible without a specific diagnosis:** Keep this fact in mind; otherwise you can search and search for someone to give you a diagnosis rather than focusing on starting to get better.

- **Structural abnormalities (such as a herniated disc) often have nothing to do with your pain:** For instance, a large percentage of adults with no back pain have bulging or herniated discs, meaning that a condition like a herniated disc is not necessarily causing your pain (see Chapter 3).

Feeling Fine with Help from Your Spine

Have you ever wondered why you have a spine and what it does? Probably not, but the subject really is fascinating. Your spine serves several purposes:

- **Supports your upper body:** Your spine supports the weight of your head and upper body, allowing you to do things like read this book.

- **Provides flexibility:** Your spine supports your upper body in a way that allows you to bend forwards, backwards, and side-to-side. Life would be a bit more challenging if your spine were a straight, rigid pole from your hips to your head.

- **Houses and protects your spinal cord and nerves:** Your spine houses your spinal cord, which is a relay station of nerves going to and from your brain to all parts of your body. Your spine also acts as a protective covering so that these nerves aren't damaged as you move around.

✔ **Serves as an attachment for muscles and ligaments:** Your spine is one of your skeleton's basic building blocks. Without your spine to provide an attachment for many of your torso's muscles and ligaments, your upper body would fall into a shapeless pile of tissue.

✔ **Serves as a platform for your head:** If you didn't have a spine, where would you put your head?

Don't take the engineering marvel that is your spine for granted. Your spine continues to provide you with all the features just mentioned when you are in pain. The following section offers a chance to become more familiar with the amazing intricacies of your spine.

Touring Your Splendid Spine

The rest of this chapter discusses the various parts of your spine. You can divide your spinal structures into the following:

✔ The spinal column

✔ The vertebrae

✔ The discs

✔ The facet joints

✔ The ligaments

✔ The spinal canal (which is nowhere near the Panama Canal)

✔ The sacrum and coccyx

✔ The sacroiliac joints

✔ The nerves

✔ The muscles

The spinal column

As shown in Figure 2-1, your back divides into three natural curves that form an S-shape: the *cervical curve,* containing your neck bones; the *thoracic curve,* containing the bones of your middle back; the *lumbosacral curve,* containing the bones of your lower back.

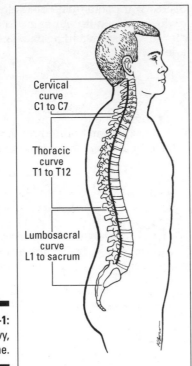

Cervical
curve
C1 to C7

Thoracic
curve
T1 to T12

Lumbosacral
curve
L1 to sacrum

Figure 2-1:
Your curvy,
boney spine.

The bones of your spine are called *vertebrae* (just one of these bones is a *vertebra*). You have a total of 24 vertebrae in your back:

✔ The cervical part of your spine contains seven vertebrae, which support the weight of your head and protect the nerves that come from your brain to the rest of your body. In technical terms, medical people refer to these vertebrae as C1 through C7, with C1 being the vertebrae just under your head. The next time someone says you've "lost your head," blame your cervical vertebrae; they literally keep your head on your shoulders.

✔ The thoracic part of your spine contains 12 vertebrae, making up your mid-back. Those in the know refer to these as T1 to T12.

✔ The lumbosacral spine contains the five vertebrae in your lower back and sacrum. No surprises here — the lumbar vertebrae go by L1 through L5. The lumbosacral curve is your spine's workhorse, moving more than the rest of your spine (except your neck) and carrying the majority of the weight.

As Figure 2-1 shows, when all of your spine's curves are in balance, your ear, shoulder, and hip align to make a straight line, even though your back curves between these points. *Good posture* means keeping your back curves in balance (more about posture in Chapter 13).

Vertebrae: The bones of your back

The vertebrae are one of the most important parts of your spine. A vertebra has three parts: the vertebral body, the transverse process, and the spinous process.

Figure 2-2 shows two vertebrae with a disc in between (see the following section for more about discs). The *vertebral body* is the large front part of the vertebra that is cushioned by the discs. The *spinous process* is the part of the vertebrae that you can feel as the bony bumps on your back. The *transverse process* provides an area of attachment for the muscles that control your spine's movement. Also notice the opening through which the spinal cord passes which is termed the *spinal canal*.

The discs

Lying in between each of the vertebral bodies, the *discs* are your spine's cushioning pads or "shock absorbers." Figure 2-2 shows two vertebrae with a disc in between. These three parts (two vertebrae and a disc) are also known as a *functional unit*. Figure 2-3 shows a cut-away view of a functional unit.

As shown in Figure 2-4, two parts make up the disc:

✔ **Nucleus pulposus:** This spongy center provides lubrication and shock absorption for your spinal column, allowing some flexibility in between each vertebra while also providing shock absorption to the structures of your spine (including the nerves). The nucleus pulposus is mostly made up of water, making it very flexible.

✔ **Annulus fibrosis:** This outer layer actually attaches to the vertebrae, holding them together. The annulus fibrosis is very tough (but also very friendly) and has a crisscrossed design like the layers of a radial tire.

The disc's design allows the bony vertebrae to move back and forth, giving your spine great flexibility (like the links of one of those jointed toy snakes).

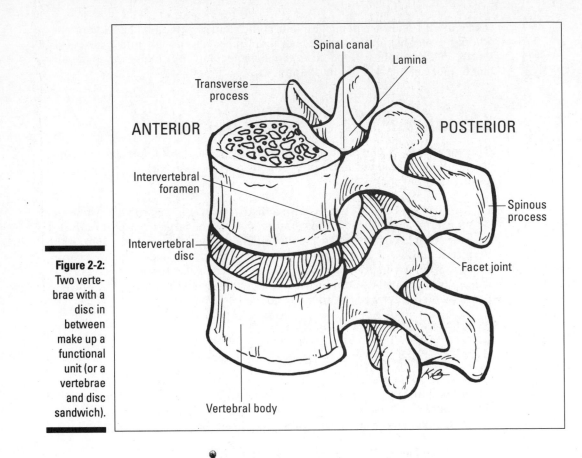

Transverse process

Spinal canal

Lamina

ANTERIOR

POSTERIOR

Intervertebral foramen

Spinous process

Intervertebral disc

Facet joint

Figure 2-2:
Two verte-
brae with a
disc in
between
make up a
functional
unit (or a
vertebrae
and disc
sandwich).

Vertebral body

The facet joints

If you refer to Figure 2-2, you can see a *facet joint* — a gliding joint — between each vertebra. Facet joints help keep the vertebrae in alignment as your spine moves around. In between the facet joints are joint capsules that consist of a smooth lining called *synovium*. The synovium produces synovial fluid in the joint capsule, which helps lubricate the joint for smooth movement and also provides nourishment.

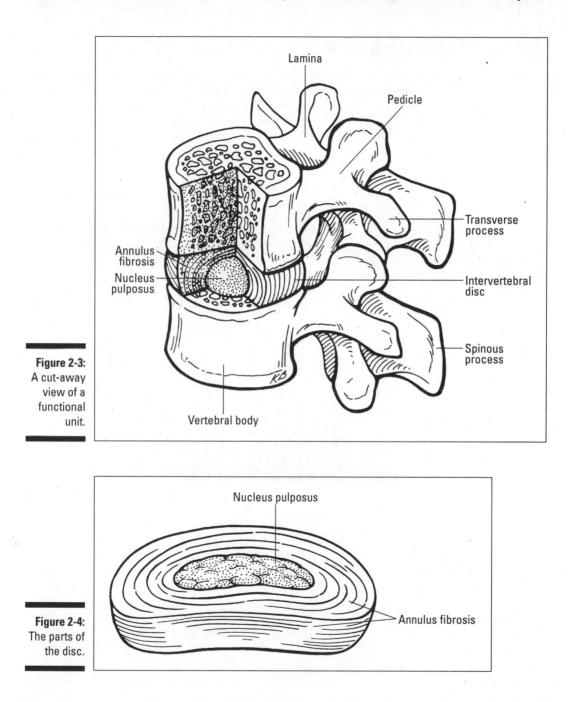

Lamina

Pedicle

Transverse process

Intervertebral disc

Spinous process

Annulus fibrosis

Nucleus pulposus

Vertebral body

Figure 2-3:
A cut-away view of a functional unit.

Nucleus pulposus

Annulus fibrosis

Figure 2-4:
The parts of the disc.

The ligaments

As shown in Figure 2-5, your spine has more ligaments than anyone cares to know about — except maybe a back doctor. *Ligaments* are strong bands of fibrous tissue that "knit" your spine together and also contain pain fibers. At this point, we discuss just two of the ligaments that may be implicated in back pain problems:

- ✔ The anterior (toward the front) longitudinal ligament
- ✔ The posterior (toward the rear) longitudinal ligament

These ligaments connect the functional units together and go up and down the entire length of your spine. They also help control the motion of your spine while providing flexibility. If you think of all the ligaments in your spine as sailors, then these two are the captain and first mate. Hopefully, yours behave better than the Skipper and Gilligan.

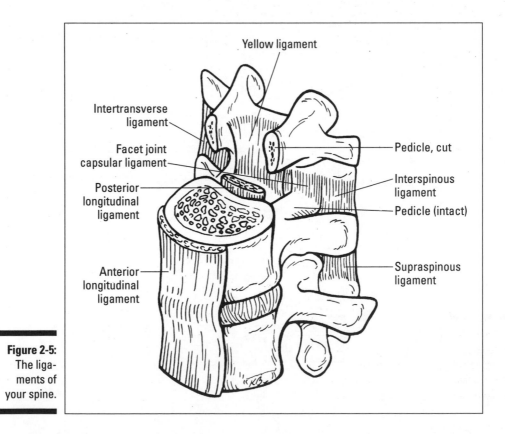

Yellow ligament

Intertransverse ligament

Facet joint capsular ligament

Posterior longitudinal ligament

Anterior longitudinal ligament

Pedicle, cut

Interspinous ligament

Pedicle (intact)

Supraspinous ligament

Figure 2-5:
The liga-
ments of
your spine.

The spinal canal

Because your vertebrae are aligned on top of one another, they form an opening, which is the spinal canal (refer to Figure 2-2). The spinal cord passes through this opening and is protected by the boney vertebrae.

The sacrum and coccyx

Below the five lumbar vertebrae, five more vertebrae are fused together. These five vertebrae make up the *sacrum* (see Figure 2-6), which forms the back part of your pelvis and the lowest part of your lumbosacral curve. Most people have five lumbar vertebrae and five fused sacral vertebrae. But in some people, the sixth vertebrae does not fuse with the sacrum, resulting in six lumbar vertebrae and four fused sacral vertebrae. If you are one of these unique people, don't worry; this condition is rarely the cause of any back problems.

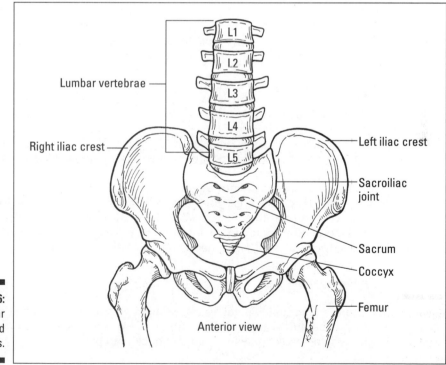

Figure 2-6:
The lumbar
spine and
pelvis.

The *coccyx* — the very bottom structure of the bony part of your spine — consists of three to five small vertebrae that are attached to the bottom of the sacrum. You may be more familiar with the coccyx as your *tailbone*. Injury to this very sensitive area can result in a painful condition called *coccydynia,* which we discuss in Chapter 3.

The sacroiliac joints

The *sacroiliac joints* are the joints that attach the sacrum to the *iliac bones* — or hip bones — of the pelvis (see Figure 2-6). The hip bones are attached to the sacrum by a number of ligaments on either side. To feel your iliac bones, just place your hands on your hips.

The nerves

The spinal cord is made up of nerves that extend from the brain into the spinal canal and then out to the various parts of the body. As we mention earlier, the spinal canal is formed by the large part of the vertebrae as well as other structures. *Cerebral spinal fluid* (CSF) — the same fluid you find in the center part of the brain — partly fills the tube-like spinal cord. CSF helps protect the spinal cord within the spinal canal.

Figure 2-7 shows the *nerve roots* (where nerves exit your spine) at various places along the spine. The nerves exit the spinal cord at different points and go out to the various parts of the body.

Figure 2-8 shows a close-up view of the spinal cord, nerve roots, and the spinal nerve branches. The most common nerve pain problem is caused by a *disc bulge* or herniation. In this condition, part of the disc bulges or herniates out of its usual space and ends up pressing on one or more nerves. If herniation occurs in the neck area, you often feel pain down your arms and in your fingers. This pain is often described as sharp, shooting, electrical, or tingling. If a disc herniation occurs in the lower back, it may cause pain and/or tingling in the buttocks, legs, or feet. This is called sciatica.

The muscles

The spine's functioning involves a great many muscles, including those in the back and abdominal areas. This section reviews only the most important muscles involved in spine function and back pain problems.

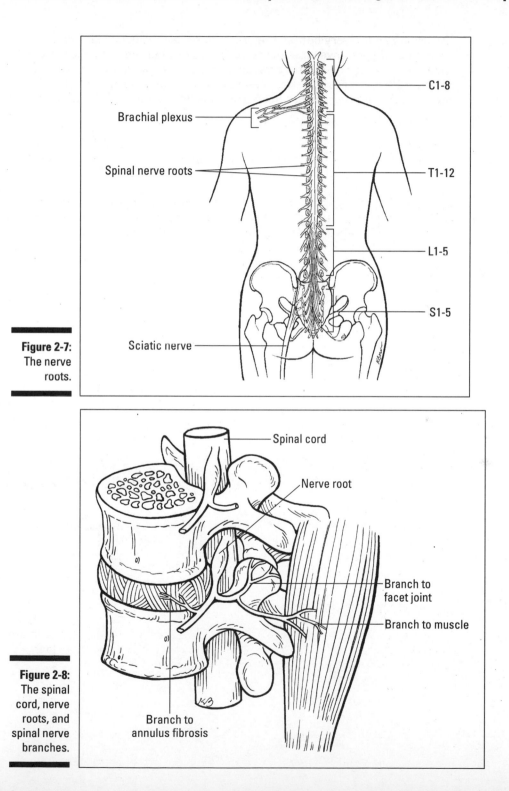

Figure 2-7:
The nerve
roots.

Brachial plexus

Spinal nerve roots

Sciatic nerve

C1-8

T1-12

L1-5

S1-5

Figure 2-8:
The spinal
cord, nerve
roots, and
spinal nerve
branches.

Spinal cord

Nerve root

Branch to
facet joint

Branch to muscle

Branch to
annulus fibrosis

The *erector spinae* muscles (see Figure 2-9) are the ones you can feel on either side of your lower spine. When your doctor talks about muscle spasms in your back, these muscles are usually the culprits. Just under these long muscles are medium length muscles that extend from one vertebra to the next. Underneath these are even shorter muscles that attach to the facet joints.

On the front part of your body, the *psoas muscle* is important. This muscle runs from the front and sides of your lower spine, goes across the hip joint, and attaches to the very upper part of the thigh bone (femur).

The very front of your body houses the all-important *abdominal* muscles. These muscles are critical to your spine's forward movement. They provide support as well, which is why physical therapists often instruct you to focus on strengthening your abdominal muscles as part of a back pain rehabilitation program.

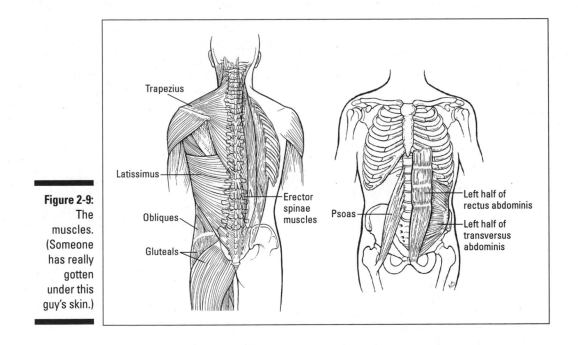

Figure 2-9:
The muscles. (Someone has really gotten under this guy's skin.)

Chapter 3

The Root of All Back Pain

Contrary to popular belief, all pain is real. Seems obvious, right? Unfortunately, many people with back pain are treated as if their pain is imaginary or exaggerated. We've seen patients whose pain has been dismissed so often by friends and family that they feel the need to "prove" it to us when we first meet them. Some doctors even try to convince patients that because they can't see a physical cause for the pain, the pain "can't be that bad." If this happens to you, run — don't walk — to get a second opinion from a doctor who takes your pain seriously.

Why all the misunderstandings about back pain? No medical tests are available to measure pain levels, so doctors can't test for pain the way they test for a broken leg (with an X ray) or an infection (with a blood test). To make matters more challenging, in back pain cases there's often little or no physical evidence to explain the pain. Back pain sufferers go from one doctor to the next, searching for explanations. They struggle through one unnecessary evaluation after another and never-ending treatments. We have seen patients who were actually harmed by well-meaning but poorly informed healthcare professionals who treated back pain incorrectly.

Doctors are subject to many of the same biases as the general public — and that includes all the usual misunderstandings about back pain.

Understanding why you hurt is a useful tool in learning to control your pain and the first step to recovery. We first look at one view of how pain works: the gate control theory.

A New Idea About Pain: The Gate Control Theory

Why do some people with serious injuries experience little pain, while others with relatively minor injuries suffer far more? How do mind-body techniques such as hypnosis work to control pain? How is it possible that negative thoughts (being pessimistic) and emotions (like being depressed) can make your pain worse? And, how is it possible that being optimistic and happy can make your pain better? These difficult questions were answered by the *gate control theory of pain,* developed in the early 1960s by Doctors Ronald Melzack and Patrick Wall. The gate control theory explains that pain can be influenced by your thoughts, emotions, and physical factors (such as inactivity). As illustrated in Figure 3-1, nerve or *pain gates* in your spinal cord can open and close depending upon messages coming down from your brain (along the descending spinal nerves). If the pain gates are more open, the pain message flows freely, and you experience more pain. If the gates are more closed, your pain is reduced or even stopped.

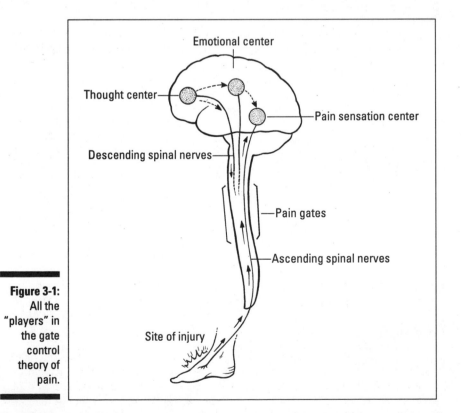

Figure 3-1:
All the "players" in the gate control theory of pain.

Test the gate control theory on yourself

To experience the gate control theory in action, try this exercise. (Don't worry, we're not going to have you walk across hot coals or lie on a bed of nails!)

Go to your laundry room, get a clothespin, and put it on your arm. Now, imagine that you've been instructed to leave it there the entire day. At first, the pain of the clothespin pinching your skin and muscles should be quite strong. But as

your brain begins to assess the situation, it decides the clothespin pain is not harmful. Why? The clothespin is not causing tissue damage — and besides, you know it's going to be there all day. The brain therefore gives less attention to the pain message, and the pain signals brought to consciousness are much less. In fact, in about thirty minutes, you should hardly feel any pain at all. (Just remember to take the clothespin off before you leave the house!)

While a full understanding of the gate control theory is complex, the message it offers is simple and empowering: You can control your experience of pain. The gate control theory is also extremely important because it explains how all the different kinds of remedies for back pain work, including both mental and physical techniques.

In the gate control theory of pain, the pain signal (in Figure 3-1 the pain signal starts in the foot) is transmitted through the *peripheral nervous system* (the nervous system outside of your brain and spinal cord) to the *central nervous system* (which includes the spinal cord and brain). In the spinal cord, the pain gates determine how much of the pain message gets through to the "pain sensation center" of the brain where you actually "feel" the pain (refer to Figure 3-1). After a pain signal reaches your brain, it can be amplified or minimized depending upon your thoughts, emotions, and physical factors (such as your overall health and conditioning). Figure 3-1 shows how the thought and emotional centers of the brain influence the pain gates and the pain sensation center.

The pain gates are opened and the pain signal amplified (more pain overall) by such things as pessimistic thoughts, fear of the pain, hopelessness, depression, anxiety, and inactivity. The pain gates are closed and the pain signal minimized by such things as optimistic thoughts, distracting yourself from the pain, outside interests, taking control of your life, and physical conditioning.

Understanding and applying the gate control theory to your experiences of pain can be a powerful tool for managing and relieving back pain. Allowing negative emotions such as anger, anxiety, frustration, hopelessness, and helplessness to overwhelm you can fling your pain gates wide open. Focusing on your pain, having no outside interests, worrying about the pain, and thinking that you have no future are all thoughts that greatly increase your pain.

Open pain gates create a crisis

Dr. Sinel had a patient at Cornell University Medical Center who came in complaining of headaches, which she described as severely painful and debilitating. She couldn't make it through the day without narcotic pain medicine. A thorough neurologic examination and history was entirely normal.

Speaking further with the patient, she revealed that her husband had recently been diagnosed with an inoperable brain tumor. She said his initial symptoms were headaches, for which he had failed to seek medical advice for three months. A brain tumor was ultimately diagnosed, and the patient's husband died shortly afterwards.

In this case, the patient's extreme fear that she, too, had a brain tumor made her pain gates open up, causing intense suffering. After we reassured her with an MRI of her brain that the headaches were not the result of something harmful, her symptoms dissipated. Within two days, she was managing the headache pain with nonprescription medicine, and after taking stress-management training over the next few weeks, the headaches disappeared.

Conversely, you can get your pain gates to close by increasing your activity, using short-term pain medication, exercising aerobically, and taking relaxation training. Combine those tactics with positive thinking to distract you from the pain, and you can be well on your way to recovery.

Understanding Categories of Pain

Understanding how pain is defined is important in order to learn how to better control it. Healthcare professionals and researchers separate pain into three categories. Treatment approaches for each type of pain differ:

- ✔ **Acute pain:** *Acute pain* lasts less than one month or is directly related to tissue damage or injury. This is the kind of pain that you experience when you cut your finger. Acute pain is usually proportional to the amount of injury — a cut finger hurts less than a broken arm.

- ✔ **Chronic pain:** *Chronic pain* is generally described as pain that lasts more than three to six months, or beyond the point of tissue healing. Chronic pain is usually less directly related to tissue damage or injury. Examples of chronic pain problems include such things as long term back pain and headaches.

- ✔ **Recurrent acute pain:** *Recurrent acute pain,* or intermittent pain, is an acute pain episode that occurs over and over again. Examples of recurrent acute pain include acute back pain episodes that come and go, the cramps and pain associated with menstruation, and migraine headaches.

As we discuss later in this chapter and in Chapter 12, the longer your back pain goes on, the more susceptible it is to influences such as negative thoughts and emotions as well as physical inactivity.

The Need to Diagnose: Helpful or Harmful?

Doctors are trained to give them. Patients are conditioned to expect them. But when it comes to back pain, the medical system's need for diagnoses can do more harm than good.

In many cases, there is little evidence that whatever diagnostic explanation your doctor gives you is the cause of the pain. In trying to comply with the medical establishment's system of examine, diagnose, and treat, healthcare professionals often focus on some supposed abnormality discovered on a new imaging study or other high-tech approach. They may tell you that the abnormality is the cause of your pain even when it may have nothing to do with it.

Most patients with back pain would rather hear, "Your pain is due to a bulging disc," or "Your spine is out of alignment," than "We don't know what is causing the pain." You'd probably be more attracted to a doctor who says, "I know what is causing your pain," although in reality, many back pain problems are never specifically diagnosed. See A.L. Nachemson, "Newest knowledge of low back pain: A critical look" in *Clinical Orthopedics and Related Research* 279 (1992), 8–20.

The need to diagnose can lead to incorrect and unnecessary treatment. In many cases, your back pain would improve whether or not the treatment was administered.

Don't despair if your doctor can't make an exact diagnosis — only about 10 to 15 percent of back pain cases find a specific diagnosis. Even without knowing the source of the pain, you can be treated effectively. About 90 percent of back pain sufferers recover, most within a week or so. Just realizing that an episode of back pain is not unusual is the first step on the road to recovery.

In this section, we discuss how the medical establishment diagnoses your condition and why the process can short-change back pain sufferers who aren't well-informed. (After reading this chapter, that certainly won't be you!) We also tackle emotional and psychological factors and their role in back pain.

Before proceeding, take a look at the cautions we discuss in the beginning of Chapter 2 on spinal anatomy. The same cautions apply when discussing causes of back pain.

Diagnosing based upon an imaging scan

Doctors commonly make a diagnosis based upon an imaging scan. Some believe that showing you an alleged "problem" on an X ray will provide a diagnosis. What many doctors don't realize is that telling you these findings are significant can lead you to believe that your spine is damaged when it isn't. In most cases, the findings have absolutely nothing to do with your pain.

An all-too-typical case is that of a 40-year-old patient of Dr. Sinel who had been told by another doctor that his low-back pain was due to "arthritic" changes seen on an X ray. This unfortunate person thought that his spine had deteriorated so much at the age of 40 that he was experiencing back pain. He also assumed that things could only get worse, even if the doctor didn't explicitly make that statement.

The truth is, arthritic changes are seen on the X rays of the vast majority of 40-year-old men (and women) who do not have back pain. The tragedy is that although these "findings" probably have nothing to do with the person's back pain, some doctors pinpoint them as the source of the back pain in order to satisfy the medical establishment's need for a diagnosis.

The role of psychological and emotional factors

Never underestimate the role of psychological and emotional factors in back pain. Some doctors — including us — think that emotions and stress cause a great many back pain cases. In common conditions such as stress-related back pain and chronic back pain syndrome, which we discuss later in this chapter, psychological factors play a key role in exacerbating and extending back pain.

When doctors are not aware of emotional influences on back pain, the likelihood of an incorrect diagnosis and inappropriate treatment is great. If you suspect that emotional factors may be a part of your back pain problem, be sure to discuss it with your doctor. Don't be deterred if your doctor minimizes or discounts that possibility — keep searching until you find a doctor who treats you as a whole person, both mind and body.

Understanding the Deconditioning Syndrome

Deconditioning or *deactivation syndrome* occurs when you try to alleviate your back pain by limiting normal activities, restricting exercise, or resting more. Deconditioning syndrome can be part of any of the diagnoses that we discuss later in this chapter.

Deconditioning syndrome begins when you avoid activity — often on the recommendation of a healthcare professional. Rather than helping, inactivity may make a bad situation worse. By reducing your activities, you eventually decrease the size, strength, and flexibility of your muscles and ligaments, as well as your cardiovascular and muscular endurance.

If you're experiencing deconditioning syndrome, getting active again to strengthen those muscles is important. Let us reassure you that your back pain is not harmful (even though it may hurt). We strongly encourage you to resume normal activities as soon as possible.

Conditions that Cause Back Pain

Back pain is notoriously difficult to diagnose: The cause is rarely just physical, in the way that a broken leg has a clear-cut physical cause. Because of the close relationship between the mind and body in general — and the mind and the back in particular — psychological factors strongly influence back pain. Various emotional, mental, and physical factors can cause back pain, as shown in Figure 3-2.

Herniated disc. Pinched nerve. Bulging disc. Because back pain is so common, you've probably heard all these diagnoses — and they often provoke unnecessary anxiety. Fear not! Most back pain diagnoses aren't as awful as they sound. In this section, we discuss common back pain diagnoses. We look at the full range of conditions — from common to more rare — and answer the questions: What are the symptoms of each condition? How is the condition diagnosed? What are the treatment options and outlook for recovery?

A few very rare but serious conditions require aggressive medical treatment: cauda equina syndrome, a spinal tumor, and a spinal infection. Your doctor can diagnose these conditions quickly with modern testing techniques. Because they often require surgery, we discuss these conditions more fully in Chapter 8.

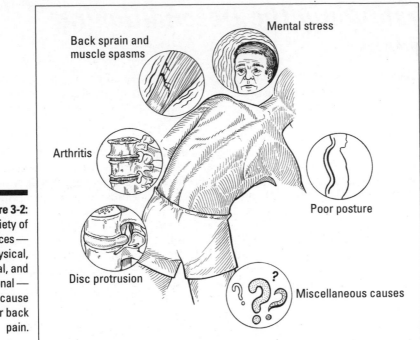

Figure 3-2:
A variety of influences —
physical, mental, and emotional —
can cause your back pain.

Herniated disc/sciatica

As we discuss in the anatomy chapter, the discs lie between the vertebrae (the bones of your back) and act as cushions for the spine. A disc bulge or herniation occurs when the inner part of the disc, which is soft and gel-like (refer to Figure 2-4), pushes out from between the vertebrae in one of two ways:

- ✔ A **bulge** occurs when the fluid inside a disc bulges out but doesn't actually break through the disc wall. Figure 3-3 shows a bulging disc. Bulging discs are commonly seen on MRIs. Bulging discs don't usually cause any symptoms because the nerve roots of the spine aren't irritated or compressed.

- ✔ A **herniation** occurs when the fluid inside a disc bulges toward the back of your body and breaks through the disc wall's outer ring, called the annulus fibrosis (see Figure 3-4).

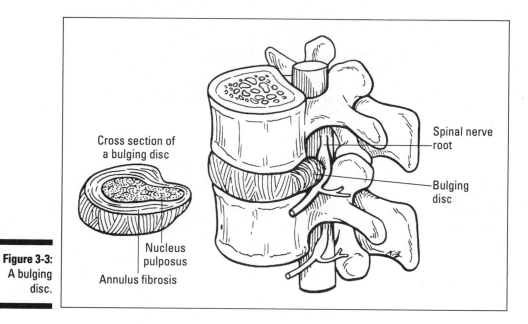

Cross section of
a bulging disc

Spinal nerve
root

Bulging
disc

Nucleus
pulposus

Annulus fibrosis

Figure 3-3:
A bulging
disc.

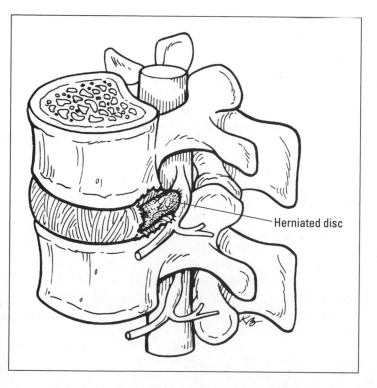

Herniated disc

Figure 3-4:
A herniated
disc.

When a disc is herniated, the disc material that has moved out of its usual space may press against a nearby spinal nerve, producing pain. *Sciatica* pain, commonly called a "pinched nerve," occurs when a herniated disc compresses the nerves of the lumbar spine (lower back). Because these nerves supply the sensation and strength to your legs and feet, a disc problem in your lower back can cause symptoms in your legs, such as weakness or numbness. (You can also have sciatica when a nerve is irritated without being compressed.)

- ✔ More than 90 percent of all lumbar herniated discs occur in between the last two levels of the lower spine (between L4 and L5 and between L5 and S1). Refer to Figure 2-1 for a picture of the lower spine.

- ✔ Sciatica pain typically occurs in the buttocks, back of the thigh, and calf, and occasionally down to the foot and heel.

- ✔ A disc herniation usually "compresses" but doesn't "compromise" the nerve as it leaves your back and goes down your leg (see Figure 3-5 for a view of how a herniated disc can compress against a nerve). While the nerve is irritated, it still works. Occasionally, however, the nerve is so compressed that it causes a decrease in strength, feeling, and reflex. In this case, surgical treatment may be more likely.

If your doctor believes you may be suffering from a disc herniation, the following checklist can help you get a proper diagnosis:

- ✔ **Be sure that your doctor gives you a careful physical exam:** This exam should include a thorough examination of your lower extremities (hips, thighs, legs, and feet); a testing of how your nerves are working in these areas; and a strength test for all the individual muscle groups of the lower extremities. A good physical examination tells the doctor whether you have a disc problem and what nerve roots are being affected. Based upon this evaluation, your doctor can determine whether high-tech imaging studies are necessary.

- ✔ **Sophisticated testing such as an MRI is not always necessary even if you have a suspected herniated disc:** Doctors are generally too quick to order high-tech studies even when they know it will not change the treatment plan. In the vast majority of cases, a herniated disc and sciatica can be diagnosed and treated successfully without imaging studies. High-tech studies are generally only needed if your condition is getting worse or you're considering surgery.

- ✔ **Do not allow your doctor to diagnose a herniated disc as the cause of your pain based simply on an MRI:** Your doctor should give you a careful physical examination. Also, if you do have an MRI and it shows a herniated disc, your doctor should be able to determine that there is a high correlation between your symptoms and the location of the disc herniation. Otherwise, the MRI finding may mean absolutely nothing.

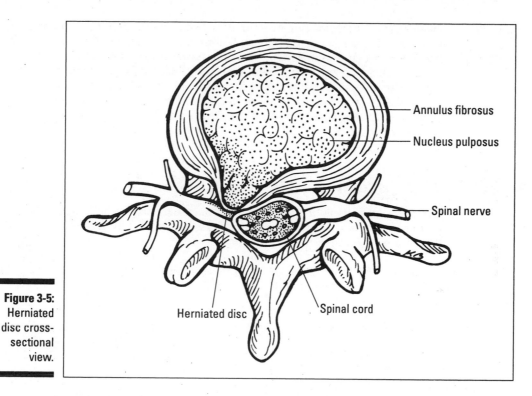

Annulus fibrosus

Nucleus pulposus

Spinal nerve

Spinal cord

Herniated disc

Figure 3-5:
Herniated
disc cross-
sectional
view.

If you've had symptoms of a disc herniation for less than one month, your doctor can reasonably begin conservative treatment such as physical therapy, exercises, and anti-inflammatory medication or epidural steroid injections to reduce swelling. Some alternative medicine procedures, such as yoga, acupuncture, or massage, can also be useful.

The natural healing pattern of a disc herniation is very favorable. The great majority of disc herniations can be treated using nonsurgical, conservative management such as a combination of physical therapy, exercises, epidural steroids, nerve blocks, medications, and healing time (which we discuss in Chapter 7). Most people get better within two to three months of conservative treatment. Don't get panicked about mild sensory loss, reflex loss, or weakness associated with a herniated disc: These functions usually return to normal as you recover.

Even if your symptoms become chronic (lasting more than three months), you can still choose to continue conservative management. Ongoing pain and symptoms are not necessarily reasons to have surgery, and you still may improve, even after three months. While your doctor may recommend surgery as an option, don't automatically assume it is your only course of action. Surgery is sometimes suggested in an effort to "try something." Surgical decisions should be made according to very specific rules, which we discuss in Chapter 8.

The sprain-strain diagnosis

Sprain-strain injury is the most common diagnosis used in the medical treatment of back pain. This diagnosis also has the greatest number of different definitions. A sprain-strain is an injury to the muscles, ligaments, or tendons of the lower back and is caused by an injury (due to a sports activity or lifting a heavy object, for example) or poor posture or lack of physical conditioning over time (or any combination of these).

Pregnancy and back pain

One of the more common side effects of pregnancy is back pain. Some women describe the back pain as simply a "discomfort" while others find it almost unbearable. If you have a history of back pain, you may be concerned about how pregnancy may affect your pain. Thankfully, you can effectively manage your back pain while you go through your pregnancy.

Why is back pain so prevalent during pregnancy?

As your abdominal muscles expand, they lose some of their ability to keep your spine erect and stable. This lack of stability, in addition to changes in your center of gravity, can cause your posture to change in a way that is conducive to back pain.

Fortunately, there are some things you can do to help prevent or minimize back pain during pregnancy. First, pay attention to your posture as much as possible (see Chapter 13 for details). Also, practice the exercises we describe in Chapter 14. A specialized yoga class for pregnancy can also be an excellent option. Of course, you should always check with your doctor prior to beginning any exercise program during a pregnancy. Lastly, be aware that inadequate calcium in your diet can cause muscle spasms. You may require more calcium while you are pregnant and if you subsequently breast feed. Check with your doctor to determine whether you're getting adequate calcium.

A sprain-strain is not a serious condition. We can't emphasize this point enough! It will heal just like any other injury. An ongoing exercise and conditioning program can help prevent sprain-strain injuries from recurring. Tempting as it may be to spend a few days on the couch, one of the worst things you can do for a sprain-strain injury is to rest too much.

Typical symptoms of a sprain-strain injury include:

- **Pain, tightness, and spasms in your lower back area:** Pain may occur quickly (such as in response to an injury), or the pain may build slowly over time (in which no specific injury is identifiable).

- **Tenderness:** The muscles on either side of your spine and down to the upper part of your buttock area may be more sensitive.

- **Pain that worsens by bending forward or to the sides:** In severe cases, this pain may be associated with a muscle spasm.

- **Pain that is worse in the morning and then improves with activity over the course of the day:** This is a common pattern in sprain-strain injuries: The muscles seem to warm up as you move around and the discomfort subsides.

There is no specific test (such as a blood test or X ray) for a sprain-strain injury. The diagnosis of sprain-strain is usually based upon history and the absence of other findings that suggest any type of nerve root irritation.

Doctors often link a sprain-strain diagnosis to some type of activity associated with its onset. We try to avoid doing this. If a doctor pinpoints certain activities as the cause of your pain, you may develop a phobia about these movements. We've seen patients develop a serious fear of almost any movement. They begin to limit their activities, and they soon develop a full-blown case of deconditioning syndrome.

In the majority of sprain-strain cases, a simple treatment approach alleviates symptoms and returns you to full functioning and activities. Treatment includes:

- Initially, you should temporarily stop or reduce any activity that produces an increase in symptoms while trying to maintain some lower level of activity. You can then gradually increase your activity over several weeks.

- Use ice on the painful areas during the first 24 to 48 hours after injury. To avoid ice burn of your skin, you should limit ice use to 20 minutes every two hours. Don't allow ice to have direct contact with your skin.

- Take Tylenol or a nonsteroidal, anti-inflammatory medication if Tylenol isn't helping.

✔ Allow for one or two days of bed rest and use muscle relaxant medications for three to four days in the case of a severe sprain-strain injury.

✔ Gradually resume normal activities, light stretching, and movement on the third or fourth day to prevent you from becoming fearful of movement and to keep your muscles conditioned.

In some cases (for example, if a patient has developed a very strong fear of re-injury) additional formal treatment may be necessary. Physical therapy can help by providing support and guidance as you return to activity as well as reducing acute pain and spasms.

Stress-related back pain

Stress-related back pain is not a traditional medical diagnosis. Based on our experience, we believe stress may be one of the most common causes of back pain. Typical symptoms include diffuse muscle aches (including back pain), sleep disturbance, depression, anxiety, and fatigue.

Be aware that because many traditional medical doctors aren't familiar with the stress-related back pain diagnosis, you may need to raise the possibility if you believe stress may be causing your back pain. As in a sprain-strain, stress-related back pain is diagnosed based on history and the absence of structural causes of back pain such as a herniated disc.

Most people with back pain are naturally inclined to focus on the physical problem. If your back pain is stress-related, looking at the emotional issues is essential for improvement. Part of your treatment for this condition may include psychotherapy or stress counseling to help get control of the emotional issues that are causing the back pain. We often make the recommendation to "think psychological, not physical" when the pain occurs. A therapist is often useful in providing the necessary reassurance as you begin to increase activities and "challenge" the pain.

Arthritis of the spine

Arthritis is a general term that means "inflammation of a joint or joints" in any part of the body, including the spine. Arthritis has many different causes and comes in many types. Some are part of the natural aging process and cause no pain symptoms, while others can be quite severe in terms of deformation of the joints and pain.

Many people associate the term "arthritis" with rheumatoid arthritis, which causes pain and malformation of joints in the body. That can make the diagnosis of arthritis associated with your back pain very scary. The good news is that rheumatoid arthritis rarely affects the spine.

CLINICAL INFO

Psychosomatic pain: Not just "in your head"

When emotional issues are thought to cause physical problems, the condition is called *psychosomatic* or *psycho-physiological.* People generally think that psychosomatic medical conditions are imaginary. This is not true. *Psychosomatic* means that an emotional issue has caused a real physical problem.

Psychosomatic conditions include certain types of asthma, neck pain, headaches, ulcers, skin problems, and back pain. No one would argue that these are not "real" physical and medical problems. They cause very real stress, discomfort, pain, and disability.

Simple changes in your lifestyle can go a long way in preventing and treating psychosomatic back pain. The first step toward a full recovery is to work with a therapist who can help you identify the source of your psychosomatic pain and provide support and encouragement as you work through the pain.

When discussing "arthritis of the spine," doctors are most often referring to findings on X rays and MRIs that are actually part of the natural aging process. Arthritic changes in joints occur naturally with age and do not produce pain symptoms.

In our opinion, the term "arthritis" should rarely be used when discussing joint changes in the spine. We frequently see young to middle-aged patients who say, "My previous doctor told me that I have the spine of an 80-year-old." A message like this can create great suffering and fear for no reason.

Degenerative disc disease

Degenerative disc disease is a condition in which the soft, central portion of the disc loses some of its water content and begins to dry out. The first image in Figure 3-6 shows a normal disc. The second image in Figure 3-6 shows that disc degeneration has occurred, which decreases the disc's height, narrows the *foramen* (or opening), and misaligns the facet joint.

You can think of degenerative disc disease as being similar to getting gray hair. The condition isn't really a disease at all, but a term that describes the wear-and-tear of aging that begins at about age 20. Degenerative disc disease is simply a part of the aging process in those unfortunate humans who get older — and that includes all of us!

Sometimes this condition can lead to a mechanical type of low back pain in people who are not physically fit and attempt strenuous activity. Degenerative disc disease is treated with appropriate exercise, body mechanics, and anti-inflammatory medication. This disease rarely requires surgical treatment.

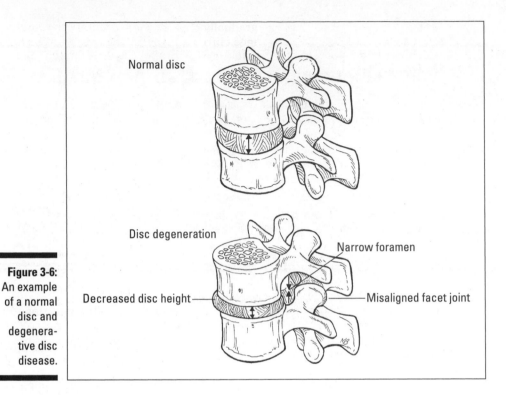

Normal disc

Disc degeneration

Narrow foramen

Decreased disc height

Misaligned facet joint

Facet syndrome

A *facet joint* is the technical name for a joint between two vertebrae. Facet joints allow your vertebrae to move while keeping your spine in proper alignment. Like all joints, they are subject to wear and tear and begin to look abnormal as you age. If you suffer from *facet syndrome,* you have an inflammation of one or more of your facet joints. Inflammation of these joints can produce *referred pain,* which is pain that you feel some place other than where it is being caused.

Facet syndrome may cause tenderness in an area of about one and one-half inches to the side of your spine in your lower back. Pressure in this area may cause discomfort and sometimes pain down into your buttock or thigh area. You may notice that the pain gets worse when you bend sideways, backward, twist your waist, or stand on one leg.

This syndrome is not serious. Although it can produce pain, the pain usually goes away within two to three weeks. Treatment for facet syndrome is the same as for a sprain-strain: temporarily stopping or reducing the activity that produces an increase in symptoms; using ice on the painful areas in the first 24 to 48 hours after injury; taking anti-inflammatory medication; using a back brace to reduce movement; and gradually resuming normal activities and movement. If the condition becomes chronic, it may be treated by an injection of anti-inflammatory and anesthetic medication into the irritated joint known as a facet block.

Arachnoiditis

Arachnoiditis is scarring of the connective tissue (the spinal arachnoid) around your spinal nerve roots. *Arachnoid* literally means "like a cobweb" and describes how the condition looks on your imaging studies. The most common cause of arachnoiditis is a previous surgery in that area. Arachnoiditis symptoms can include pain, numbness, and tingling in your legs. You may have no pain or symptoms at all, despite an MRI finding of arachnoiditis in some cases.

High anxiety: A new theory about stress-related back pain

Dr. John Sarno popularized the notion of stress-related back pain in several books. He believes that a person's emotions — espccially pent-up anger and anxiety, which have serious negative effects on the body — cause stress-related back pain. We work with Dr. Sarno and have personally witnessed some dramatic results.

Sarno suggests that certain personality types are likely to get stress-related back pain. According to Sarno, the following personality characteristics interact with stressful life situations to cause stress-related back pain:

✔ Strongly driven to succeed

✔ Hold a strong sense of responsibility

✔ Self-motivated and disciplined

✔ Harshly critical of yourself

✔ Have perfectionist and compulsive tendencies

Sarno believes that your mind, when faced with a stressful emotional situation, may push emotional tension and stress out of your awareness and into your unconscious. This unconscious tension from emotional stress causes muscle tension, spasm, and pain in your lower back and elsewhere. Your mind chooses the distraction of physical pain instead of dealing with the actual emotional issues that your mind perceives as more threatening.

Sarno says awareness and understanding of how your mind can deal with emotional stress is the first step toward healing stress-related back pain. He warns against repressing your anger or emotions and says you shouldn't let back pain intimidate you. He also says to not think of yourself as injured, because psychological conditioning can contribute to ongoing back pain.

Sarno suggests resuming physical activity; "talking back" to your brain and telling it you won't take it any more; and stopping all treatments for your back, as they may be blocking your recovery.

Arachnoiditis can be difficult to resolve because its symptoms are not very responsive to traditional back pain treatments. You may be treated with pain medicines, physical therapy, or a cortisone injection. In severe cases, a spinal cord stimulator may be recommended for you. For more information on spinal cord stimulators, check out Chapter 7.

Arachnoiditis does not always mean that you shouldn't undergo spinal surgery if doing so is necessary for some other spine problem. Often spine surgeons try to avoid spine surgery for any reason when arachnoiditis is present because surgery can make the condition worse. If you're diagnosed with arachnoiditis, proceed very cautiously. The condition itself cannot be treated by surgery, and there is always the risk that any spinal surgery may make arachnoiditis worse.

Spondylolisthesis and spondylolysis

Spondylolisthesis literally means "slipping vertebrae" and describes a condition in which one of your vertebrae "slips" over another (see Figure 3-7). What causes the vertebrae to slip? Often, it's a fracture or crack (called a *spondylolysis*) in part of the vertebrae, often due to degenerative changes.

A spondylolysis often results from trauma occurring over a period of time during your teenage years. Sports activities that involve repeated *hyperextension* (bending over backwards) are often the culprit. Although you can get this condition for many reasons, both in childhood and adulthood, spondylolisthesis is most often seen in gymnasts, ballet dancers, and football players. Typically, a single episode of hyperextension does not cause a problem, but repeated episodes can result in an actual break.

Figure 3-7: Notice how the two vertebrae are slipping (Spondylolisthesis) due to the fracture (spondylolysis).

Lateral view — Defect — Amount of vertebral slippage

Posterior view — Superior articular facet — Transverse process — Inferior articular facet — Defect

Spondylolisthesis can cause pain in the lower back and occasionally, sciatic pain if the nerve roots are involved. A very common indicator of this condition in a young person is a backache that lasts for more than one or two weeks.

If your doctor suspects that you have this condition, you should have a bone scan, which can detect very fine cracks in your vertebrae. (We discuss bone scans in Chapter 7.) If the problem is diagnosed at the time the fracture occurs (usually when the patient is 13 to 16 years old), the condition can be treated effectively and completely. Treatment usually includes a brace and restriction of activities for about four months to allow the fracture to heal. In severe cases of "slipping," spinal fusion surgery in which two adjacent vertebrae are fused together may be necessary. We discuss fusion surgery in Chapter 8. If this condition goes unrecognized when it occurs in childhood, it can cause back problems later in life.

The other common type of spondylolisthesis is called *degenerative spondylolisthesis.* This condition is caused by severe wear and tear changes in the facet joints or connecting joints of your lower back due to a variety of reasons. The most common location for this condition to occur is between the fourth and fifth lumbar vertebrae, with the fourth vertebra slipping forward (toward your stomach) over the fifth vertebra. Treatment is the same as in spondylolisthesis.

Coccydynia

Coccydynia literally means "pain in the coccyx." The *coccyx* is the bone at the very bottom of your spine. Coccydynia most often occurs as a result of trauma, usually a direct fall on the buttocks (or in technical terms, your bottom). A fall of this type can sometimes result in a broken tailbone. In other cases, you may have no evidence of a break in the tailbone, but you have pain near your tailbone for unknown reasons. Coccydynia can also result in persistent pain and tenderness just above your rectal area. Coccydynia is often diagnosed simply by the symptoms, because in many cases, nothing unusual is seen on X rays. Diagnosis is made by physical exam, history of pain in the coccyx area with or without trauma, and sometimes X rays. Coccydynia can be a real pain in the you-know-what!

If you have coccydynia, you can expect the treatment to include several things. First, the painfully obvious: You must avoid sitting on hard surfaces. Using a donut-shaped cushion can help control the pain. If you have a more resistant case, you may receive anti-inflammatory medication or a local injection of anesthetic and cortisone. Recent research suggests that a special type of biofeedback that teaches you to relax local muscle spasms can also help. See Chapter 12 for a detailed explanation of biofeedback.

Surgery to remove the coccyx may be considered as a last resort if you have a severe and chronic case of coccydynia. If your doctor recommends surgery for this condition, we recommend that you get a pre-surgical psychological evaluation from a qualified psychologist to insure that the pain is not due to a stress-related problem. We have seen many cases in which surgery was done only to have the pain continue. We recommend getting a second opinion before considering surgery for this problem. To find out more about what coccydynia surgery entails, what to expect, and its risks and benefits, see Chapter 8.

Spinal fractures

Spinal fractures, diagnosed through an X ray, are almost always caused by one of the following:

- A severe trauma such as a motor vehicle accident or fall
- A disease that causes weakening of the spinal bones, including osteoporosis and cancer of the spine

Typical warning signs of a possible spinal fracture is back pain that

- Occurs suddenly in middle-aged or elderly persons after bending or lifting
- Is worse with activity
- Is so severe it wakes you up at night
- Does not go away within a week or two

If you suspect a spinal fracture, you should be evaluated immediately by a physician who is familiar with spinal problems. An X ray can detect a fracture. *Compression fractures,* which are more common in people with diseases that weaken the spinal bones, are easily detected through an X ray because these fractures often cause a pie-shaped appearance to the vertebral body.

Subluxation

Subluxation, or a limitation of movement in a joint, is a term frequently used by chiropractors to explain the cause of low-back pain. Various chiropractic treatments are used to restore a joint that is supposedly "subluxed" or restricted.

This diagnosis is controversial among physicians who treat spinal problems. Not all doctors are convinced that subluxed joints actually exist and cause pain. We discuss getting appropriate chiropractic treatment in Chapter 10.

Treatment can include the use of narcotic analgesics for pain relief in the first two to three weeks. Sometimes, a spinal fracture requires long-term use of narcotic analgesics, restricted activity, and the use of a brace for up to three months as the fracture heals. The prognosis is excellent for the fracture to heal and result in a return to normal activities.

Lumbar spinal stenosis

Lumbar spinal stenosis is a narrowing of the spinal canal that causes a compression or "pinching" of the nerves that go to the buttocks and legs. Stenosis occurs because of:

- Disc bulges
- Wear and tear change that creates boney spurs
- Overgrowth of the facet joint
- Congenital (meaning "from birth") narrowing of the spinal canal

Lumbar spinal stenosis most typically presents itself as pain in the buttocks and legs that

- Limits your ability to walk for any great distance or at a fast pace.
- Goes away if you lean forward at the waist as you walk. For example, someone with pain from lumbar stenosis would find relief by leaning on the shopping cart as they shop for groceries.
- Is relieved if you sit down for a short period of time or until your symptoms subside.

Lumbar spinal stenosis is diagnosed based on your medical history, a physical examination, and imaging studies. This condition is seen more frequently as you pass age 65, due to aging of the spine.

Although lumbar stenosis usually gets worse over time, it does not lead to paralysis, a shortening of life, or a loss of life. The most common consequences are limitations in your activities. In most cases, the progression of symptoms is slow. Sometimes, the condition actually improves even though your MRIs look worse — and doctors don't know why!

Treatment consists of three phases going from least invasive to most invasive:

- First, depending on your symptoms, your doctor may recommend an exercise program combined with use of oral medication such as anti-inflammatory medicine.

✔ Second, your doctor may recommend a special type of epidural steroid injection into the space surrounding the spinal nerves. This often provides dramatic relief and may last for several years before being repeated.

✔ Third, you may be asked to consider a surgical widening of your spinal canal. The procedure includes a *laminectomy,* or removal of the bony part of each vertebra (see Chapter 2 for all the anatomical details). Remember that undergoing surgery for this condition is also your decision to make, depending on your tolerance of the symptoms and your quality of life.

Chronic back pain syndrome

The *chronic back pain syndrome* is a group of symptoms that occur when your back pain lasts for more than about three to six months — beyond the point of tissue healing. The chronic back pain syndrome goes beyond simple physical deconditioning as we discuss earlier in this chapter (see Figure 3-8). According to Dr. Robert Gatchel, physical and mental deconditioning cause chronic back pain syndrome. In other words, if you don't use it, you'll lose it.

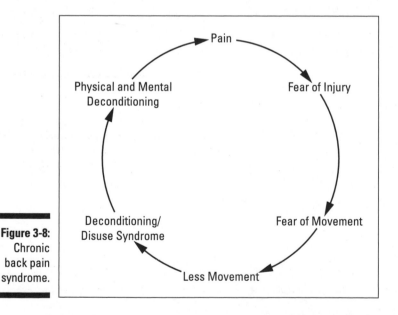

Figure 3-8: Chronic back pain syndrome.

Research has shown that the physical findings in chronic back pain patients are no more serious than in those patients whose back injury heals in the normal amount of time. That's why we believe stress and other emotional factors probably contribute to chronic pain. Changes to blood flow patterns to the back muscles and anxiety about the pain may keep the muscles perpetually in spasm. Overtreating with rest and passive therapy can lead to deconditioning and chronic pain syndrome.

The failed back surgery syndrome

In our opinion, *failed back surgery syndrome* occurs most commonly when the wrong patient is selected for a spine surgery. Unfortunately, failed back surgery syndrome is all too common. The symptoms are similar to chronic back pain syndrome, except that they arise *after* spine surgery. You can get failed back surgery syndrome due to:

- Early infection after spine surgery

- Spine surgery that is done at the wrong level or that does not heal properly

- Psychological distress

- Inadequate re-conditioning after a spine surgery

- Some other structural problem (stenosis, arachnoiditis, and so on)

The best treatment for failed back surgery syndrome is to avoid creating it in the first place. Be very wary of spinal surgery and make the decision to undergo it only after careful consideration of all the alternatives. We discuss this issue further in Chapter 8 on surgical decision-making.

If you already have failed back surgery syndrome, your treatment should never be just more spine surgery. Instead, try a conservative, nonsurgical approach similar to that used for chronic back pain syndrome. Focus on treating your physical, psychological, and emotional issues simultaneously.

Chronic back pain syndrome often gets worse over time and includes physical and psychological symptoms. By the time chronic back pain syndrome is fully developed, many of the symptoms are not related to the original pain problem. Rather, they are due to deconditioning, overuse of pain medication, depression, anxiety, and social isolation.

If you have chronic back pain syndrome, treatment most likely needs to be multidisciplinary in order to treat all aspects of your problem simultaneously. Treatment may include:

- Physical exercise and reactivation to address your deconditioning

- Psychological intervention to address mental deconditioning and emotional issues

- Detoxification to address medication dependence and substance abuse problems (not an issue in all cases)

- Return to work or other activity that provides you with a sense of purpose

- Various medications including antidepressants, which are often prescribed as part of a comprehensive treatment program

Other Conditions That Cause Back Pain

The conditions described in this section usually aren't the primary cause of significant back pain. If you have one of these conditions, you may have some associated back pain — or none at all. We include these diagnoses because we get frequent questions about them.

Discitis

Discitis, or "inflammation of the disc," is a rare condition. Although the exact causes are unknown, discitis may be caused by a bacterial or viral infection in the disc space. The result is inflammation and pain. You are more likely to develop discitis if you have diabetes or immune system problems. If bacteria is the cause of your discitis, the treatment will include antibiotics. In children, discitis is treated in part with a back brace, if needed.

Fibromyalgia

Fibromyalgia, a diagnosis often made if you're suffering from chronic low-back pain, is characterized by sleep disturbance, multiple tender joints, fatigue, diffuse pain, and limitations of activity.

Fibromyalgia may have associated symptoms such as bowel problems, tingling and numbness, chronic headaches, chest pain, problems with memory, anxiety, and depression, among others. Your doctor will assess all these symptoms to make the diagnosis, especially the area (or areas) of your body where you experience pain. There is no medical test (such as blood or X ray) for fibromyalgia.

Several terms have been used to describe this pain problem, including myofascial pain syndrome, myositis, fibrositis, and tension myalgia, just to name a few. There continues to be no clear understanding of the cause or cure for fibromyalgia, but a large number of treatments are purported to be beneficial.

Current treatment programs generally include anti-inflammatory medications to relieve pain, antidepressant medications for their effect on sleep and depression, and a gradual increase in activities through appropriate exercise. You can also use various complementary medicine approaches to augment this general treatment approach.

In our opinion, if you have been diagnosed with fibromyalgia, you must choose your treatments carefully. Fibromyalgia patients often go from one treatment to the next in search of a cure. Sadly, they rarely get any real benefit.

REMEMBER

We strongly believe psychological and emotional issues are part of fibromyalgia. Whether these issues cause fibromyalgia or are a reaction to fibromyalgia is unknown. One thing is clear: If you do not address psychological and emotional issues as part of the treatment, it is unlikely to be successful.

We advise fibromyalgia patients to keep the treatment simple and recommend that they consider the following treatments: a brief trial of anti-inflammatory medications for your pain; an antidepressant medication to help improve your sleep, relieve depression, and provide pain relief; an exercise program that gradually increases your activities and encourages you to return to a normal lifestyle; complementary medicine approaches to help with the overall goal of managing your symptoms and returning you to a normal life; attention to psychological and emotional issues that may be increasing your level of suffering and preventing you from recovering; and trying to keep a positive mental attitude.

Osteomyelitis

Osteomyelitis is a rare infection in the vertebrae or bones of the spine. Symptoms include back pain while resting, weight loss, and fever. Osteomyelitis is detected on a number of tests, one of which includes abnormal blood findings. This condition is treated with a brace and appropriate antibiotics for three to six weeks.

Spina bifida occulta

Spina bifida occulta is a technical term that means there is a defect in the *lamina,* or the back part of the vertebrae. (See Chapter 2.) In this condition, the boney ring that forms the back of each vertebra fails to close completely leaving a tiny gap in the rear (usually less than a sixteenth of an inch). The condition occurs during early development of a baby in the mother's uterus and is present in approximately 8 percent of the population. Spina bifida occulta is not a cause of lower back pain.

Scoliosis

Scoliosis is a term that is used to describe a curvature of the spine. Scoliosis, which occurs in several different varieties, rarely causes low-back pain in people under 40 years old, unless it is very severe. Watching out for scoliosis in young people, especially teenage girls, is important, because early treatment with a brace can help avoid surgery later on. For this reason, many schools have scoliosis screening programs.

The key to managing scoliosis is determining if it is progressive (curving more and more over time). A small percentage of scoliosis in the lower back is progressive and needs to be treated through an exercise program, brace, and possibly spine surgery. In the majority of cases, however, a finding of scoliosis is not a reason for back pain or any symptoms and requires no specific treatment.

You should be warned that:

- Scoliosis is commonly given as a reason for low-back pain with recommendations for extensive treatment to straighten out the spine. In these cases, your back pain may actually be due to a disc, sprain-strain, deconditioning, or stress-related problem.

- If you have a scoliosis curve less than 20 degrees — as in the majority of cases seen clinically — you probably need no treatment.

Transitional vertebrae

A transitional vertebra is either one extra or one fewer lumbar vertebra than normal and is often seen on X rays. Transitional vertebrae are found at the base of the lumbar spine where it connects to the sacrum (refer to Figure 2-6). The condition usually is not associated with a greater frequency of low-back pain. If you have this condition, simply consider yourself unique and ignore it.

Osteoporosis

Osteoporosis can cause a weakening in the bones of the spine, making them susceptible to spinal fractures. Elderly, post-menopausal females are most likely to suffer from this condition. If you experience pain from a fracture caused by osteoporosis, it is usually minimal and may last three to six weeks.

Treatment usually consists of limiting your activities, taking mild painkillers, and using an appropriate brace for your lower back. Your family doctor should evaluate the condition of osteoporosis that caused the weakening. Appropriate medications such as supplemental calcium or estrogen therapy may be helpful.

Chapter 4

Out of Your Hands: When to Seek Help and from Whom

● ●

In This Chapter

▶ Understanding the medical community

▶ Knowing what to ask

▶ Getting safe alternative treatments

▶ Developing a positive relationship with your doctor

● ●

*I*n searching for relief from your back pain, you may consult a variety of healthcare professionals. Listing all of the providers who treat back pain is beyond the scope of this book, but the common ones include your family doctor, general practitioner or internist, osteopath, orthopedist, physiatrist (like Dr. Sinel) neurologist, or neurosurgeon. Chiropractors, acupuncturists, and massage therapists are among the other professionals who are also involved in back treatment. All these titles and different folks who treat back pain can be confusing, but we explain the differences among these professionals later in this chapter.

Along with reviewing many types of professionals who treat back pain, we give you some questions to ask your doctor so that you can become an informed and smart consumer when working in partnership with your healthcare provider.

Who Treats Back Pain?

Finding your way in today's confusing medical culture can be like visiting a foreign country in which you don't speak the language or know the lay of the land. You can easily become scared and confused, especially if you don't have a map or translation guide. Don't end up being the bewildered tourist without a clue as to what's going on around you.

The medical community is arranged by levels of specialization:

- **First level:** Your family doctor or general practitioner handles a variety of medical problems. These doctors have a good understanding of all aspects of medicine and often act as coordinators or managers of your treatment program.

- **Second level:** Specialists in disciplines such as orthopedics, neurology, neurosurgery, and physiatry provide a more detailed evaluation of your back pain problem along with more specific treatment approaches. These specialists see patients with problems that fall within their area of expertise, in addition to back pain problems. For example, an orthopedist treats a variety of orthopedic problems (such as knees, elbows, and hips) along with back pain. We discuss these specialists later in this chapter.

- **Third level:** *Subspecialists,* including orthopedists, neurosurgeons, neurologists, and physiatrists who have further specialized training in back pain and spine disorders, provide even a more focused evaluation and treatment approach. Subspecialists often see only back pain or spinal problems. Another doctor (your family doctor or a specialist you have seen) usually refers you to a subspecialist.

Primary care doctors

General practitioners, internists, and family practitioners often bear the term *primary care physicians.* These doctors are usually the first people you consult for any type of medical problem, including back pain. These professionals are usually comfortable and confident treating a variety of medical problems, including back pain.

Healthcare reform and managed care plans discourage the use of specialists, so these primary care doctors are likely to treat more back pain problems in the future. If your primary care doctor has been treating your back pain problem for more than a few weeks and you're not seeing a benefit, you should ask about a referral to a specialist.

Find out whether your family doctor is comfortable treating a back pain problem by asking the questions that we present later in this chapter. Generally, these doctors make certain that your spine has nothing seriously wrong and then treat you during the first six to eight weeks. Your doctor may refer you to a specialist if other symptoms occur or if the pain lingers.

Specialists

Orthopedists, neurosurgeons, neurologists, and physiatrists are the medical specialists most likely to evaluate and treat back pain at the specialist level, as part of a general practice in these areas. Specialists in these areas may or may not focus on back pain and spinal disorders. General specialization in these areas requires a residency after general medical or surgical training, as well as board certification. Subspecialization requires even more training and focus on spine problems as we discuss later.

You're probably familiar with the specialties of orthopedics, neurology, and neurosurgery, but physiatry may be new to you. *Physiatrists* are medical doctors with special training in physical medicine, rehabilitation, and *musculoskeletal* (the muscles and bones) problems. These doctors use non-surgical, conservative treatment approaches for musculoskeletal and other medical problems, including back pain.

Osteopaths also commonly treat back pain problems. Osteopaths can become qualified to practice in any area of medicine, similar to physicians trained at traditional medical schools. Osteopaths can prescribe medicine and do surgery of any type (if they complete an appropriate residency). Osteopaths are also trained in other musculoskeletal and spinal manipulative techniques, similar to chiropractors.

If you need to see a specialist, confirm that the doctor has competency in treating back pain. The questions we present later in the chapter can help you gather this information. Also, make sure that the doctor is familiar with a conservative approach (one that doesn't use surgery). Orthopedists and neurosurgeons complete a surgical residency and are primarily trained in surgical approaches to solve medical problems (including back problems). If you see a neurosurgeon or orthopedic surgeon, you should be sure that she has been trained in (or at least understands and prescribes) conservative treatment approaches to back pain.

Subspecialists

The specialists we mention in the preceding section can further specialize in the areas of spinal disorders and back pain. Although orthopedists, neurosurgeons, and physiatrists most often subspecialize in spinal disorders, other areas of medicine may also focus on back pain.

Our top recommendation is to see a physiatrist who specializes in spinal disorders. For more info, see Appendix B.

Asking Your Doctor the Right Questions

Use the following questions to find a treating professional for your back pain problem so that you get the highest quality of care and avoid unnecessary and harmful treatments.

Checking board certification

The following organizations can help you gather information on board certification, including what training and expertise is required, whether your doctor is board-certified, and how to go about finding a board-certified doctor in a certain discipline. We list additional organizations in Appendix B, and you may get referrals to other resources by calling the following groups:

✔ **Physicians:**

American Board of Medical Specialties, 1007 Church Street, Suite 404, Evanston, IL, 60201-5913; phone 708-491-9091 or 1-800-776-2378

American Medical Association, 515 N. State St., Chicago, IL 60610; phone 312-464-5000 or 800-621-8335

Canadian Association of Physical Medicine and Rehabilitation, 774 Echo Drive, 5th Floor, Ottawa, Ontario, K1S 5N8; phone 613-730-6245

Canadian Orthopaedic Association, 1440 Ste-Catherine Street, West, #421, Montreal, Quebec, H3G 1R8; phone 514-874-9003

Canadian Neurological Society, 906-12th Avenue SW, #810, P.O. Box 4220, Station C, Calgary, Alberta T2T 5N1; phone 403-229-9544

✔ **Osteopaths:**

American Academy of Osteopathy, 3500 De Pauw Blvd., Suite 1080, Indianapolis, IN 46268; phone 317-879-1881; Fax 317-879-0563

American Osteopathic Association, 142 East Ontario St., Chicago, IL 60611; phone 312-280-5800

✔ **Chiropractic:**

American Chiropractic Association, 1701 Clarendon Blvd., Arlington, VA 22209; phone 703-276-8800

British Chiropractic Association, 29 Whitley St., Reading, Berks, U.K. RG2 0EG; phone 17-34-757-557

✔ **Health Psychology:**

American Board of Professional Psychology, 2100 E. Broadway, Suite 313, Columbus, MO, 65201; phone 573-443-1199

American Psychological Association, 750 First St., NE, Washington, DC 20002-4242; phone 202-336-5700

Most back pain problems don't require the care of either a specialist or sub-specialist. A family doctor or chiropractor can safely manage the majority of acute back pain problems. In working with any doctor, you need to have a good idea about the answers to the following questions. You don't necessarily need to grill your doctor; rather use these questions as guidelines for the kind of information you should know about your doctor. You can get much of this information from the office staff — you can ask the doctor directly any remaining questions.

- ✔ **What is your degree?** Determining the treating practitioner's professional degree is important. Many professionals go by the term "doctor" even though they aren't medical physicians. Groups who are referred to as "doctor" but are not physicians include such degrees as Ph.D. (for example, exercise physiology, physical therapy, and nursing), D.C. (Doctor of Chiropractic), and a variety of "doctorates" in alternative medicine practice. Although you may choose to get treatment from a doctor without medical training, you need to know what type of evaluation and treatment the doctor is qualified to provide.

- ✔ **Where did you do your training?** Know where your doctor did his or her training in terms of medical school education, internship, residency, and any subspecialty training.

- ✔ **Are you a board-certified specialist?** Completing a multi-year residency and passing a national board certification examination is usually necessary for board certification in a medical specialty. Ask where your doctor did his or her residency and when he or she passed the specialty board certification examination.

   Distinguishing between the terms *board-eligible* and *board-certified* is important. *Board-eligible* means that the doctor has completed the required training but has not yet passed the examination. *Board-certified* means the doctor has completed the entire certification process, including the examination.

   Board certification also occurs in areas other than medicine. Most professional groups have a certification process. For instance, chiropractors, osteopaths, psychologists, and physical therapists, as well as many other disciplines, all have board certification. Almost any healthcare practitioner can train to be a specialist in areas beyond general practice.

   In areas other than medicine, ask how the board certification was completed. Many so-called board certification credentials are available simply by filling out a form and sending it in with an appropriate dues payment. These "credentials" can mislead you because you may assume that board certification actually documents a higher level of specialized training. You can double-check any doctor's board certification by checking with the organizations listed in the sidebar at the beginning of the section and Appendix B.

✔ **To what medical and professional societies do you belong?** Ask about the types of medical and/or professional societies in which your doctor has membership, because this information can give you an idea of his or her treatment focus. General medical and professional societies are relevant to each discipline. Beyond those groups, doctors can belong to specialized societies in the area of spinal disorders and back pain problems. Membership in specialized societies usually indicates that the healthcare professional is obtaining continuing education in the area of spinal problems and back pain.

✔ **How long have you practiced in this area?** A doctor who has practiced a number of years in the community can help in terms of *treatment networking*. A treatment network may lead your doctor to recommend other local specialists or a potentially helpful exercise program. Even though all doctors have to start out new in practice at some point, a well-established practice is more likely to have a good understanding of community resources available.

✔ **Do you have special training in treating back pain problems?** Subspecialization in the area of back problems includes having further training or having a practice limited primarily to spine and back pain. Subspecialization usually isn't common in smaller communities and is most often available through university medical schools.

✔ **Are you comfortable treating back pain by using a conservative approach?** Find out whether your doctor is comfortable and competent using a conservative approach to back pain. (As we discuss in Chapter 7, a *conservative treatment approach* is one that does not involve surgery.) You especially need to ask this question in the case of specialists who have trained primarily as surgeons.

✔ **What percentage of patients do you see with back pain problems?** This important question is often best directed at the office manager rather than the doctor. Going to a doctor who specializes in spinal disorders would ensure that his or her practice is primarily made up of back pain sufferers.

You can obtain many of the answers to the preceding questions by looking at a copy of your doctor's *curriculum vitae,* or résumé. Most offices have this document on file and are more than willing to provide you with this information prior to scheduling your first appointment. You can look it over in the doctor's office or request a copy of your own.

Be reasonable when asking the preceding questions. Don't expect a doctor to take the time to answer all of the preceding questions prior to scheduling an initial appointment (or even as part of the initial appointment). Obtain all the information you can from the doctor's résumé and then ask any remaining questions you still have.

Dealing with Chiropractors and Other Practitioners

Chiropractors and other practitioners (for example, homeopaths and naturopaths) treat a great number of back pain cases. This treatment is either primary or in addition to medical care. In this section, you find out how to obtain these treatments in an informed manner.

Address the following issues whenever you obtain chiropractic or other non-traditional care for your back pain:

✔ **See your physician first:** Your medical doctor should evaluate your back before you obtain non-traditional care. Your doctor can rule out any serious causes of back pain such as a tumor or infection. Even though these causes of back pain are extremely rare, they do occur. Your medical doctor can also determine whether other treatments are safe for you.

✔ **Get a referral from a dependable source:** To investigate a referral, gather information from an appropriate professional society. You may also get referrals from family and friends who have had positive treatment experiences. When getting referrals from non-professionals who have had treatment, ask about the nature of the treatment provided and the outcome.

✔ **Ask questions:** When seeking non-traditional care for your back pain, you can use many of the questions that we outline in the section, "Asking Your Doctor the Right Questions." Other specific questions include

• **Do you treat primarily back pain problems?** You want to be sure that your practitioner is qualified to treat back pain problems and treats patients with problems similar to yours on a frequent basis.

• **Will you work with my medical doctor?** Your non-medical practitioner needs to be willing to work and communicate with your physician. Although communication may not always be necessary, you want to know that your practitioner would contact your physician or coordinate care if you, your physician, or practitioner felt it was necessary.

• **Will you recommend exercises and other things I can do at home?** Similar to working with your physician, you need to know whether a non-traditional practitioner can give you something that you can begin to do on your own to help with your back pain.

• **Can you tell me how long and how often I should expect to be treated?** This question is appropriate for anyone providing you with treatment. You should have an idea as to how long and how often you will be treated based upon the practitioners' work with patients similar to you.

The warning signs of poor practice: Watch out!

You are more likely to find the following signs of poor practice in the nontraditional arena. However, be concerned if *any* doctor

✔ Doesn't complete a history and clinical examination before beginning treatment

✔ Tries to get other family members to begin treatment

✔ Wants you to sign a contract for long-term care

✔ Promises to prevent back pain or disease through regular check-ups or manipulation

✔ Discourages getting a second opinion

Building a Positive Relationship with Your Healthcare Provider

Your relationship with your doctor or other healthcare professional (traditional or non-traditional) treating your back pain problem is critical to your getting better. Significant problems with treatment can occur if your expectations and your doctor's don't match. You may, for example, expect your doctor to simply diagnose your problem and then fix it. Being a passive patient can have negative results. For instance, if you're given an exercise program and don't practice it properly, it won't work.

Back pain treatment is most effective when you *and* your doctor take an active role in seeking solutions. Being active in your treatment can be challenging because you may have to deal with potentially intimidating people, including your doctor (see Chapter 22 for more information). Also, doctors are sometimes uncomfortable with patients who want to be fully involved in their treatment. Some doctors become defensive when you try to be active in your treatment by asking questions, thinking that you are questioning their judgment rather than trying to get yourself the best care possible. Use the tips in this book (especially Chapter 22) to help you be active in your treatment and work successfully with your doctor.

Part II
Conventional Treatment Options

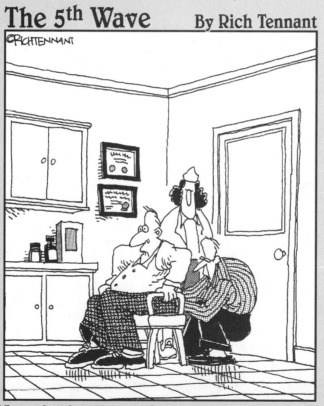

The 5th Wave   By Rich Tennant

"I don't think the crackling sound coming from
your lower back is as serious as you thought.
Just relax, and I'll have this Rice Krispie Square
out of your back pocket in no time."

In this part . . .

*W*hen back pain strikes, your first reaction is probably some very basic self-care, such as ice packs or heating pads, bed rest, and over-the-counter pain relievers. If the pain continues for more than a couple of days, your next stop is most likely your family doctor, who, depending on the type and severity of pain you're experiencing, may or may not refer you to a specialist.

This part explores all these traditional treatment options. We also explain common medical tests and treatments, and we spend a chapter discussing back surgeries, concentrating on whether and when they may be appropriate for you.

Chapter 5

Home Remedies: First Aid for Your Back Attack

· ·

In This Chapter

▶ Knowing when you need to see a doctor

▶ Managing your own back attack

▶ Working the steps to recovery

· ·

So, things seem to be going along relatively smoothly. You have your job, you have your family, and you make time to have a little fun. Then, like a blind-sided tackle in a football game, the *back attack* hits. Your back attack may consist of a slight pain and stiffness in your lower back area. Or the pain may significantly restrict your movements and cause you distress. You may even have pain running down one or both legs.

Perhaps you have just hit the perfect drive on the eighth hole of your favorite golf course. Maybe you lifted a heavy piece of equipment at work. Maybe you bent over to pick up a pencil. Or, maybe you just woke up with back pain one morning. In any case, the back pain hit and got your attention in a major way.

Fortunately, all is not lost (not even close!). Whatever your situation, you can choose from several techniques — which we discuss in this chapter — to help you manage your back attack successfully.

Heading for the Doctor

You can manage and treat most episodes of back pain on your own. But, you also need to recognize a few warning signs that mean you should skip the home remedies and head straight to the doctor for an evaluation:

✔ **You can't control your bowel or bladder.** If you suddenly lose control of your bowel or bladder, you should either see a physician who specializes in spinal problems or go to the emergency room *immediately*. Bowel or bladder problems include the following:

- You can't control or initiate urination or bowel movements

- You have no feeling in your groin and/or anal area

- You're male, and you can no longer get an erection

Any of the preceding symptoms indicate possible *cauda equina syndrome*. In cauda equina syndrome, some of the nerves that control bowel, bladder, and other functions become compressed. If this compression isn't corrected surgically within about 24 to 48 hours, these problems may become permanent due to nerve damage. (Chapters 3 and 8 offer a more detailed discussion of cauda equina syndrome.)

✔ **Your legs are weak or you experience foot drop.** If you experience weakness in your legs and feet, then you should see a spinal specialist within 24 hours or go to the emergency room. Weakness that occurs in your foot is called *foot drop* because you have trouble flexing your foot and toes up toward your head. You also have trouble walking because your foot is weak and has a tendency to drag.

✔ **Your back pain awakens you at night.** Back pain that awakens you from sleep at night can indicate a tumor or spinal infection. This type of pain is called *rest pain* and involves severe throbbing and aching that worsens with rest. Although many people with back pain report being awakened at night by pain, this pain is different from the constant throbbing that a tumor or spinal infection causes. Although a tumor or spinal infection may not be quite the emergency that cauda equina syndrome can be, you should still see a specialist fairly quickly or go to the emergency room.

✔ **You experience a significant trauma such as a car accident or a fall.** In general, if you suffer a significant trauma such as a car accident or fall that causes back pain, you should see a doctor. Depending on how bad the pain is, you may go to the emergency room, see your family doctor, or see a spinal specialist. Although most back pain doesn't require imaging studies, your doctor may recommend an x-ray or other imaging test to check for fractured vertebrae if you've had a trauma.

✔ **Your back pain is excruciating.** If your back pain is simply excruciating and unbearable, then you need to go to the emergency room or to your doctor *immediately*. Also, a physician should check any significant increase in pain to an excruciating level right away. *Excruciating* is a subjective term; however, if your pain is so bad that you can barely move or are on the verge of tears, don't be a tough guy (or girl) — have it checked out.

Using Home Remedies

The following home remedy techniques can help you manage your own back pain in the initial stages or during a back pain flare-up. Keep the warning symptoms we discuss in the preceding section in mind when determining whether you need to see a physician.

If your back pain appears to be worsening as you use any of the home remedies, visit your physician or spine specialist.

Other home remedy treatments you may consider include wearing a brace or corset, applying a topical anti-irritant to sore muscles (Ben-Gay or Sports Cream, for example), having your muscles *lightly* massaged and stretched, and engaging in deep breathing and other relaxation exercises. Always avoid placing direct pressure on or over the spine.

Climb into bed — but not for too long!

In the early stages of back pain or during a significant flare-up in your chronic back pain, the pain may be signaling you that something is wrong — perhaps you're having a muscle spasm, sprain-strain, or something else.

The best course in the early stages of back pain is to *let pain be your guide*. In other words, listen to the pain signal and stop what you're doing. For instance, if you're in the middle of a sporting activity, you may want to call it a day after doing some cooling down movements such as stretching or gentle walking. Or, if you're at work, you may want to tell your supervisor and either take a break or head home for the remainder of the day. Your response to the pain you're experiencing depends on the degree of the pain. For the sake of this discussion, we assume that your pain is fairly severe, requiring you to stop your activity and go home to bed.

In the old days (about ten years ago!) doctors recommended weeks of strict bed rest for a back pain problem. The idea was to rest your back until the pain resolved. That thinking has changed, and bed rest is considered one of the worst things you can do. Limit your overall bed rest to about two or three days. (Up to five days maximum of rest may be appropriate in some cases.)

Extended bed rest for back pain promotes muscle weakness, decreased flexibility, stomach and bowel problems, and ultimately, an overall increase in your pain. You can avoid these negative aspects of too much rest by staying somewhat active even in the initial stages of back pain. For instance, in the first day or two of a back attack, you may only be able to walk from your bed to the bathroom and back. Shortly thereafter, though, try to increase your out-of-bed time and walk some more, even if you just walk around the house. Expand this activity as you feel able or as your doctor guides you.

Resting the right way

Getting bed rest for your back pain isn't as straightforward as it sounds. You should still feel free to get up occasionally to go to the bathroom and take a lap or two around your home. In fact, you should try to get some movement at least two to four times per day.

You may be tempted while resting in bed (possibly due to significant boredom!) to prop yourself up on some pillows and either watch TV or read. However, propping yourself up actually causes more pressure on your discs than if you are standing.

You can assume two optimal positions for your painful back when you're in bed (see Figure 5-1):

✔ Lie on your side and bend at your hips and knees to 90 degrees. Place a small pillow between your knees.

✔ Lie on your back with your legs elevated by pillows to put your body in a position similar to the second image in Figure 5-1. In this position your hips and knees are bent, and the stress and pressure on your spine is at a minimum.

If you're like some people, you may be more comfortable sleeping on your stomach. Unfortunately, sleeping on your stomach places your spine in a slightly extended position that can cause more pain. If you can't avoid sleeping on your stomach, consider placing a pillow or a towel under your stomach to straighten out your spine. Doing so can help relieve the pressure on your spine if you just can't sleep in any other position.

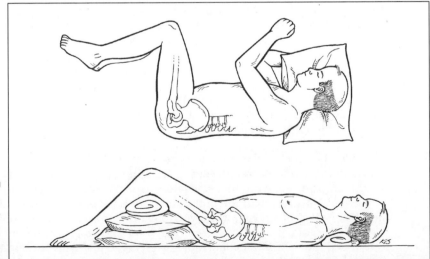

Figure 5-1:
Two healthy resting positions.

Getting out of bed

You may need a special technique to help you get in and out of the bed without significantly increasing your back pain.

1. **Lie on your side while facing the side of the bed from which you plan to get out.**

   See the first image in Figure 5-2.

2. **While lying on your side, work your way to the edge of the bed, taking care not to fall out of bed and onto the floor.**

3. **While keeping your back straight, use your lower arm and then the palm of your hand to push yourself slowly up to a sitting position.**

   As you push yourself up, allow your legs to fall over the bed and gently to the floor. You should now be in a sitting position on the bed with your feet planted firmly on the floor. (See the second image in Figure 5-2.)

4. **From this position, you can make a smooth transition from the sitting to the standing position.**

   If you have trouble going from the sitting to the standing position, you may want to hold on to the headboard or other stable piece of furniture (such as a dresser or nightstand) while you stand up.

   If you feel weak or unsafe going from sitting to standing on your own, have someone help you or use an *assisting device* (a walker or cane) per your doctor's recommendation.

   Try to do this entire movement without twisting or bending your spine. Keeping your abdominal and gluteal (buttocks) muscles tight can help you safely perform this movement.

To get into bed, simply follow the preceding steps in reverse. Remember to move slowly and smoothly.

After about two or three days of bed rest, try to increase your level of activity. You may want try more walking or being up and out of bed for more time during the day. You should also try some gentle knee to chest stretches. To increase movement, you may also want to try doing some other special back exercises. See Chapter 14 for some exercises we recommend. If your back pain is so severe that you don't feel that you can increase your movement after about two or three days of bed rest, consult your physician if you haven't already done so.

Cool down and heat up

Ice and/or heat can go a long way in relieving your back pain, but you should understand how and why they work:

✓ **Ice reduces inflammation** initially (due to decreasing blood flow from constricted blood vessels) and provides pain relief.

✓ **Heat causes blood vessels to expand,** allowing more blood to flow to the affected area, thereby encouraging healing.

You have a number of ways to apply ice and heat to your back pain. For instance, you can place ice cubes in a plastic bag and then place that in a towel; you can use an ice pack purchased over-the-counter from a drugstore; or you can try using a bag of frozen peas. (No kidding!)

Never apply ice directly to your skin for more than five minutes at a time because it can freeze the skin and cause soft-tissue damage. If the ice isn't directly on the skin or is not making you uncomfortable, then apply ice for up to 20 minutes every two hours.

You can also apply heat in a number of different ways. For instance, you can heat a moist towel in the microwave, use a heating pad, or select from a variety of moist heating pads at your drugstore.

Don't make your towel or heating pad so hot that you risk burning your skin or that it makes you uncomfortable.

Figure 5-2:
How to get out of bed if you have severe back pain.

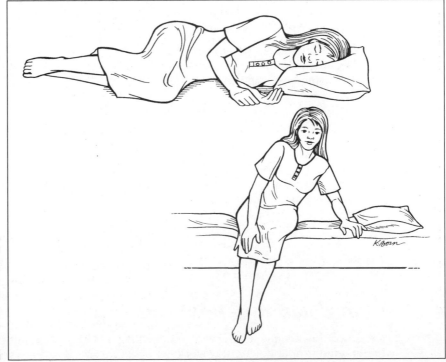

One of the most common questions patients ask us is when to apply cold and when to apply heat. Take a look at two common tenets about when to apply ice and heat:

- Most doctors say to apply ice or heat as feels best for you. This decision may include predominantly one or the other, whichever seems to provide the most benefit for you. Also, you can alternate ice and heat.

- Other doctors recommend ice in the first 48 hours after the injury and then heat thereafter. The rationale behind this belief is that the ice helps reduce inflammation and provides more pain relief. After the initial swelling decreases, applying heat can then help healing by causing more blood flow to the area.

Either of these methods works just fine. Both ice and/or heat can reduce muscle spasms.

Try anti-inflammatory drugs

In addition to bed rest and applying ice and heat, anti-inflammatory medications can help your back pain in the initial stages. Anti-inflammatories include such readily available medicines as aspirin, ibuprofen (Advil, Nuprin, Motrin), and naproxyn sodium (Aleve). See Chapter 7 for more on these and other medications. Any over-the-counter anti-inflammatory medication can help decrease inflammation associated with your back pain, and can provide some pain relief. To avoid side effects, we recommend trying Tylenol first.

Take your medicine according to the directions on the bottle. An important note: If you think your moderate to severe back pain may go on for more than a day, then continue taking the medicine for several doses. Don't stop the medication because you feel slightly better. Taking medication at regular intervals, according to the directions, for about one or two weeks builds a level of the medication in your blood that can continue to fight inflammation and provide pain relief over the course of your acute back pain flare-up.

On the other hand, do not believe that "if a little medicine is good, then more must be better." Follow the directions on the medication bottle unless your doctor says to do otherwise. Taking more medicine than is recommended can have serious side-effects such as liver and kidney damage, among other things.

Many anti-inflammatory medications that are now available over-the-counter were previously prescription drugs. As with all medication, you must take care to follow the directions and read warning information on the label. For instance, one of the most common side effects of anti-inflammatory medications includes stomach upset, abnormal bleeding (especially with aspirin), and ulcers. If you have problems with your stomach or gastrointestinal system, you should check with your doctor before taking any of these medicines. Acetaminophen generally does not have the stomach and gastrointestinal effects that the other medicines can cause. But beware that acetaminophen can cause liver damage at higher doses (more that 4g per day or about 8 tablets that contain 500mg of acetaminophen each).

If your back pain does not improve after taking these medications for one or two weeks (and following our other recommendations in this chapter), consult your doctor (if you haven't already). If you're on other medications for different medical problems, or if you have a medical problem in addition to your back pain, you should always consult with your physician before self-medicating. Talking with your doctor can help you avoid any serious drug interactions.

Starting to move and returning to normal activity

After a few days of bed rest, you should start gradually increasing your activity and overall time out of bed. Walking is an excellent exercise that is safe for your back, gets your blood flowing, and stretches out your stiff muscles. Moving around also helps you feel like you're starting to return to a normal life.

You can begin by walking around the inside of the house and progress to walking around the block or further. Adjust your speed depending on your back pain, starting out very slowly and eventually working your way up to speed walking. Make sure that you begin your walking program on a level surface. When you're in the midst of a back attack, walking up and down hills can aggravate your back pain.

If you have trouble with a walking program initially, consider doing mild exercises in a pool if that option is available to you. This workout may involve simply getting into the pool and walking across the shallow end. This mode of exercising is easier on your body because it is almost weightless in the water. You're placing minimal stress on your back. Also, the water prevents you from doing any jerky or rapid movements. We discuss water workouts further in Chapter 7.

If your walking is going relatively well, you can add the back exercises we discuss in Chapter 14. As you start to feel better, you can also begin to engage in more normal activities, usually beginning with doing things around the house.

So you don't have any of the initial warning signs that we discuss at the beginning of the chapter, and you have completed the Four Step program for your acute back attack. If you aren't experiencing significant relief or if your back pain isn't improving, you need to seek professional help from your physician or a spinal specialist. Your doctor will give you an evaluation and further treatment recommendations (see Chapters 6 and 7 for more information).

Chapter 6

Back Pain under the Microscope: Common Medical Tests

*Y*our back hurts. In fact, your back has been hurting for quite some time now. You may have seen your doctor, your chiropractor, and your massage therapist. Or, maybe you've been treating the pain on your own. Regardless, the initial treatment — such as limited bed rest, mild exercise, and possibly some medications — isn't working. So you're back at your doctor's office (probably wearing one of those breezy, open-backed gowns), ready for the next step in your treatment. But what is that next step? What are your options?

When initial treatment fails to significantly alleviate your pain, your doctor may recommend some testing. (Your first visit to the doctor, though, should always involve a thorough medical history and physical exam.) Some of these tests are very simple. Some are very high-tech. Some may not be right for you. This chapter explains the most common back pain tests (including psychological assessments) and gives you the information you need to have an informed dialog with your doctor.

Meeting with Your Back Pain Doctor

In recent years, we've seen an explosion in the number of amazing, high-technology approaches to assessing back pain. Such advances include the CT scan and MRI, both of which we discuss in this chapter.

Even with technology on your side, your doctor gains the most important information from the history of your back pain problem and a physical examination. Be aware, too, that a psychological assessment of your back pain may be an essential component in helping to determine proper treatment for your problem. (See Chapter 3 for more information about how your mind influences your pain.)

Getting personal

The most important diagnostic tool with respect to your back pain is a complete and thorough medical history. Your doctor should take this history in a face-to-face interview, in conjunction with your physical examination.

To be thorough and complete, the history should assess *at least* the following factors:

- ✔ **How your back pain started:** Did you have an accident, or did you just wake up with the pain one day?

- ✔ **The course of your symptoms:** Are your symptoms getting better or worse from the time you first noticed them? Are you experiencing any new symptoms? Have any symptoms come and gone?

- ✔ **Your current symptoms:** Mention all the symptoms you currently experience (not only the pain, but also any weakness, sleep problems, depression, and so on).

- ✔ **How the pain influences your day-to-day life:** Has your pain interrupted your work, play, family, or sexual activities in any way?

- ✔ **Whether the pain interferes with your relationships:** Are you still going out with friends or are you staying home more often because of the pain? Do you see outside family members?

Assessing on the whole

After the history and physical, a healthcare practitioner who is well-trained in spinal disorders should have a relatively clear idea of an appropriate treatment plan. Your doctor should conduct the physical examination to confirm his or her diagnostic impressions based on your history. To get a good idea of your back pain problem, the healthcare practitioner should assess both physical and emotional issues.

One of the primary problems we often see in the healthcare community is that many healthcare professionals focus almost entirely on physical factors to the exclusion of emotional factors. An assessment of the entire person — including the body *and* the mind — is extremely important.

Getting physical

A thorough physical examination helps your doctor determine whether you have any type of disc problem in your lower spine and where — at which *level* of the spine — the problem has occured. Your doctor can obtain all this information without any fancy, high-tech tests.

During the physical, your back pain specialist may conduct some standard evaluations, such as taking your blood pressure and listening to your heart and lungs. She also looks at and assesses general attributes, such as how you walk, stand, and sit. The doctor may have you get into certain positions to see if doing so increases your back pain. She may push on areas of your body where you complain of pain. She may also get out a little rubber hammer and test your reflexes.

Beyond these tests, the doctor also does special tests that focus more on your spine. These include assessments like the following:

- **Straight leg test (sciatic nerve stretch test):** In this test, you lie flat on your back with your legs and feet extended fully on the exam table. The doctor then lifts one leg at a time to see whether doing so causes pain anywhere in either leg. This test increases the tension in the nerve that goes from your back down your legs (the sciatic nerve). If this test causes pain, your doctor can get an idea as to whether you have an irritated nerve root.

- **Lasegue's test:** In conjunction with a straight leg test, your doctor may also perform a Lasegue's test. In this test (done while you are lying on your back), your doctor brings your ankle and foot up toward your knee (first one leg and then the other) to put further tension on the nerves in your back that go down your legs.

  To better understand the reasons for these tests, think of yourself as a marionette with nerves for strings. Your sciatic nerve is the string going from your spine to your tips of your toes. These tests pull on the string to see whether doing so causes pain. Pain during these tests indicates a problem at the *nerve root* (where the nerve comes from the spine) such as a disc. (See Chapter 2 for more on spine anatomy.)

- **Detailed evaluation of your lower-body nerves (hip, thigh, leg, and foot):** Your doctor checks sensations in these areas, usually by running a painless "pinwheel" device along your skin. (Though the instrument looks like a pinwheel, your doctor is not *toying* with you. Oh, we heard that groan, but even doctors are allowed to make bad jokes once in a while!) Your doctor looks for any suspicious changes in sensation, and this gives an indication of how your nerves are working. Normally, you should just slightly feel the pinwheel running along your skin. If you feel it too much (discomfort or pain) or too little (numbness), your doctor will take notice.

✔ **Reflex test:** Your doctor also carefully assesses your lower body's reflexes to be sure that the nerves coming from the spine are working properly. (Yes, your doctor will come at you with that little hammer again!)

✔ **Muscle strength test:** Finally, your doctor assesses the strength of all the individual muscle groups of your lower body. Each of these muscle groups corresponds to a specific *nerve root level* (the part of your lower spine where the nerve exits the spine). If a nerve is injured, then the muscles that it controls may show weakness because your muscles are controlled by nerves. Your doctor conducts strength tests to make sure that a nerve problem isn't causing muscle weakness.

If your doctor focuses only on finding a problem in your spine to be fixed, the diagnosis and treatment often will be incomplete and incorrect. As we discuss earlier in the chapter, your back pain problem needs to be assessed from a viewpoint of you as a whole person (mind, body, personal history, and so on) rather than you as a walking spine with nothing else attached.

After your doctor completes the history and physical examination, he usually recommends a treatment plan. In some cases, however, he recommends further diagnostic testing.

Unfortunately, some doctors suffer from the impression that advances in technology over the past several years means that they don't need to rely as much on a good history and physical examination. If your doctor falls into this category, she is likely to move straight to diagnostic testing to determine the "cause" of your low-back pain. You may be willing to quickly accept this approach if you believe that high-tech machines are more accurate and more "scientific." However, nothing can be further from the truth.

High-tech diagnostic tests, such as the MRI and CT scan, are very sensitive and enable doctors to see normal wear-and-tear changes in your spine that they couldn't otherwise. Unfortunately, many doctors interpret these normal changes as "abnormal" and proceed with inappropriate recommendations and treatments (not to mention scaring you with a horrific-sounding diagnosis).

A detailed and appropriate history and physical examination are more critical than ever. Without them, your doctor can't look at a high-tech study and properly identify clinically significant changes.

Examining Your Doctor

You should feel that you and your doctor are partners in your treatment. You have the right to address your concerns and questions regarding testing with your doctor. Like voting for president, be sure to exercise this right. If your doctor isn't interested in answering your questions, then you may want to consider another doctor. See Chapter 22 for more information about working with your doctor.

The following questions are useful to ask your doctor when he recommends testing:

- ✓ **What is the test and what does it show?** Get the exact name of the test that your doctor is recommending. What does he expect to find out from the test? Expect a response along the line of, "I am recommending an MRI, which will show all the tissues of your spine including the discs, bones, and nerves."

- ✓ **Why do you advise I have this test?** Find out what information your doctor expects to get from this test.

- ✓ **What can I expect before, during, and after the test?** Get some idea of what the test involves. For instance, how long will it take? Do you have to prepare in any way? Is it uncomfortable or painful? (Although we answer many of these questions later in the chapter, you still want to have this conversation with your doctor.)

- ✓ **What does it mean if the test is positive or negative?** This question homes in on how your doctor expects to use the test results and what those results mean for your treatment.

- ✓ **Will the results of this test change my treatment plan?** If not, then why put yourself through the test?

The results of any of your diagnostic tests without referencing you as an entire person — physical, psychological, and emotional — are of no value and can even be detrimental to you.

Exploring Your Diagnostic Testing Options

In this section, you find out about several diagnostic tests, ranging from imaging tests to nerve tests to psychological tests.

Although the actual interpretation of the tests themselves is complicated, you can still gain a solid understanding of what the test does, what it will show, and why having it makes sense in your case. You should also be aware of any potential side effects from the test.

Keep in mind that your doctor needs to assess you as an entire person — your mind and body — and not just as a spine that happens to come with a human being wrapped around it. Although these tests are very high-tech and impressive, they often still don't identify the exact cause of your back pain. Even without an exact diagnosis, you can treat and manage your back pain. Also, the results of any of these tests (except the psychological) are meaningless if they're not combined with your history and physical exam.

Plain X rays

An x-ray machine passes low-level radiation through part of your body, projecting a picture, or *radiograph,* on a piece of film. The level of radiation from an X ray is very small — less than the amount you receive on an airplane flight from Los Angeles to New York.

Your doctor may recommend an X ray if he wants to see the bones of your spine, sacroiliac joint, and pelvis. An X ray can show whether you're experiencing changes associated with normal aging, fractures, and overall alignment of your spine. (For more about alignment problems like scoliosis, see Chapter 3.) You may be an appropriate candidate for an X ray if

- ✔ You still have back pain after two or three weeks of conservative treatment.
- ✔ You have back pain even during periods of no activity.
- ✔ You have back pain that awakens you from sleep at night.
- ✔ You have back pain after a trauma or fall.

Generally, your doctor should not recommend an x-ray test on your first visit unless he has very clear reasons (like the possibility of a fracture due to trauma or if your pain has been present for a long time before you were evaluated). Although doctors often order an X ray on a patient's first visit, this practice may not be worthwhile. For instance, a research study found that only 19 percent of cases show meaningful data obtained from X rays done on the first visit to the doctor for low-back pain. See M.H. Liang, et al., *The Adult Spine,* edited by J.W. Frymoyer, (New York: Raven Press 1991).

If your back pain begins after a trauma (such as a fall or car accident), then you can reasonably expect to undergo an X ray. In all other cases, your doctor should use your history and your physical exam to determine whether or not to x-ray.

You've most likely had X rays before, so you know that the test is simple and painless; the person performing the x-ray test may cover sensitive areas with a lead shield. X rays aren't safe for women during pregnancy, but otherwise they aren't harmful and have no side effects.

Supposedly "abnormal" findings on your X ray, such as wear-and-tear changes that occur with aging (given the scary name of "degenerative changes" by doctors), usually aren't significant. In fact, in many cases they don't relate to the back pain that you're experiencing. Findings that may relate to your back pain include such conditions as a fracture, severe degeneration, or significant scoliosis.

Just because your X rays don't show anything significant doesn't mean that your pain isn't real. Remember that the majority of painful back conditions probably come from the soft tissues of your spine including the muscles, tendons, discs, and ligaments. Like Superman, X rays see right through these.

The MRI (magnetic resonance imaging)

Magnetic resonance imaging uses a strong magnetic field, radio waves, and a computer to generate a picture of your spinal structures. Figure 6-1 shows a patient about to undergo an MRI.

The MRI shows your doctor the nerves, muscles, ligaments, and discs, as well as the bones of the spine. This test gives your doctor much more information than X rays, without exposing you to radiation.

An MRI may be appropriate for you if

✔ You are a possible surgical candidate.

✔ Your still have back pain after six to eight weeks of appropriate, conservative treatment.

✔ Your doctor suspects your pain may be related to an infection or tumor. (Severe pain that awakens you from sleep is often a symptom of infections and tumors.)

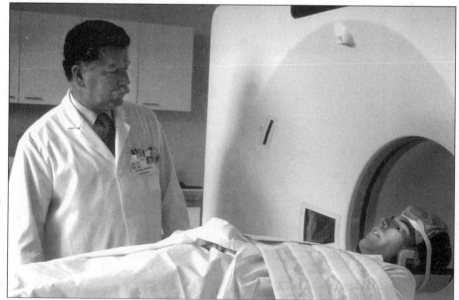

Figure 6-1:
A patient about to undergo MRI testing.

Because the MRI test is extremely sensitive, your doctor can detect subtle changes in your spine that occur naturally as you age. Mother Nature and Father Time seem to have worked out a pretty good deal with this age and change stuff. The good news is that these changes occur in people without back pain, too. So, you can be fairly confident that these changes aren't causing your pain — especially if you are over 35.

An MRI is generally safe. However, pregnant women may be at some risk. In this case, work with your doctor to determine the best course of testing for you.

Physicians frequently overuse MRI tests, a practice that leads to excessive and unnecessary costs. Reasons for overuse of MRI testing include

✓ **Discomfort in treating back pain:** Doctors who don't regularly treat back pain may order an MRI because they aren't comfortable with their diagnosis based solely on your history and physical exam. Ask your doctor the questions we mention in the section "Examining Your Doctor" to help determine whether an MRI makes sense for you. An open dialog with your doctor can save you money and stress in the long run.

✓ **Fear of malpractice:** With everybody hiring a John Grisham-esque attorney today, some physicians prefer to err on the side of caution. However, you shouldn't undergo any testing that you believe is more in the interest of protecting your doctor than alleviating your pain. If you're concerned about this issue, be sure to ask your doctor why the test is being recommended.

✓ **Means to justify unnecessary surgery or continued treatment:** Doctors can use MRI results to justify ongoing treatment, surgery, or prolonged disability following a work injury, automobile accident, or fall. Remember, though, that "abnormal" findings are often a natural part of the aging process.

Don't be frightened if your doctor recommends an MRI. The MRI procedure is safe and has almost no side effects. (Pregnant women should consult their doctors before this test, however.) MRIs require no special preparation. You lie down on a scanning table that slides into a giant magnet shaped like a large tube. (You may feel like the stuffing in a manicotti.)

If you're claustrophobic, the closeness of the tube may make you uncomfortable. In that case, your doctor can arrange for you to receive a sedative. You may also receive special glasses, headphones so that you can listen to music, or some other type of distraction during the test to lessen your anxiety.

Inside the tube, you hear several noises, including a humming sound and a thumping as the radio waves are turned on and off. Generally, the most difficult part of the test is lying still for 45 to 60 minutes, especially if your back already hurts. If your back pain is severe, you may want to ask your doctor for pain medicine prior to the test.

In some cases, you may undergo an MRI with a *contrast agent,* which is a fluid that is injected into your arm or leg prior to the test. This nonharmful substance can help provide an MRI picture that is much clearer, especially if you have had prior spine surgery. The contrast agent can help your doctor distinguish scar tissue, which may occur with prior surgery. If your doctor doesn't mention the possiblity of using a contrast agent, ask — especially if you have had prior spine surgery.

An MRI cannot show some causes of pain such as a sprain-strain in the muscles or ligaments and stress-related back pain. Therefore, you can have normal test results and still have pain.

The CT scan

CT stands for *computerized tomography.* You may know this test as a *CAT scan,* which is *computerized axial tomography.* A CT scan is a computerized recording of a slice or section of your body.

A CT scan does expose you to a greater amount of radiation than a plain X ray, but it is well within the safe range. The CT scan doesn't show your soft tissues, nerves, and muscles quite as well as the MRI, but it does show the anatomy of the bony structures of your spine, as well as your discs and nerves.

So you and your MRI want an open relationship

Many newspapers and magazines currently run advertisements for "open" MRI machines. These machines claim to solve claustrophobia problems for patients because they don't use a tube like the closed machines. Unfortunately, the resolution and quality of the MRI picture suffers greatly in most open machines.

Just recently, open MRI machines have been developed that provide high quality pictures, although these are not readily available to most people. (They are now only at large medical institutions such as UCLA in Los Angeles or select, private imaging centers.) If you're having an MRI, go for the best machine possible (currently a closed machine with the largest magnet), which provides the best results for your doctor. If you have claustrophobia, tell your doctor ahead of time so that you can work together to minimize your discomfort. If you live in an urban area that has a large medical center and you desire more information about high-quality open MRI machines, ask your back doctor about your options.

Your doctor may choose a CT scan for you over an MRI scan if

- You're very claustrophobic and can't tolerate being in the MRI machine even with a sedative.
- Your doctor needs to see the anatomy of your boney structures where the nerves exit the spinal canal.

The CT scan is also a cylinder-shaped machine, just like the MRI. You lie on your back for about 30 to 45 minutes. Unlike the MRI, the tube portion of the CT scan is much larger and less likely to make you feel closed in if you are prone to claustrophobia. Figure 6-2 shows a patient about to undergo a CT scan.

The test is painless. As with the MRI, in some cases you may have a CT scan with a contrast agent to help make certain aspects of the picture more clear.

Myelography

A *myelogram* is an X ray of the fluid-filled sack around your spinal cord. In this test, a radiologist injects dye into this sack, which helps the area show up on the X ray. *Radiologists* are physicians who specialize in the administration and interpretation of imaging tests such as X rays, MRIs, and CT scans.

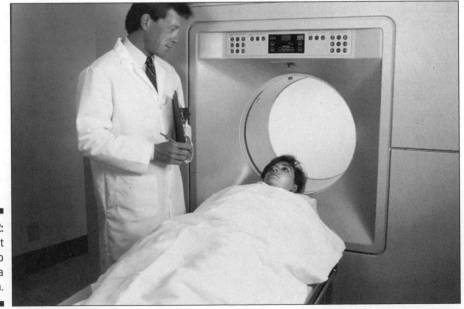

Figure 6-2:
A patient about to undergo a CT scan.

Generally, a CT scan immediately follows a myelogram. By combining the two tests, your doctor can see your bones or skeletal structure as well as neurologic structures, such as the nerves, and you have to endure only one injection.

This test generally is appropriate only if your doctor is considering surgery. The test also is helpful if your MRI or CT scan image isn't clear, your doctor cannot make a specific diagnosis from the scan, and/or there is a question about the presence of a tumor.

The myelogram procedure may cause minimal to moderate pain. Because of new technology and improved safety, this test no longer requires a hospital stay and is now done on an outpatient basis. You lie on a table as the radiologist injects dye into your spinal canal — a process that takes one or two minutes. You may feel a slight prick as the radiologist inserts the needle. After the dye is injected, the technician takes plain X rays of you in many positions including standing, partially upright, lying down, and turned to the right or left side (like a roller-coaster ride, but not nearly as fun). A CT scan may follow. The entire process takes approximately one hour.

After you complete the test, the recovery period is approximately 6 to 12 hours. You may be asked to lie with your head slightly elevated, and you will need to drink plenty of fluids. Following these recommendations keeps the contrast material or dye away from sensitive areas in your head while flushing the material from your body.

Although rare, you may experience a headache as a side effect, which can occur for one of two reasons:

- ✔ **You may react to the dye:** Less than 1 percent of people who undergo a myelogram have a reaction to the dye. The good news is that over the past five years, newer, water-soluble dyes have become available.

- ✔ **A small amount of spinal fluid may leak out into your body through the needle hole:** This situation occurs in approximately 5 to 10 percent of patients undergoing the procedure. The resulting headache lasts for one to two days following the test. Should this happen to you, your headache will almost certainly subside with a short period of rest and the intake of fluids.

You can be assured that a myelogram is considered a very low-risk procedure even though it does carry slightly more risk than the tests we discuss earlier in this chapter. Specifically, the test carries two very rare risks: infection and excessive bleeding. But, you can get an infection with any invasive procedure. If you do get an infection, your doctor can treat it appropriately with antibiotics. To prevent excessive bleeding (usually as a result of clotting problems), stop taking aspirin or any blood thinners for a period of three to five days prior to your test.

Bone scan

The *bone scan* is a test that requires you to be injected in the arm with a special radioactive dye. The radioactivity of the dye is extremely low and safe. You lie down for about two hours while the dye circulates throughout your entire body, including the bones of your skeleton.

After the dye has had a chance to circulate through your body, special X rays determine how much of the dye has penetrated into various parts of your skeleton. The scan works by detecting an increase in metabolic activity in any part of your skeleton that has an increase in blood flow. The increase in blood flow can result from a tumor, infection, fracture, or simply age-related degenerative changes. Your doctor may recommend a bone scan if she can't diagnose these conditions by plain X ray, MRI, or CT scan.

The test is relatively inexpensive and very safe. In general, the test is risk-free, although if you have moderate to severe back pain, you may have difficulty lying down for an extended period of time while the dye circulates. As with the other tests we discuss, your doctor must interpret the results as part of your entire evaluation.

The most common mistake made in interpreting a bone scan is to attribute too much significance to a "finding" that results from normal arthritic or wear-and-tear changes in the bones of the spine. See Chapter 2 for more anatomical details.

Discogram

In a *discogram,* you're required to put on a leisure suit, play some funky music, and do the Hustle under a sparkling ball while your doctor assesses your back pain. (Now, don't go out and ask your doctor about that — we're just kidding!)

Actually, in a discogram, dye is injected directly into the discs of your lumbar spine. The dye helps create a better picture of this area of your spine, and doctors can determine whether or not injecting the dye in a specific disc causes the type of back pain that you have been experiencing. You may experience moderate to severe pain during this test. Of all the tests we discuss in this chapter, our patients say that this one is the most uncomfortable, but it has almost no side effects (except the very rare infection).

Dr. Steven Waldman, M.D., an expert in discograms, says that your doctor may recommend this test if you show disc bulges or herniations at more than one level on an MRI study (see Chapter 3 for more information about bulges and herniations). In this situation, the discogram helps identify which, if any, of the disc herniations or bulges are responsible for your pain. A discogram may also help determine whether a degenerative disc is the source of your back pain.

You should agree to the test only if you're willing to consider surgical treatment based on the test results.

Electrodiagnostic studies

Electromyography (EMG) and nerve conduction studies (NCS) are the most common *electrodiagnostic studies* — tests that measure the electrical activity and function of your nerves and muscles — that your doctor may use in assessing your back pain. The tests can show whether the electrical activity of various nerves has somehow been disrupted. These tests are usually done by physiatrists or neurologists, so you may be referred to another doctor if yours does not specialize in this type of testing.

During the study, your physician inserts small needles into several of the muscles he's measuring. In an EMG, these needles are connected to a monitor that shows the electrical activity of your nerves and muscles. In a nerve conduction study, an electrical pulse "buzzes" your nerves — kind of like the guy in that kids' game "Operation" — so that special receiving electrodes can monitor the electrical activity. You may experience mild to moderate pain with this test.

These tests can help determine a variety of diagnoses that involve problems with the nervous system or assess the regrowth of nerves after lumbar disc surgery for sciatica. Because doctors can make the majority of diagnoses with a good history and physical exam in addition to the other diagnostic tests available, electrodiagnostic studies are becoming less necessary.

Moving from Body to Mind

Some people may be surprised to find that psychological testing often goes hand-in-hand with the other diagnostic tests that we discuss in this chapter. A number of psychological tests have been designed or adapted for use with back pain patients. Your doctor may recommend these tests as part of a pre-surgical screening; or to assess the emotional aspects of your pain, ongoing psychiatric problems, or your ability to cope with the pain.

Just as the history and physical exam are the most important parts of diagnosing your back pain problem, the clinical interview is the key psychological assessment tool.

Your doctor may suggest a psychological assessment of your back pain if he has the following concerns:

- ✔ You may have significant depression and/or anxiety.

- ✔ You may be abusing alcohol or other substances or overusing pain medicines.

- ✔ You are unable to cope with the pain.

- ✔ You are experiencing undue stress in your family or work situation.

- ✔ You may benefit from psychological pain control procedures.

- ✔ You would benefit from psychological preparation for surgery.

- ✔ Your back pain may be stress related.

A psychologist or psychiatrist with special training in pain problems usually conducts the psychological assessment. Your interview involves getting information about the history of your pain problem, including previous treatments, your family and work situations, litigation and compensation issues related to your back pain, history of previous psychological treatment, substance abuse problems, and history of emotional and/or physical abuse, among other factors. In addition, a special examination assesses your mood; sleep, memory, and concentration abilities; changes in your sex drive and frequency; and energy levels.

Psychological testing reveals information about many aspects of your back pain problem including the following:

- ✔ Your level of depression and anxiety related to your pain

- ✔ Your personality features and how they affect your experience of pain

- ✔ Whether you are comfortable in the sick role

- ✔ Whether you are more dramatic or stoic in showing pain behaviors

- ✔ How likely it is that that non-physical factors (emotions, family, work, and so on) are influencing your back pain

A referral for psychological assessment may feel threatening. For instance, you may feel like your doctor is "dumping" you. Or, you may believe that by giving you the referral, your doctor thinks your pain is in your head, not your back. In truth, the purpose of the evaluation is usually to help the referring doctor better determine a treatment approach. The evaluation can also determine which, if any, psychological pain control methods may help you (such as relaxation training, changing the way you view the pain, and helping family members cope with your pain).

All pain is real and includes emotional or psychological factors. Just because your physician refers you for psychological assessment does not mean that you're starring in a reenactment of *One Flew Over the Cuckoo's Nest.* If your doctor states or implies that your pain is imaginary, consider finding another healthcare professional.

Chapter 7

Going the Conservative Treatment Route

●●●

In This Chapter

▶ Exercising your way to a better back

▶ Understanding conservative medical treatment for your back pain

▶ Finding out which treatments feel good (but do they work?)

▶ Appraising pills for back pain

▶ Getting under your skin: Invasive conservative treatment

●●●

*W*hen you hear the word "conservative" in today's world, you may immediately think of politics and economics. In the world of back pain, though, "conservative" applies to any treatment that is reversible and doesn't involve major surgery on your spine. Most common medical treatments are conservative.

Conservative treatments fall into two categories: invasive and non-invasive. Non-invasive techniques are further broken into active (you administer the treatment yourself) and passive (someone else — usually a physical therapist — gives you the treatment). Most back pain treatments are non-invasive and include treatments such as physical therapy and medications. Invasive approaches include mad-scientist-sounding measures such as trigger point injections, nerve blocks, and "implantable" pain therapies. This chapter introduces you to the conservative — invasive and non-invasive — approaches that are available to you.

We admit that some of these treatments can sound frightening. Keep in mind as you read, however, that these are all reversible treatments. And remember that nothing substitutes for an open dialog with your doctor. Sharing your thoughts gives your doctor the opportunity to alleviate your fears, address your concerns, and explore other treatment options.

The doctor dialog

Having an active partnership with your doctor is one of the most important aspects of any treatment you receive for your back pain. As part of this active participation, you need to make sure that you thoroughly understand why your doctor recommends a particular treatment and what you should expect from it. The following questions can help you get this information:

✔ Why are you recommending this treatment for me?

✔ What benefit should I expect, and how long will it take to know whether it has been achieved?

✔ What, if any, possible problems can occur with this treatment? What should I do if these occur? Will they go away if I continue with the treatment?

✔ Will this treatment interfere with other treatments I am pursuing? (In fact, you may want to give a list — complete with names and phone numbers — of everyone involved in your treatment to all your doctors and treating therapists.)

The Active Therapies

Active treatments can include general exercise, conditioning programs, and special back exercises. These are treatments that you actively do for yourself (under the guidance of a professional).

Exercise

Exercise is one of the most important treatments that your doctor will recommend to help your back pain. Your doctor will most likely prescribe a conditioning program, and she may add other exercises that strengthen a specific area of your back. A conditioning program will have the goals of increasing your strength, improving your flexibility, and building your endurance. The more specialized exercise programs have fancy names like *flexion, extension,* and *lumbar stabilization.* (See Chapter 14 for more detail.)

Conditioning

Conditioning exercises, which actually focus more on total body fitness than specific back pain, should be a key component of your back pain rehabilitation program. This type of program incorporates activities such as the stationary bike, treadmill, and a walking program.

A conditioning program can help you:

- ✔ **Manage your fear of the back pain:** Exercise requires you to move around. Beyond conditioning your body and your back, exercise reassures you that you don't have to fear your back pain or protect your movements.

- ✔ **Change the "hurt equals harm" mindset:** A proper conditioning and exercise program helps you accept that increased pain does not necessarily mean injury. Your back pain may initially increase when you start to exercise, but truthfully, this type of pain is often the same that non-back pain sufferers experience when they haven't worked out for a while.

- ✔ **Get out of the sick role:** A conditioning program also helps you openly address any issues that may be forcing you to maintain the sick role. (See Chapter 3 for more information on the sick role.) If you exercise and move around, others won't think of you as a sick person. As they begin to treat you as a healthy person, your attitude and confidence tend to improve.

A conditioning program can be appropriate no matter what stage of back pain you have. Generally, your doctor will prescribe a program tailored to your specific back pain problem.

Your doctor should do a careful physical evaluation before prescribing a conditioning program to ensure that you have no physical problems (such as spinal instability or a fractured vertebra — see Chapter 3) that make exercise harmful. Medical problems such as heart disease or high blood pressure can also change the type of program your doctor recommends. Don't forget to tell your doctor if you are on any medications or if you are pregnant.

The pedometer: A simple but powerful tool

A pedometer is a small device that attaches to your belt and simply "counts" your number of steps. Walkers and joggers often wear electronic pedometers to measure number of steps taken and distance traveled. These devices are inexpensive and can be a useful means for you to keep track of your overall activity level as you try to overcome your back pain problem.

Several researchers found that using a pedometer provides an accurate assessment of the degree to which you are engaging in normal levels of healthy activity. For comparison purposes, some government statistics advise that healthy individuals aim for step levels of 19,000 steps per day. In contrast, one study of patients with rheumatoid arthritis showed an average of 5,037 steps per day with a range of 207-12,515 steps. One good way to use a pedometer is to gather baseline information over a few days to measure your usual level of activity. You can then compare your increase in activity relative to your baseline. For more about using your baseline activity to further develop your strength and stamina, see the sidebar, "Using the quota system."

You must take responsibility

Your physician, osteopath, or chiropractor usually monitors and supervises your conditioning program. In most cases, however, a physical therapist or other qualified healthcare professional actually implements the conditioning program.

You need to remember several points when you're starting a conditioning program:

- ✔ **Your pain may initially increase:** When you begin the program, you will be using muscles that you've probably been protecting for quite a while. As a result, you may experience a mild to moderate increase in pain. This pain does *not* mean that you are injuring your back, and that initial pain should decrease over time.

- ✔ **You must be willing to follow the program independently:** Your physical therapist will probably monitor you closely at the beginning of the program and then instruct you to go ahead and complete the exercises on your own. To really conquer your pain, you simply must be willing to follow through with the program on your own.

- ✔ **You must comply with the conditioning recommendations:** Cutting the conditioning exercises short can be very tempting, especially when the physical therapist isn't monitoring you — kind of like passing notes in class when the teacher isn't looking. At the risk of sounding like that same teacher, you are only cheating yourself when you take these shortcuts.

Your physical conditioning program depends on your phase of back pain

Back pain has different phases. Your conditioning program depends on which phase you're experiencing. With chronic back pain, for instance, your muscles may be weak from inactivity. In that case, your conditioning program starts out quite slowly and builds in intensity over time. (We discuss the specifics of designing a conditioning program later in this chapter.)

The following list discusses how your doctor may design your conditioning program based upon your phase of back pain:

- ✔ **Initial phase of acute back pain (one to five days):** Your pain and muscle spasms may be quite limiting during this phase. Your doctor or physical therapist will most likely recommend ice, bed rest, and some gentle knee to chest stretches on day two or three.

- ✔ **Acute back pain (less than one month's duration):** Mild exercise that you gradually increase can help you avoid the next stage of back pain altogether. Even in this early stage of back pain, mild exercise, such as limited walking, is appropriate. Over the next several weeks, you can slowly add more strenuous activities such as faster walking, swimming, or bicycling. The exact type of exercise you choose usually isn't important, but you should discuss your choice with your doctor. At this stage of treatment, avoid any severe twisting or bending motions. Let your pain be your guide — exercise until you experience more pain and then stop at that point.

✔ **Subacute back pain (one to three month's duration):** Exercise and conditioning issues become very important in this phase. Your doctor and physical therapist should be trying to keep you as active as possible, even with ongoing back pain. The exercises they give you may initially increase your pain, but, if you do the exercises as prescribed, they're designed to be safe for your spine. At this point, your doctor may monitor your physical therapy program more closely.

✔ **Chronic back pain (longer than three month's duration):** At this stage, a physical reconditioning program that includes strengthening, stretching, and aerobics should be part of your total treatment plan. As you begin to use the weakened muscles, your back pain initially will increase. Using some of the passive therapies we discuss later in this chapter may help control your symptoms so that you can complete your exercise program more effectively. At this phase of conditioning, your pain takes a hike as your guide. Instead, you take a drill-sergeant approach where you slowly work through the pain by completing a certain number of repetitions, regardless of the pain.

✔ **Recurrent acute back pain (pain flare-ups with pain-free episodes in between):** Participating in an aerobic, conditioning exercise program about three times per week can significantly decrease the frequency, intensity, and duration of your back pain episodes. You can choose any type of exercise as long as it includes aerobic, stretching, and strengthening elements. You may want to include any specific back exercises you have been given in the past.

Your back conditioning program

You should design your back conditioning program in conjunction with your doctor and physical therapist while taking into account the information contained in this chapter and in Chapter 14. Also, in this section you look at important elements of a back conditioning program. These features help increase the chances that you actually follow through on your back conditioning program on a regular basis.

One element of your back conditioning program should include aerobic conditioning. The aerobic conditioning components can be in addition to special back exercises such as those reviewed in Chapter 14 or as given to you by your doctor. Aerobic conditioning exercise can be anything from speed walking to the stationary bicycle to the treadmill. Although aerobic conditioning is not exercise that is targeted directly to your back, we find that this type of exercise helps you not only manage back pain more effectively but also can improve your mental abilities, provide stress relief, and help you sleep better.

Using the quota system

The *quota system* is a specialized approach to your exercise program. You work to a specific quota rather than being guided by your pain. Exercising in this way is especially important if you're in the sub-acute and chronic stages of back pain.

To set up a quota system for any exercise, begin by establishing your *baseline*. Your baseline for that exercise is the amount of exercise you can do until either pain or fatigue stops you. Your amount of exercise can be measured in several ways depending upon the type of exercise (for example, the time it takes, number of repetitions, or distance).

Record this figure for three consecutive exercise sessions to get a good measure of your baseline capabilities. Say, for example, that you can do your treadmill exercise for five minutes on the first session, six minutes on the second session, and seven minutes on the third session. In each of these sessions, you would have stopped when the pain or fatigue became uncomfortable.

In this example you take the average of the three sessions to establish your baseline of six minutes (5+6+7=18, divide by 3 to get 6). After you establish the baseline, subtract 20 percent. The remaining number sets your *initial quota*. In this example, 6 – 20% = 4.8. Your initial quota, then, is approximately five minutes.

After you establish your initial quota, you complete that goal regardless of your back pain. You then set increasing quotas for yourself based on discussions with your physical therapist or doctor. One example may be to increase your quota by 10 percent each week or every third exercise session.

You can use the quota system for any of your exercises or activities: the number of blocks you can walk, laps you can swim, amount of time you can sit at a desk, and time on the treadmill, for example. The important point to remember about quotas is that the goal is to *work to the quota* rather than pain. As such, don't make your quotas too difficult or potentially unachievable. If you can't achieve a particular quota, simply back off a little for a couple of sessions and then return to your previous quota goals.

Pacing your activities

Pacing your activities involves a gradual increase in activity according to a specific plan. This concept also involves taking a rather extensive activity and breaking it up into small pieces (with breaks in between) to help prevent any flare-up in your back pain problem.

Pacing your activities prevents a common pattern that involves *overdoing* and *crashing*. You may experience the overdoing and crashing pattern if you vigorously engage in an activity when your back pain is minimal only to have it cause a flare-up that sets you back. The overdo and crash pattern is an unhealthy approach to your back pain problem, and you should replace it with a pacing approach. Pacing involves doing a reasonable amount of exercise or activity, with breaks in between so that you keep your back pain under reasonable control.

Don't confuse pacing yourself with letting pain be your guide. If you pace your activities you will notice that you can do more rather than less and you will not experience the overdo and crash pattern.

Getting your family and friends involved

One of the best ways to implement your conditioning program is to get your family and friends involved. Your family and friends may be inclined to tell you to "take it easy" and not be so active even when your doctor has told you to exercise more. In this situation, your family and friends are inadvertently reinforcing your being in the sick role.

Educate your family and friends about the importance of your back conditioning exercise program. Explain pacing to them and ask them to encourage you to maintain a regular, healthy regimen and to warn you if they think you're entering overdo-and-crash mode.

Include your family and friends in your efforts to become more active by doing the following:

- ✔ **Make a public commitment:** Tell as many people as possible about your plan to increase your activities and your exercise program to help ensure that you follow through with your program.

- ✔ **Get an exercise buddy:** Setting up a regular exercise program with your exercise buddy makes you less likely to cancel or drop your exercise program.

Pain programs, functional restoration, and work hardening programs

Your doctor may suggest that you try a pain program if the usual treatments (physical therapy, exercise, medicines, and so on) aren't helping, and your pain is quite debilitating (for instance, if you can't work).

The terms *pain program, functional restoration,* and *work hardening program* describe treatment programs that have slightly different focuses. The three programs, however, do share a few characteristics:

- ✔ **Multidisciplinary approach:** A number of different specialists work on your case at the same time.

- ✔ **Structured approach:** You receive various treatments at a specific time for a specific reason.

✓ **Common goals:** Each program works to decrease your pain, increase your functioning, and improve your quality of life.

✓ **Motivation driven:** Each program relies on a high level of motivation and involvement from you, the patient.

We define various other types of pain programs in the sidebar.

A *functional restoration program* focuses on helping you eliminate any disability your back pain causes and restore your function by increasing your physical and mental abilities. The theory behind these programs is that your back pain diminishes when your ability to participate in day-to-day activities increases. The treatments are primarily exercise-oriented, with a "hurt does not equal harm" attitude. Instead of trying to "fix" your back pain (by the time you get to one of these programs the fix-it approaches have fallen flat), these programs focus on what you can do to help you work through your back pain safely and gradually.

A *work hardening program* is similar in philosophy to a functional restoration program except that it focuses almost exclusively on return-to-work issues. In a work hardening program, you do work simulation activities (not much different than being at the office, huh?) at the treatment center under the guidance of a specially trained physical therapist. You start slowly (maybe one hour a day) and gradually work up to full-time (eight hours per day). When you reach your maximum level of work ability at the treatment center — even if that's less than eight hours — you return to actual employment.

Well, the IASP says . . .

No official body oversees the operation of pain programs, but the International Association for the Study of Pain (IASP; see Appendix B) defines the various pain programs in the following manner:

✓ **Multidisciplinary pain center:** Usually associated with a medical school or teaching hospital, this organization of healthcare professionals provides patient care, research, and teaching on both an outpatient and inpatient basis.

✓ **Multidisciplinary pain clinic:** These clinics are the same as pain centers, but they don't

do research or teach, and they aren't necessarily associated with a university, medical school, or hospital.

✓ **Pain clinic:** A center or doctor's office that specializes in only one diagnosis (such as back pain).

✓ **Modality oriented clinic:** A center or doctor's office that uses only one *modality* or treatment approach (such as biofeedback, massage, acupuncture, or nerve blocks).

Most programs (including ours) have a screening evaluation that looks at the type of back pain you have (they usually treat chronic back pain syndrome and failed back surgery syndrome — see Chapter 3) and your willingness to try such an approach, among other things.

 These programs can be quite expensive and getting insurance approval for them can be challenging. (*Challenging* is the only word our editors would let us use.) The pain organizations in Appendix B can give you the success rates of these types of programs, which may help with insurance coverage.

These programs have been found to be highly successful if you're a good candidate and you're interested in a quality program. You can check the quality of the program in the following ways:

- **Get referrals from your doctors:** Your doctors will be familiar with local programs.

- **Check with pain organizations:** You can find a listing for several organizations, including IASP, the American Pain Society (APS), and the Commission on Accreditation of Rehabilitation Facilities (CARF), in Appendix B.

- **Ask about the screening evaluation:** A good program screens you carefully and takes you only if they feel you have a good chance of success. A poorer quality program takes everybody.

The Passive Therapies

Passive treatment is something that a physical therapist or other professional does to you. In these treatments, you're essentially a passive recipient of the treatment. This section looks at the most common passive physical therapy treatments.

Hot and cold packs

The use of *hot and cold packs* (or some other method of alternating heat and cold) is one of the most common techniques to treat the symptoms of back pain. The overall action of hot and cold packs (other than the obvious temperature difference) is similar. Hot packs help relax your muscles, increase local blood flow, and relieve your pain. (Too bad they don't make hot packs for in-law visits!) Cold packs also help relieve your back pain and decrease muscle spasm. After causing an initial decrease in blood flow, cold packs eventually cause an increase in blood flow to the affected area.

Generally, applying hot and cold packs to your back provides only temporary relief. No existing evidence shows that hot or cold application results in any long-term benefits; however, by using hot and cold packs to manage your back pain symptoms, you can more effectively complete appropriate back exercises. (See Chapter 14 for more information on back exercises.)

Ultrasound

Ultrasound waves are nothing more than high-frequency sound waves. Various tissues in your body can absorb ultrasound waves, even though the frequency is too high for the human ear to actually hear. (Too bad you can't say the same about some forms of music!) This absorption produces heat deep at the tissue site, below the surface of your skin. Heating the tissues in your back area helps relieve your pain, increase blood flow, and promote muscle relaxation — just like hot packs.

Physical therapists often use a combination of hot packs, cold packs, and ultrasound to help relieve your back pain. The relief you feel is usually temporary, and the therapies have no long-term benefits by themselves. We recommend that you use these types of treatments in conjunction with an appropriate exercise program.

Ultrasound requires special equipment and training, so a trained technician must administer it. To keep you from becoming dependent on your physical therapist or doctor for pain relief, we recommend that you seek these treatments only on a short-term basis (the first few weeks of your back pain treatment, for instance). After that time, you should be able to apply hot and cold packs yourself on an as-needed basis to help manage your back pain as you increase your exercises.

Massage

Massage is thought to increase the blood flow to the massaged area and to relax your muscles, causing a decrease in spasm and pain. We have many patients tell us that massage is helpful for their back symptoms, and you may find similar results — at least on a temporary basis. And as an added bonus, massage feels great! Any massage treatment you undergo, however, should be part of an overall treatment plan that involves an active, appropriate exercise program. We don't recommend massage as a treatment by itself. (See Chapter 9 for more information about massage.)

Depending on the intensity of the massage approach, your pain may increase during the massage. Usually, though, muscle relaxation and pain relief quickly follow. Applying heat before massage or deep tissue work helps loosen up your muscles. After a massage or deep tissue work, applying ice can help relieve pain.

As with the other passive physical therapy approaches, don't become dependent solely on massage as a way to manage your back pain over the long-term. Massage can become expensive and not address your underlying problem.

Bed rest

Doctors often prescribe bed rest and limited activity, although these aren't technically physical therapy treatments. Bed rest may sound great to you, because at the very least, it doesn't increase your pain. However, we believe that too much bed rest and limited activity puts you at risk for developing *physical deconditioning syndrome.* In this syndrome, your muscles weaken, which actually contributes to and prolongs your back pain problem. (See Chapter 3 for more information about the deconditioning syndrome.)

Research indicates that, in most cases of back pain, you should limit your bed rest to about two to five days after onset of severe back pain and then begin to gradually increase your activities. Let your physician or physical therapist guide you into gradually resuming your activities. See R.A. Deyo, et al., "How many days of bed rest for acute low back pain? A randomized clinical trial," *The New England Journal of Medicine,* 315 (1986): 1064–1070 and A.L. Nachemson, "Newest knowledge of low back pain: A critical look," *Clinical Orthopedics and Related Research* 279 (1992): 8–20.

Water therapy

Water's physical properties make it a good source of treatment for back pain. In water, you're buoyant and essentially weightless, which takes the pressure of gravity off your body, specifically your low-back area. Water also provides resistance to your movements, forcing your movement to be slow, rhythmic, and smooth. Exercises done in water often produce less pain and tend not to cause pain flare-ups either.

Water therapy can be either active or passive. In active therapy, you actually exercise in the pool. Starting in the pool can be an excellent way to begin an exercise program, especially if you're out of shape or afraid to exercise your back. After a few weeks in the pool, you can graduate to a land program.

In passive therapy, you simply sit in a whirlpool. Treatment using a whirlpool is essentially a passive physical therapy treatment, and we recommend that you limit your use of a whirlpool, although this treatment may help manage your symptoms while you engage in a more active therapy.

Transcutaneous Electrical Nerve Stimulation (TENS)

Transcutaneous Electrical Nerve Stimulation (TENS) is a procedure in which you or your physical therapist apply a mild level of electrical stimulation to the painful area of your back. Basically, you place bandage-like electrodes on your skin. Wires attach the electrodes to a small, battery-operated unit, which passes low-level electricity between the electrodes. When the unit is on, you may feel a tingling going between the electrodes. (You may also feel like an extra in Dr. Frankenstein's lab.) A variety of TENS units are on the market; they emit electrical patterns of differing amplitude, frequencies, and pulse widths. Ask your doctor or physical therapist about the rationale behind the differences.

The theory behind TENS is that the mild electrical stimulation that the unit supplies overrides the pain signal coming from your back. As the TENS unit blocks the pain signal, you begin to feel a decrease in pain.

TENS therapy is strictly for pain relief; it does not cure the problem.

The only way to determine whether a TENS unit will work for your pain is to try it. These units can be costly, so we recommend that you try TENS initially at your doctor's or physical therapist's office. If you notice some benefits in terms of pain relief, you may want to consider renting one for a month or so. Only then should you consider purchasing one of these units.

As with all the other treatments that focus only on pain relief, we recommend that you use a TENS unit in conjunction with an exercise program and increased activities.

Traction

Traction (used mainly in low-back pain cases) is an apparatus or manual treatment that applies *tension of distraction* to your spine in order to pull the vertebrae away from each other. Slightly separating the vertebrae of your lower spine is thought to relieve some of the pressure on your disc. In pelvic traction, an apparatus wrapped around your hips applies distraction tension to your lower spine.

Traction is a passive treatment. Like other passive treatments, traction can provide temporary pain relief. Most research indicates that traction has no long-term benefits. However, traction may have some promising applications for low-back pain in the near future based on yet unpublished research.

Corsets and braces

At some time during your treatment for back pain your doctor may suggest that you try a corset or brace for your back pain. A brace can restrict motion, provide abdominal support, and correct your posture. Certain conditions — such as recovering from a spinal fusion surgery (see Chapter 8) or the fracture of a vertebra (see Chapter 3) — require you to wear a brace for a short period of time.

In most back pain cases, wearing a brace or corset provides temporary pain relief, especially during increased activity or while sitting for long periods of time. We recommend that you use braces or corsets in conjunction with an ongoing exercise program as prescribed by your doctor (see Chapter 23 for more info).

Medications

Medication and back pain don't necessarily go hand-in-hand. In conjunction with an overall treatment plan that includes such remedies as appropriate exercise, medications can help decrease your pain, reduce inflammation, and relieve muscle spasms. Still, you and your doctor should decide together whether medication is a good option for you.

Any time you take medication, you need to be an informed consumer. You need to be aware of any potential side effects or drug interactions. To make sure that your treatment with medications goes well, ask your doctor the following questions about your medications:

- ✔ Why are you recommending this medication?

- ✔ What benefit should I expect, and how long before I know whether the medication is achieving the goal?

- ✔ How do I take this medication? (Morning or night, with meals, on an empty stomach, every four hours, and so on.)

- ✔ What side effects should I be aware of? What should I do if these occur? Will they go away if I decide to stay on the medicine?

- ✔ Is it okay to use the generic version of this medication?

- ✔ Can I take this medication in addition to the other medications I am on? (Make a practice of giving all your doctors a list of your current medications for their records.)

- ✔ How do I stop taking this medication safely?

Always check that the medication you get from the pharmacy is the same one that you and your doctor discussed. Although rare, the pharmacy can make mistakes in the dispensing of medications. Also, some pharmacies or managed care insurance plans may automatically use the generic version of a medicine unless instructed otherwise on your prescription. Ultimately, you are responsible for asking whether you're being given a generic and if that is okay with your doctor. Also, be aware that there may be different levels of coverage from your insurance company for generics versus name-brand drugs.

The following sections explain the various types of medications that doctors commonly prescribe to treat back pain. In the following discussion of medications, each section contains guidelines for use. These are *general guidelines,* and you should always be clear about what your doctor is recommending for your unique back pain problem. Follow your doctor's usage recommendations carefully.

The following medication categories are generally listed from the most commonly used to the least commonly used. Therefore, you may expect your doctor to start with medications at the beginning of the list and move towards the end of the list if necessary.

Analgesics

Doctors commonly prescribe *analgesics* — a fancy name for painkillers — for back pain. Analgesics vary from over-the-counter preparations, such as aspirin and Tylenol, to very strong narcotics, such as morphine. Many anti-inflammatory medications (which we discuss later in this chapter) can also help relieve pain.

Among the most commonly prescribed analgesic medications that have no anti-inflammatory actions are codeine, drugs derived from codeine, narcotics, or synthetic narcotic compounds. These medicines include Tylenol with codeine, hydrocodone (Vicodin), oxycodone (Percoset), and dihydrocodeine.

Regular over-the-counter Tylenol should be the first analgesic you try for your pain before trying anti-inflammatories or prescription analgesics. Painkillers are strictly for pain relief. Use these medicines for only a short time unless your doctor has other reasons for using them long term.

In most cases, you can expect to get analgesics only in the early phases of acute back pain. Doctors generally prescribe a time-limited course of pain medication along with other methods of pain relief such as limited bed rest, ice, and heat. You usually take analgesics on a *PRN (pro re nata),* or as-needed, basis. If you're experiencing short-term, acute back pain, analgesics may help — but don't wait until the pain is unbearable before taking the pain

Addiction

The latest research shows that when given for a legitimate pain problem, addiction to analgesics rarely occurs. With appropriate use, narcotics are a safe and effective way to control your back pain. See R.K. Portenoy, "Chronic opioid therapy for persistent noncancer pain: Can we get past the bias?" in *APS Bulletin* (1992): 1–5.

Opioid-based medications (narcotics) are one of your doctor's primary weapons against moderate to severe back pain. The fear of addiction may cause you to avoid or even refuse these narcotics. Because of this fear, you may end up not taking adequate doses to provide relief or waiting to take the medicine until you can't bear the pain. To ease these fears, you need to understand the difference between tolerance, dependence, and addiction.

- ✔ **Tolerance** is a well-known property of all narcotics. Over time, your body gets used to the medication's effect, which sometimes means that you have to increase the dose to maintain effectiveness.

- ✔ **Dependence** is also a well-known and understood physical process. If you suddenly stop taking the medicine, you may experience physical withdrawal symptoms such as diarrhea, agitation, and stomachaches.

- ✔ **Addiction** is a *psychological craving* for the medication even when you don't need it for pain relief.

Your doctor can manage tolerance by adding other non-addictive medicines that help the narcotics work better and by using the other pain relief techniques that we discuss in this chapter. Your doctor can manage dependence by slowly tapering the pain medication (adding other medication to control withdrawal) when the time is appropriate.

medicine. At that point, your back pain may be so severe that the medication will do little to relieve your pain. And that means that you then need more pain medicine to get the pain under control. As this pattern repeats, you may find yourself experiencing higher levels of pain overall while actually taking more pain medicine.

If your doctor prescribes stronger analgesics on a long-term basis, take them on a *time-contingent schedule* rather than as-needed. In a time-contingent schedule, you take your medication on a fixed schedule — perhaps every four hours — regardless of your level of back pain. This approach keeps the pain-relieving effects of the medicine constant and avoids the ups and downs of the as-needed approach. Time-contingent medication scheduling can help prevent you from having severe pain episodes by "catching" the pain early. In addition to using a time-contingent schedule, you need to utilize the lowest level of pain medicine possible to stay comfortable. Doing so helps avoid tolerance and dependence, and keeps side effects to a minimum.

Usage: In general, the pure narcotics are quite safe and have minimal side effects *in limited use*. You may experience dizziness, trouble focusing your thoughts, constipation, sedation, and lethargy, but these side effects tend to go away after a week or two.

Anti-inflammatory medications

Anti-inflammatory medications reduce inflammation. (How's that for obvious?) Aspirin is probably the most common anti-inflammatory medication. In addition to reducing inflammation, aspirin and most other non-steroidal anti-inflammatories also help relieve pain. A number of different types and classes of anti-inflammatory medications are currently on the market. Some of the common anti-inflammatory medications include ibuprofen (Motrin and Advil) and naproxen sodium (Naprosyn and Aleve).

These medications are standard back pain treatments, especially if your pain is possibly due to an inflammatory component such as muscle sprain-strain and injuries to the soft tissues. Your doctor may also recommend anti-inflammatory medication for many other types of spine problems including conditions such as degenerative disc disease, arthritis, and disc herniations.

Your doctor will probably prescribe anti-inflammatory medications on a regular dosing schedule, which allows the medicine to establish and maintain a therapeutic level. You should plan to take the anti-inflammatory medication for approximately two weeks, unless your doctor instructs you otherwise. Resist the temptation to stop taking the anti-inflammatory medication when you start to feel better after a couple of days (unless your doctor tells you to stop) because you may actually start to feel worse. As with all of the other medications, you should use anti-inflammatories in conjunction with other treatments for your back pain and pain relief.

Usage: Be aware that you may bruise more easily while taking anti-inflammatories because these medicines make your blood clot more slowly. Less common side effects include ringing in your ears, light-headedness, and stomach upset. You can help avoid any nausea and gastrointestinal upset by taking this medication with meals. Contact your doctor if you have any of these side effects.

If you use anti-inflammatory medication for a long period of time (more than two months), there is greater risk of kidney and liver problems, in addition to ulcers. If you've taken anti-inflammatories for an extended period of time, talk to your doctor about your other options. When you take anti-inflammatory medications you should avoid alcohol as it can increase the risk of bleeding ulcers.

There's a new kid on the block

Nonsteroidal anti-inflammatory drugs (NSAIDs) such as aspirin and ibuprofen are prescribed millions of times per year for back pain. Chances are that you have taken these medicines at some time for your back pain problem. Although NSAIDs can be quite effective, they can cause serious side-effects such as stomach and intestinal upset, bleeding ulcers, and kidney problems.

Because of these side effects, scientists have been searching for an alternative type of anti-inflammatory medication that is safer to take. This search is now complete with the development of anti-inflammatories called *COX-2 inhibitors,* recently approved by the Food and Drug Administration. This is a completely new type of medicine that provides an anti-inflammatory benefit without the same degree of stomach and intestinal side effects. Check out the hot topics in Chapter 23 for more information and then talk to your doctor.

Muscle relaxants

If your doctor believes that some type of muscle spasm or tightness is contributing to your back pain, she may prescribe muscle relaxant medication. We believe muscle relaxants are appropriate only when muscle spasm is clearly a prominent feature of your back pain problem.

Muscle relaxants calm anxiety and agitation because of the way they affect your brain. Don't come to rely on these medications for their emotional calming effects.

No one knows exactly how muscle relaxants work. One thought is that the muscle relaxants operate on your brain and then secondarily on the muscles of your back. Alternatively, the medication may also act directly on the back muscles themselves.

Among the more common muscle relaxants are Soma, Robaxin, Flexeril, Valium, and Skelaxin. Doctors generally prescribe these medications on an as-needed basis. You should use these medications in conjunction with other techniques for reducing muscle tension and spasm including ice, heat, stretching, or biofeedback.

Unless your doctor has a specific reason for prescribing these drugs over a longer time, you should take them for only two weeks. In the initial stages of your back pain, your doctor may prescribe these medications to help you sleep at night. This treatment should be short-term because these medications have a tendency to disturb healthy sleep patterns in the long run. In addition, long-term use of muscle relaxants can promote depression.

Usage: Common side effects of muscle relaxants include sleepiness during the daytime, difficulty with coordination, and depression. Avoid alcohol use if you're taking muscle relaxant medications as it can worsen side effects.

Sedatives

If you're having trouble sleeping, your doctor may prescribe *sedatives* (also known as *hypnotics* — "you're getting verrry sleeepy"). Before you use sleeping medications, discuss your sleep problem with your doctor.

- ✔ If your sleep problem relates to depression, then a sedating antidepressant may be more appropriate than a sedative.

- ✔ If your sleep disruption is due to pain, then an evening dose of a pain medication may be more appropriate.

- ✔ If you are neither depressed nor in pain, then short-term use of sedatives may be helpful for you.

Use sleeping medication only on an as-needed basis and for as little time as possible. For long-term improved sleep, focus on other techniques such as relaxation training. Practice *good sleep hygiene,* which is not sleeping with a bar of soap but creating good sleep habits including:

- ✔ Go to bed and wake up on a consistent schedule.

- ✔ Don't nap during the day.

- ✔ Do stressful things — like paying bills — someplace other than your bed (or bedroom if possible).

- ✔ Get up if you don't fall asleep after 30 minutes. (You can try again when you feel more tired.)

In choosing a sedative, try the least addictive first. Ask your doctor about trying Tylenol PM or Benadryl (25 to 100mg at bedtime) before taking prescription sleeping medications. If these are ineffective, ask your doctor about trying a prescription medication such as benzodiazepine. Barbiturates (Amytal, Nembutal, and Seconal) have fallen into disfavor because of the potential for abuse and the availability of much safer medications.

Usage: Any sedative should be used only when you need it and for as short a time as possible. You should use the smallest dose that is effective in helping you to get to sleep. Although you can experiment with what works best for you, generally you should take the medication about 30 minutes before bedtime so that you are drowsy and ready to fall asleep when you "hit the sack." The most common side-effects are difficulty getting up the next morning (hangover) and sleepiness during the daytime. Do not use alcohol in conjunction with these medications.

Anti-anxiety agents

If your back pain is acute and associated with anxiety and trouble sleeping, your doctor may prescribe an anti-anxiety medication. Benzodiazepines such as Xanax, Ativan, Valium, Tranxene, and Centrax are widely used anti-anxiety agents.

You may notice that we mention some of these medications in the preceding section. Medicines can fall into more than one category of use depending on their properties. Many of the anti-anxiety agents (and the antidepressants as we discuss later) are also good for sleep. Take these medications for a very short time when anxiety, specifically, is making your back pain worse, and use these medications in conjunction with other treatment approaches. If, along with your back pain, you're prone to anxiety or panic attacks, consider working with a psychiatrist or other doctor who has special expertise in prescribing anti-anxiety medications.

Usage: Common side effects of the benzodiazepines include drowsiness, sedation, and short-term memory loss. You can eliminate many of these side effects by working with your doctor to adjust the dose of the medications. Be aware that tolerance and dependence may develop when using these medications. (See the sidebar, "Addiction," in this chapter.) Avoid taking alcohol with these medications. You should never abruptly stop taking the benzodiazepines or attempt to adjust the dosage yourself. Abruptly stopping the benzodiazepines can cause agitation and anxiety, sleep disruption, and, rarely, seizures. Taper off of these medications under your doctor's guidance.

Antidepressants

Antidepressants are becoming more and more common in the treatment of chronic back pain problems. Extensive research now confirms that certain antidepressant medications can actually provide you with some pain relief, even if you are not depressed.

Even though your pain is in your back, it is actually *experienced* in your brain. For this reason, researchers believe that the effect antidepressants have on certain chemicals in the brain provides not only an antidepressant effect but also pain relief. Antidepressant medications appear to be particularly helpful in nerve pain problems and chronic pain.

Your doctor's choice of antidepressant medication for you depends upon your specific back pain problem and associated symptoms. Some of the antidepressants have sedating properties, while others have more of an energizing effect. In addition, different antidepressants affect different brain chemicals (such as seratonin and norepinephrine). Your doctor takes all these factors into account when choosing an antidepressant for you. You may need to try two or three different antidepressants before you find the one that works best for your situation.

The sedating properties of some of the antidepressants can be helpful in normalizing sleep patterns, while at the same time helping reduce your pain. Antidepressants seem to provide more restful sleep than sedatives, along with other positive benefits such as pain relief. Antidepressants also help with the depression commonly associated with chronic back pain problems.

As you can see in Table 7-1, the dosage range for pain relief and the dosage range for antidepressant effect is quite different. Even so, considering that depression is about four times more prevalent in people with chronic back pain than it is in the general population, these medicines are certainly appropriate if you have significant depression with your ongoing back pain.

Table 7-1	Dosage Ranges for Antidepressant Medications When Used for Pain and Depression	
Antidepressant	*Dose for Pain*	*Dose for Depression*
Elavil	10 to 150mg	150 to 300mg
Desyrel	25 to 75mg	150 to 400mg
Norpramine	25mg	75 to 200mg
Pamelar	25 to 100mg	75 to 150mg
Sinequan	10 to 100mg	150 to 300mg
Tofranil	25 to 75mg	150 to 300mg

Prozac, Zoloft, Paxil, and other antidepressants that work differently are also being used and studied for their effects on pain.

Antidepressants are usually effective only after they attain certain blood levels. If your doctor prescribes an antidepressant, you must take the medication every day (either at bedtime or in the morning, depending on the drug) in order to reach and maintain that effective level.

Usage: Antidepressants vary in their side effects, but the most common include dry mouth, blurred vision, constipation, difficulty urinating, sedation, and nausea, among others. These side effects frequently occur in the first week or two that you take the antidepressant medication. If you can tolerate the side effects during this time period, they often go away. If side effects are causing problems for you, talk to your doctor about other options. These medications are not addictive, and you do not develop tolerance to them; you may need to take antidepressants for three to twelve months or longer. As with all medications, you need to employ other techniques such as psychological pain management, counseling, relaxation procedures, meditation, biofeedback, and exercise that will ultimately become substitutes for these medications.

Invasive Conservative Treatments

Invasive conservative treatments are those in which your doctor actually pierces your skin as part of the treatment. These treatments are still considered "conservative" because they are reversible. Doctors usually reserve these treatments for those patients whose back pain problems do not respond to the non-invasive conservative treatments. We discuss invasive conservative treatments in the order of most common (and least invasive) to the least common (and most invasive).

Trigger point injections

A *trigger point injection* involves injecting a small amount of anesthetic into certain muscle points, or *trigger points*. Your doctor may give you trigger point injections if you seem to have areas of muscle that "trigger" pain throughout a region of your body such as your lower or mid-back. (Gives a whole new meaning to the phrase "trigger happy," doesn't it?) For instance, you may be able to point to certain specific areas in your back that, when pushed with your finger, seem to cause pain not only in that local area but also throughout an entire region of your back.

We recommend that you undergo trigger point injections on a time-limited basis (such as a few weeks or during times of back pain flare-up) and — usually — only in conjunction with an overall active rehabilitation program.

Facet injections

If your doctor thinks that your pain is coming from your facet joints (see Chapter 3), she may recommend facet injections. These injections use steroid or anesthetic to decrease the inflammation of the facet joint and provide pain relief. These injections are usually done on an outpatient basis in a center that has special radiology equipment called *fluoroscopy*. This equipment allows your doctor to see exactly where the injection is going into the facet joint. You may not notice the full benefit of a facet joint injection for at least one week after the injection, although you may get immediate relief from the anesthetic (which wears off).

How's that for a multi-faceted explanation?

Spinal epidural steroid injections

In an *spinal epidural steroid injection,* your doctor — usually a physiatrist or anesthesiologist pain specialist, although other doctors can undergo special training to do these procedures — uses a needle to inject steroid and sometimes an anesthetic into a specific area of your spinal canal. The doctor injects the steroid, which helps decrease inflammation and pain, into an area (or *epidural space*) around the space that contains the disc and spinal nerves. Your doctor may recommend epidural injections if some type of disc or nerve root irritation problem is contributing to your back pain and leg pain.

Spinal epidural steroid injections should be done under fluoroscopy with contrast to assure proper needle placement. Epidural steroid injection can be diagnostic and therapeutic.

Epidural injections are often done in series of three. In fact, most doctors won't give you more than three epidural injections per six month period because too much steroid in your spine is not a good thing. Whether you will have more than one epidural injection really depends on your response to the first and the amount of steriod used. Recent research suggests that the full benefits of an epidural injection may not occur for a period of seven to ten days.

We feel that you should agree to epidural injections if your doctor has a good medical reason for them and you do them in conjunction with an overall exercise-oriented rehabilitation program. We use them quite often on patients with back and leg pain (sciatica) due to disc herniation. They can be extremely helpful in relieving pain and inflammation long enough to avoid surgery and allow natural healing to occur.

Selective nerve root blocks

Selective nerve root blocks are similar to spinal epidural steroid injections, but are directed more specifically to the exact source of your pain. Selective nerve blocks should not be performed without fluoroscopy and are often diagnostic and therapeutic. They can be more effective than spinal epidural steroid injections in some cases.

The steroids used in selective nerve root blocks and spinal epidural steroid injections will not make you look like Arnold Schwarzenegger. In other words, they are not anabolic (muscle building) steroids. They are steroids that reduce inflammation of the disc or nerve root.

Implantable Pain Therapies

Implantable pain therapies are the most invasive of the conservative treatments. Implantable pain therapies consist of two different types: spinal cord stimulation and intraspinal drug infusion therapy. Both of these procedures involve minor surgery to place the devices in your body. Even though implantable therapies involve minor surgery, they are considered conservative because the treatment is reversible. These devices don't cure the problem but are designed to relieve your symptoms.

Consider these treatments only after you exhaust all other treatments for your pain and none have been adequately beneficial.

Implantable pain therapies are not a good idea for you in certain situations. Your doctor will complete a screening evaluation (which we discuss next) that helps determine whether implantable pain therapy can work for you. Do not consider these treatments if

- Your symptoms do not match your physical findings.

- Emotions such as depression and anxiety are clearly contributing to your back pain or leg pain. In fact, many insurance companies require a psychological evaluation before authorizing an implantable pain device.

- You show any signs of drug addiction or other problems including a pattern of using pain medicines for purposes other than pain or not as prescribed by your doctor.

- You aren't motivated to combine implantable pain therapy with appropriate treatments to address other aspects of a chronic pain syndrome (exercise, psychological pain management techniques, decreasing pain medication use, and so on).

- You have psychological or emotional factors (such as severe depression, anxiety, or other psychological problems) that may hinder a successful response to these types of treatments.

The preceding list includes some of the things that your doctor assesses as part of your screening evaluation. In addition, your screening includes: a history to determine the reason that your other treatments did not work, a physical examination including evaluation of your pain, a psychological evaluation by a doctor familiar with pain problems, and a trial of any conservative therapy that has not been previously tried and your doctor thinks may be useful.

If your doctor adheres to the preceding screening criteria, he rarely recommends these types of implantable pain therapies for your back or leg pain. A team of doctors, including a physician and a psychologist trained in this area, usually conduct this screening. Even the manufacturers of these devices recommend a thorough assessment! That said, assuming that you have a condition that one of these implantable therapies can help and you pass the medical and psychological screening criteria, you may be a candidate for this type of treatment.

Spinal column stimulation

Spinal column stimulation was developed more than 30 years ago to manage chronic pain. In simple terms, *spinal column stimulation* involves surgically placing a set of electrodes along the nerve fibers of your spinal cord in your lower back in order to block pain signals going through that area. (Sounds pleasant, doesn't it?) The idea behind this treatment is similar to the rationale we discuss for TENS earlier in this chapter. Your doctor may use spinal column stimulation as a last resort for failed back surgery syndrome, arachnoiditis (see Chapter 3), or for nerve root injuries that haven't responded to other treatments.

Although first implemented more than three decades ago, spinal cord stimulation did not begin to gain true popularity until just recently due to technological advances. Advances that have increased the success of this treatment include making the surgery much less invasive through the use of new equipment, developing parts of the unit that are much more durable, designing microprocessor technology that allows the power source to be tiny (similar to pacemakers for your heart, the entire assembly is easily implanted, self-contained, and under the skin), and improving patient selection which has lead to much better outcomes.

You may be an appropriate candidate for the spinal cord stimulator if you have the following characteristics:

- ✔ Your pain is primarily in one or both legs. Spinal cord stimulators are generally not appropriate if lower back pain is your only complaint.
- ✔ Your symptoms and spine condition are stable and neither worsening nor improving.
- ✔ Your pain is primarily due to a nerve problem and radiates from your lower back to your legs.
- ✔ Your pain is primarily a burning, stinging, tingling, and radiating sensation.
- ✔ You have tried conservative treatments (such as physical therapy, psychological interventions, nerve blocks, medication management, and multidisciplinary rehabilitation), and they haven't helped.
- ✔ Your complaints are consistent with your physical findings.

If you're a possible candidate, your doctor places a temporary electrode to determine whether you should receive a permanent device. The test phase for the temporary electrode is approximately two to three days, although some surgeons may require a test phase of up to two months. Your surgeon will also require anywhere from a 50 to 70 percent reduction in pain with the temporary electrode in order to consider permanent placement.

You must be truthful with your physician as to the amount of pain relief you are actually experiencing during the test phase. No matter how high your hopes, if the device doesn't work for you during the test phase, it won't work after it is permanently implanted, and you will have undergone an unnecessary procedure and a treatment failure. The latest research indicates that about 50 to 60 percent of qualified patients can expect greater than 50 percent pain relief with permanent implantation of the spinal cord stimulator. Complications of spinal cord stimulation treatment are relatively infrequent and insignificant.

Implanted drug infusion therapy

If you have chronic back pain due either to a failed back surgery syndrome or some other reason and your pain has been unresponsive to any previous treatments, you may be a candidate for *intraspinal drug infusion therapy.* This treatment's primary use is for chronic, intractable, low-back pain.

Intraspinal drug infusion therapy involves surgically implanting a "pump system" in your body that delivers pain medicine by a small tube directly to a specific area of your spine. The rationale behind this approach is that you need much less pain medicine if the medicine is delivered in small quantities directly to your spine (actually about 1/300ths of the same dose taken by mouth!). When you take pain medicines orally, their results and effects occur throughout your entire body, and only a small portion of the medicine is actually working where you need it. The intraspinal drug infusion method is designed to make the medicine more effective and have fewer side effects.

The screening criteria for an intraspinal drug infusion device is similar to that for spinal column stimulators, which we discuss in the preceding section. Other criteria that may lead your surgeon to choose this method over a stimulator include:

- ✔ Your pain is primarily in your lower back and buttocks with only minimal radiation down one or both legs.
- ✔ You have multiple pain sites in your lower back and buttocks.
- ✔ You don't describe your pain primarily as nerve pain.
- ✔ You haven't responded to all other available conservative treatments such as medications, physical therapy, nerve blocks, or psychological interventions.

After meeting all the preceding criteria, you undergo a test phase before your doctor considers a fully implantable pump system. In the test phase, you wear a pump outside of your body that delivers pain medicine to your lower spinal area. The test phase lasts for one to three days, and you must notice at least a 50 percent increase in pain relief. You must be truthful about the pain relief during this test phase because it accurately predicts the success of the permanently implanted device.

The permanently implanted system involves placing a small reservoir and pump under your skin. The pump has a tube that delivers the pain medicine to your lower spine. You need to refill the reservoir with pain medication at least every 90 days, although you may require more frequent refills. Refilling is a relatively painless procedure that is done at your doctor's office by placing a needle through your skin into the reservoir.

Complications related to intraspinal drug infusion devices include infection, contamination of the pump reservoir, cerebral spinal fluid leak, headache, mechanical pump failure, catheter failure, and side effects to the medication. Most of these complications are minor and reversible.

For more information on the latest advances in spinal cord stimulation and pump systems, check out the discussion in Chapter 23.

Chapter 8

Choosing to Have Back Surgery

· ·

· ·

We have some great news and some good news. The great news is that spine surgery is almost always your choice — yes, you read that right, *your choice.* Only about one percent of all spine surgeries are truly medical emergencies, which means that approximately 99 percent are elective!

Even if your doctor recommends surgery, most of the time you can safely opt to try a different treatment method. Throughout this book, we offer you many alternatives for a more conservative (or nonsurgical) approach. You may very well be able to manage your pain without surgical treatment for your spinal condition.

Now the good news: In some instances, spine surgery *is* your best bet for pain resolution. In fact, in our practice, we see better than a 90 percent success rate with surgery due to our careful selective process and other techniques, which we review in this chapter. And because surgery is usually elective, you have time to do things in preparation — getting a second opinion, doing surgical preparation, and so on — which we also discuss in this chapter.

This chapter gives you information on deciding whether to undergo surgery, choosing a spine surgeon, and preparing for surgery. We also discuss the most common spine surgeries.

We realize that the information in this chapter is frightening — surgery usually is. But we also believe that the more you understand about the procedures and their inherent risks, the better equipped you are to make that decision. In our practice, we treat surgery as a last resort. In this chapter, we give you the tools to make the best choice for you and your back.

Choosing Surgery

Your doctor may suggest (and you may consider) spine surgery in several situations.

- ✔ You have a certain condition (such as a spinal tumor or other emergency) that makes surgery medically necessary.

- ✔ You've completed a course of conservative treatment without getting better (see Chapter 7).

- ✔ The correlation between your symptoms and what appears to be causing your pain is high.

Spine surgery is elective in virtually all cases except emergency situations such as cauda equina syndrome, tumors, progressive neurologic deficits, and some infections (see Chapter 3).

You may think that undergoing spine surgery would be a fairly straightforward decision, based primarily on your medical need. You may also expect that spine surgeons generally agree upon what conditions are appropriate for surgery. However, the definitions of surgical or medical need are as numerous as the surgeons who perform spine operations. Whether or not your doctor recommends spine surgery depends on a number of factors:

- ✔ **Your symptoms and diagnostic test findings:** As we discuss in Chapters 3 and 6, your test findings (from such procedures as MRI) must match your symptoms. Your doctors shouldn't consider surgery unless they're confident that they've identified the condition causing your pain.

- ✔ **How and where your surgeon was trained:** Research studies show that where your surgeon trained can influence how often he recommends surgery for a spine problem. Some medical schools emphasize surgical treatments for back pain problems while others emphasize a more nonsurgical approach. See *The Adult Spine,* edited by J.W. Frymoyer, (New York: Raven Press, 1991).

- ✔ **The country you live in:** The rate of spine surgery is much higher in the United States than in other industrialized countries like Great Britain. Sometimes the region of a particular country also influences the rate of surgery. Although exact statistics are not available, as much as a ten-fold regional variation may exist across parts of the United States.

✔ **The type of insurance you have:** If your insurance doesn't cover your spine surgery, chances are that you won't have the surgery (due to the costs). Also, HMOs tend to proceed with spine surgery very cautiously, focusing on more conservative treatments instead.

✔ **How much you want the surgery:** Your desire to have the surgery influences your surgeon, whether either of you realize it. If you constantly ask about having surgery and don't give conservative treatment a chance, your doctor is more likely to agree to surgery.

Determining When Surgery Is Necessary

Although sometimes medically necessary, spine surgery is usually elective. Unfortunately, doctors don't always present surgery to you as a choice. Therefore, you need to have a good understanding of those rare cases where spine surgery is your only option, versus the majority of cases in which surgery is only one of several alternatives.

Medically necessary spine surgery

Spine surgery may be medically necessary in the following cases:

✔ **Cauda equina syndrome:** In this extremely rare condition, important nerve roots in your lower spine, critical to bowel and bladder function and responsible for sensation to the groin and anal areas, are compressed (usually due to a herniated disc).

Symptoms of cauda equina syndrome include numbness in the genital region, around the anus, and in your feet; an inability to urinate; and the loss of sexual function. Without quick surgical treatment, you may end up with permanent loss of bowel, bladder, and sexual function.

Having a disc herniation does not mean that you're going to get cauda equina syndrome. Sadly, some spine surgeons bring up the possibility without emphasizing how rare this condition is — they scare the patient into agreeing to have spine surgery. If your surgeon mentions the possibility of cauda equina syndrome, then you need answers to several questions:

• What is the likelihood that I will get cauda equina? (Remember that it is extremely rare.)

• What symptoms should I look for?

• What should I do if they occur?

✔ **Tumors:** Surgery is frequently necessary to remove a spinal tumor. Even though a tumor may be noncancerous and slow-growing, it can press on important parts of your spine, especially if the tumor is in your neck or mid-back area. A spine tumor may produce pain that awakens you from sleep, and/or you may be more comfortable sleeping in an upright position.

If your tumor is slow-growing, noncancerous, and not pressing on any important spinal areas, you may not need surgery. Only a spine surgeon can make a proper recommendation regarding the management of a spinal tumor. As always, getting an independent second opinion is a reasonable course of action.

✔ **Infections:** Just like any other part of your body, you can get an infection in your spine. How this happens isn't exactly clear. You may be more vulnerable to a spinal infection if your immune system is weakened or you have diabetes and bacteria gets into your bloodstream, ultimately spreading to your spine.

Pain from a spinal infection is an intense, throbbing, aching kind of pain. It is often present at rest and awakens you from sleep. Diagnosing a spinal infection can include the use of imaging tests, bone scans, and blood tests. Doctors treat these infections with intravenous antibiotics. Some patients may need surgical treatment to clean out the infected area in addition to the antibiotics.

Choosing to have surgery

In most cases, you are the one who ultimately decides whether to have spine surgery, so engaging in healthy surgical decision-making is important. Your surgeon begins the process by suggesting that you are a candidate for surgery. After that is done, your surgeon may or may not assist you in the rest of your decision-making process.

You may be drawn to the quick-fix appeal of surgery, but we almost always tell patients to avoid the surgical option if their condition is improving. You have no guarantee that surgery will take care of your pain better than a conservative approach and the natural course of healing.

Because most spine surgeries are elective, you have time to make an informed decision; therefore, don't make the decision to have surgery on your first visit to a spine surgeon. Consider the following issues in your surgical decision-making process:

✔ **You have leg pain rather than back pain:** Doctors commonly recommend spine surgery to treat a disc herniation with symptoms that may include any or all of the following: pain in the buttocks, one or both legs, and (sometimes) the lower back. Although a herniated disc can take 12 to 16 weeks to heal, remember that 85 to 90 percent of people can be treated effectively without surgery. The herniated portion of a disc is mostly water, so the piece of disc that is causing the problem tends to shrink and be reabsorbed by your body over time. As the disc heals and shrinks, generally the irritation or pressure on the nerve is relieved and you feel better.

If you have a lower back problem that is appropriate for surgery, the symptoms almost always include pain down one or both legs because the nerves that supply your legs pass through your lower back. So, you can have a lower back problem (such as a disc herniation) without actually having symptoms in your lower back.

In a recent study, we found that even very large disc herniations can be treated conservatively. Our research has shown an average of a 62 percent decrease in disc herniation size on follow-up MRIs after six months.

✔ **You haven't responded to conservative treatments:** Conservative treatment is always an option, but if you've tried it and it hasn't worked for you, then a surgical approach may be appropriate. Surgery may also be indicated in some cases where conservative treatment has been only partially successful. Before you agree to surgery, though, make sure that you give conservative treatment enough time to work. *Note:* Using only passive therapies like hot packs and ultrasound (see Chapter 7 for more information) is not an adequate course of conservative therapy.

Even if your conservative therapy is not entirely successful, the decision to have surgery is still your choice. We have patients with residual symptoms (such as leg pain, numbness, and back pain) who have decided they would rather live with the symptoms than have spine surgery. These symptoms are not dangerous, and as long as they don't worsen, living with them over the long-term does not cause any problems.

✔ **Your symptoms match your test findings:** Spine surgery can be highly successful when the reason for your pain is clearly established through testing and your symptoms correspond to those results. For instance, if you have sciatica or leg pain due to a disc herniation, your pain should be in a very specific area of the buttock and leg that matches your imaging studies and other diagnostic test results.

You and your surgeon may be tempted to give surgery a try if conservative treatment hasn't worked completely, even though your symptoms don't correlate with your examination findings. Resist the temptation: You risk an unsuccessful surgery.

✔ **You refuse to accept the symptoms:** If your symptoms are worsening in the face of appropriate conservative treatment and you find the symptoms unacceptable, then exploring a surgical option may be reasonable.

Many spine surgeons try to dictate when surgery is best for you by telling you that your symptoms are unacceptable to them. However, you have to live with the symptoms, so you need to determine whether they are unacceptable to *you*. We recommend that the surgery take place within two to three months.

Addressing Psychological Issues and Surgery

Your surgeon may recommend surgery based solely on the physical aspects of your problem, including such things as your MRI and other diagnostic test results, your physical exam, and your overall medical condition. A good doctor also takes your psychological and emotional health into account.

Several psychological and emotional issues may make you a poor surgical candidate by increasing the risk of an unsuccessful outcome:

- **Depression, anxiety, or other emotional problems:** Make sure that you address any depression or anxiety before considering spine surgery.

- **Lack of support from family members or significant stress in family relationships:** Lack of emotional support can cause problems with the entire surgical process. This kind of stress in your environment can make your back pain worse, which means that you may not make a good decision about surgery.

- **Fear of pain and of hospitals:** If thinking about post-operative pain or the hospital environment gives you the willies, talk to your doctor about ways to help you prepare for surgery. (We discuss preparing for surgery later in this chapter.)

- **Negative surgical experiences:** A bad surgical experience can certainly make you nervous about going through another surgery. Preparing for surgery can help.

- **Unrealistic expectations:** Talk with your doctor about what you can reasonably expect from the surgery. If you have unrealistic expectations, you can end up unsatisfied with the results.

As you prepare for surgery, make sure that you address any of the preceding issues that apply to you. Your doctor or a mental health professional can help you. (We also list some resources later in this chapter.) Some of our patients actually decide to forego surgery after successfully dealing with their emotional issues.

Some doctors believe that back pain causes some of these emotional issues. They reason that if surgery fixes your physical pain, you'll no longer be upset and the emotional issues will go away. Unfortunately, ongoing emotional and psychological issues affect your perception of pain and level of suffering. Surgery can repair a structural problem in your spine, but your psychological factors may continue, and so, likely, will your pain.

Other factors can also influence the outcome our your spine surgery. These include the following psychological and social issues (arranged here from what we believe are the most common to the less common):

✔ **Chronic pain syndrome:** The more symptoms of chronic pain syndrome you have (see Chapter 3 for a list of symptoms), the less likely you are to respond positively to spine surgery. You must treat all elements of your chronic pain syndrome simultaneously. If you respond adequately and show improvement, you may not need surgery. Fixing a structural spine problem with surgery, without addressing the other issues that come with this syndrome, almost invariably causes a failed back surgery syndrome.

✔ **Compensation and litigation issues:** Compensation and litigation issues (such as getting disability payments or being involved in a lawsuit because of your back pain) can cause psychological stress that impacts your surgery outcome without your even being aware of it. If you're engaged in litigation related to your back pain, or get compensation for it, you're at greater risk for a failed spine surgery. This is not to say that you aren't a surgical candidate; rather, you have another risk factor requiring pre-surgical assessment.

CLINICAL INFO

Factoring risks

If you don't address emotional and psychological conditions prior to undergoing surgery, you can have a surgery that is a technical success but a clinical failure. An example would be the patient who has a surgery for a disc herniation and the post-operative MRI looks great (technical success) even though the patient is having continued, debilitating pain (clinical failure).

The medical community is only now beginning to understand the power of emotional and psychological factors on surgical success. For instance, a recent study demonstrated how childhood psychological trauma influenced spine surgery outcome. The study looked at 86 patients who underwent spine surgery as adults but had experienced between zero and five psychological risk factors as children. (Psychological risk factors included physical abuse, sexual abuse, alcohol or drug abuse in a primary caregiver, abandonment, and emotional

neglect or abuse.) The study assessed the outcome from the spine surgery by looking at the following:

✔ Whether repeat surgery was necessary

✔ MRI of the spine six months after surgery

✔ Continued use of pain medicines more than six months after surgery

✔ Inability or failure to return to work

As the number of risk factors increased, the probability of a successful outcome from surgery decreased. The probability of a successful outcome for a person with zero risk factors was 95 percent. Alternatively, if a patient had four risk factors, the probability of a successful outcome was 7 percent. A person with five risk factors had 0 percent probability of a successful outcome.

✔ **Drug use:** If you take high levels of pain medication or other drugs, you risk a poor surgical outcome (especially if you use your pain and disability as an excuse to abuse pain medication, drugs, or alcohol). You also may have other non-physical risk factors such as depression or anxiety. Seek treatment for your drug abuse first, and then reassess the surgery option.

Finding a Spine Surgeon

Being actively involved in your own surgical treatment is essential. After determining that you're an appropriate surgical candidate, you need to find a good spine surgeon — a process that can be frustrating, scary, and expensive. Use the following guidelines to help you find a good spine surgeon and ensure that you get the highest quality of care.

Gathering information

You can gather information on spine surgeons from a number of sources:

✔ **Your family doctor or healthcare provider:** He can usually provide you with two or three referrals and give you an idea about how the different surgeons approach patients.

✔ **Family members or friends:** They may have personal experience with physicians or surgeons who treat back pain.

✔ **Physician referral service:** Many local hospitals and universities offer these services, but they only give names of physicians who are associated with their hospital or medical center.

Evaluating your referrals

After you have a number of referrals, how do you decide which surgeon to use? Theodore Goldstein, MD, Clinical Chief of Orthopedic Surgery at Cedars Sinai Medical Center in Los Angeles, has developed excellent guidelines to help you find the best surgeon and recognize red flags when working with your spine surgeon. The following sections discuss what to take into account when selecting a surgeon.

Consider your surgeon's approach

Ideally, your spine surgeon is the kind of person who

✔ Makes you feel comfortable and establishes a good rapport

✔ Is not threatened by your questions

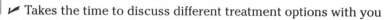

✔ Is willing to educate you with meaningful and appropriate answers to your questions

✔ Takes the time to discuss different treatment options with you

Beware of the surgeon who sees you only as a walking spine. You should feel that your surgeon is working with the whole you — not just looking on you as Mr. Bone Spur or Ms. Herniated Disc.

Consider your surgeon's specialty

Consider the training of the surgeon you select. Many neurosurgeons and orthopedic surgeons have a general practice in which they perform a wide variety of surgical procedures on many different parts of the body and may do spine surgery only occasionally. Therefore, the orthopedic surgeon who did a great job on your friend's broken arm may not be the best person to do your spine surgery. Your best bet is to find a surgeon who

✔ Has a practice limited to spinal surgery

✔ Has a great deal of experience in spinal surgery

✔ Has had fellowship training in spinal surgery

Depending on where you live, you may not have the luxury of these choices. Still, exploring a surgeon's training and experience does help you decide among those available to you.

If your spine problem is particularly complex, consider traveling to an academic medical center or to a center with physicians who specialize in spine treatment.

Recognizing Red Flags in Working with Your Spine Surgeon

After you find a spine surgeon you can work with, certain red flags may alert you to re-examine your decision. If you notice any of the following warning signs, either address — and satisfactorily resolve — the issue with your surgeon or seriously re-evaluate your choice.

Your surgeon allows no questions

A good surgeon shows compassion, tries to educate you about other methods of treatment, and discusses reasons for choosing a particular kind of surgery. You can't expect your surgeon to answer pages and pages of questions, but he should allow time for questions and should treat those questions respectfully. We recommend that you use the following approach:

- ✔ On your first visit, get answers to some of your general questions and get an idea of what the surgeon may recommend.

  Note how the surgeon makes you feel during this meeting. Does he seem like the right kind of person for you? How do you feel when you are with the surgeon?

- ✔ Schedule a second visit, where you should expect to get answers to more of your questions (especially those that arise in response to what the surgeon told you on the first visit).

Questions to ask during your first visit

You can ask the following questions on either the first or second visit:

- ✔ What is my diagnosis and what does it mean for me?
- ✔ What is the natural pattern of my problem if left untreated?
- ✔ What are my treatment options?
- ✔ What are the risks and benefits of these options?
- ✔ Why are you recommending this specific course of treatment?

Questions to ask after you decide to have surgery

After you decide to have surgery, ask the following questions — and make sure that you receive satisfactory answers:

- ✔ What does the surgery entail?
- ✔ What are the possible complications and how do you treat them?
- ✔ How will I feel after the surgery?
- ✔ How long will I be in the hospital?
- ✔ What will my recovery and rehabilitation be like?
- ✔ What preparations should I make to ensure that the surgery is as successful as possible?

Your surgeon does not allow a second opinion or is threatened by it

In virtually all cases, you should get a second opinion regarding a proposed spine surgery.

If your doctor seems to find your request for a second opinion threatening, either ask why or get a new doctor. Although your spine surgeon may not specifically recommend that you seek a second opinion, he should certainly agree that you get one if the idea makes you feel more comfortable and should welcome the opportunity to benefit from a colleague's experience.

Your surgeon says "I can cure you"

Any surgeon who presents surgery as a "cure" is not being realistic and not giving you full, informed consent. If the surgery doesn't completely alleviate all your symptoms, the surgeon may then tell you that no other options are available. Or, the surgeon may offer you yet another surgery to try to "cure" the problem again.

Your surgeon suggests exploratory spine surgery

With today's technology (see Chapter 6), we strongly feel that exploratory spine surgery is *never* appropriate. If your doctor says, "I'm going to open you up and find out what's going on and then take care of the problem," seriously consider finding a new doctor. You should not be in an operating room unless the surgeon — and hopefully you — knows almost exactly where the problem is and how to correct it.

Your surgeon uses scare tactics

Beware if you feel your surgeon is using scare tactics to influence the surgical decision-making process. We've heard patients say, "I was told that without immediate spine surgery, I may be paralyzed." Another scare tactic is a statement like, "Without immediate surgery, your back pain will never go away."

Needless to say, these statements are false — and scare tactics are inappropriate even when the need for surgery is pressing. Scare tactics are frequently very subtle. If you sense that your surgeon is trying to scare you into surgery, get a second or even third opinion.

Your surgeon doesn't consider conservative treatment

Don't consider spine surgery without first thoroughly investigating non-surgical treatment options. Both research and clinical evidence support conservative management of most spine problems (see Chapter 7). Your surgeon must be familiar with conservative approaches in order to give you the best care possible. This doctor should ask you about previous attempts at conservative care to make sure that they were carried out in an appropriate fashion. These conservative treatments typically include physical therapy, exercise, medications, and spinal epidural block, to name a few.

Different Types of Spine Surgery

In the following sections, we review the most common types of spinal surgery, starting with the least invasive and moving on to more invasive surgeries.

Chymopapain injection or chemonucleosis

In cases of disc herniation and related sciatica (leg pain), you may undergo *chemonucleosis*. In this outpatient procedure, the surgeon injects an enzyme (chymopapain) into the affected disc that chemically dissolves some of it. You're under local anesthesia during this surgery because both you and your surgeon need to be aware if the needle touches a nerve so that the needle can be redirected. You must make absolutely sure that you are not allergic to chymopapain prior to the procedure.

The risks of chymopapain injections are

✔ A disc space infection

✔ An allergic reaction to the enzyme chymopapain

✔ Paralysis due to a reaction to the enzyme

Unfortunately, doctors can't predict the risk of paralysis with certainty, so the procedure is rarely done in United States.

The FDA approved chymopapain injections for use in the United States in 1982; the procedure was popular until the mid-1980s. Because of unpredictable neurologic complications and allergic reactions to the enzyme, it fell out of favor. The procedure is still common in Canada and many European countries. The success rate for relief of sciatica is 65 to 80 percent in properly selected patients.

Percutaneous discectomy

In *percutaneous discectomy,* a portion of the disc is surgically removed by using a laser or suction device. During this outpatient procedure, you are awake in order to avoid nerve injury during placement of the probe into your disc. The surgeon uses *fluoroscopy* (a special type of X ray) as a guide to properly place the probe and in some instances it can also be monitored arthroscopically. If you undergo this procedure, you can usually return to sedentary types of work and limited activities 48 to 72 hours following the procedure.

This surgery may be appropriate if you have sciatica (leg pain) due to disc herniation, or if you have intermittent, severe attacks of low-back pain associated with *sciatica scoliosis,* a condition in which a disc herniation causes a severe spasm in the muscles on one side of your spine resulting in *scoliosis,* or a curvature of the spine.

Percutaneous discectomy is a low-risk procedure, but can lead to disc space infection, or blood vessel or nerve injury. Some patients experience a recurrence of symptoms within three to six months of the procedure. Some doctors and hospitals heavily advertise this treatment; however, we feel its usefulness in treating sciatica is limited. Conservative treatment will often serve you better than a percutaneous discectomy.

Microsurgical discectomy

In *microsurgical discectomy,* your surgeon, through an incision less than one inch long and using a microscope, partially removes some of the disc in question, as well as a small amount of the bone covering the spinal canal (see Chapter 2 for more information on spinal anatomy). You will be admitted to the hospital the morning of the surgery for a one day stay. The procedure is done under general anesthesia and generally involves only a very small incision. The process can take anywhere from 45 minutes to several hours depending on what has to be done.

Generally, you should try conservative treatment before agreeing to microsurgical discectomy. However, you may consider the procedure if you

✔ Have a herniated disc with sciatic (leg) pain.

✔ Have progressive neurologic loss (such as weakness) causing you significant problems in daily functioning.

✔ Are older and have *spinal stenosis* (a narrowing of the spinal canal) associated with a disc herniation, which is causing the sciatica pain.

✔ Have a recurrent disc herniation.

Most likely, you'll be walking by the morning after surgery. You shouldn't be in a great deal of pain after this surgery and any pain you do have can usually be controlled with appropriate pain medicines.

The local discomfort from the surgery usually goes away within several days. However, the sciatica can take some time to disappear, depending on factors including how long the nerve was irritated prior to surgery and the rate of nerve recovery, a process that can take up to two to three months or longer.

The risks of microsurgical discectomy include infection, injury to the nerve root, problems with the anesthesia, a blood clot, and recurrent disc hernia- tion. In order to prevent infection, you receive an intravenous antibiotic at the time of surgery infrequently. The nerve root is manipulated during surgery, which can cause numbness and/or weakness in the nerve distribution. In spite of how frightening this side effect sounds, it goes away in most cases.

During surgery, your surgeon removes only the portion of your disc that is irritating or compressing the nerve root. Because the entire disc isn't removed, you have a 5 to 6 percent chance of recurrent herniation. If reherniation occurs, you usually experience a sudden recurrence of your sci- atic pain after being pain free. If you're one of the unfortunate few, we must warn you that the pain is often much more intense than the original sciatica. If the reinstitution of conservative therapy fails, repeat surgery is almost always successful.

Laminectomy

During a *laminectomy*, the surgeon removes a herniated disc by first remov- ing the *lamina* (the back part of the vertebra) and associated ligament. Removing the herniated disc alleviates the pressure and/or irritation of the affected nerve roots.

Surgeons may use a laminectomy to take pressure off the spinal canal in cases of *spinal stenosis*, (a narrow spinal canal). If you have recurrent and residual problems from a previous surgery, your doctor may recommend laminectomy to remove some additional bone, which makes more room for the nerves.

You can normally expect a two to five day hospital stay. (*Note:* If you are elderly, you may need additional rehabilitation and recovery time, so you may want to plan to stay in an extended care facility for several weeks.) Complete recovery can take four to six months or sometimes even longer, but you can start physical therapy approximately two to three weeks after the operation.

The risks associated with a laminectomy are similar to that for a microsurgi- cal discectomy, but greater due to the longer operating time and the greater extent of the procedure.

Spinal fusion

A *fusion* is an operation in which the surgeon attempts to stop the motion that normally takes place between two adjacent vertebrae. Sometimes, a spinal fusion may involve the use of *instrumentation* or *fixation devices* like metal rods, screws, or newer devices that look like small cylinders called *cages* and are placed between the vertebrae. Because the spinal fusion technology is changing rapidly, we can only give an overview of what it encompasses:

- **Posterior fusion:** The majority of fusions are done from the *posterior approach,* or from the back. In these procedures, the surgeon removes part of the bone of the two vertebrae. The surgeon then places fresh bone (taken from your iliac crest or hip) in your back with the hope that these elements will eventually grow together. As the vertebrae grow together, they form one solid unit with almost no motion between them. Screws and rods can enhance fusion rates and allow you to be more active, sooner.

- **Anterior fusion:** The surgeon makes an incision near your belly button to access the front of the spine. Anterior fusion may make use of fixation devices called cages. If you undergo this very complex procedure, we feel that a spine surgeon and either a general surgeon or a vascular surgeon should do the surgery together whenever possible. A team of different surgical specialists increases the surgery's safety.

- **Combination:** In rare instances, surgeons do both a posterior *and* an anterior fusion. You may require both if prior surgeries failed, if you smoke (see the sidebar, "Smokers and fusions"), or if you have had prior complications such as infection. In these cases, you have two separate surgical procedures, either under a single anesthetic or several days apart.

Spinal fusions are much less common than disc excisions. Surgeons primarily recommend fusion to alleviate *mechanical* low-back pain (pain that is made worse by activities such as bending, twisting, and lifting is usually alleviated by rest) when X rays show some type of instability between two vertebrae.

Even though spine fusion involves significantly greater risks than the other surgeries that we discuss in this chapter, the relative risks are still low. They include:

- The fixation device can fail or break
- Pain in the hip area from where the bone graft is obtained
- The vertebrae fail to grow together

You need to weigh the risks and benefits as you consider spine fusion surgery, given the greater length of time off work, the significant costs, and the longer rehabilitation time associated with this major surgery. In our experience, you should rarely have a fusion for sciatica simply due to a disc herniation.

Always get at least one second opinion from a qualified spine surgeon if a doctor recommends an elective spinal fusion for you (an exception would be trauma requiring emergency surgery to stabilize your spine). We strongly recommend that only a surgeon who specializes in spine surgery do this procedure. (Also, pay particular attention to the preparing for surgery issues in the next section.)

Preparing for Surgery

You can divide preparing for spine surgery into medical, psychological, and psychosocial aspects. Most surgeons focus on the medical aspects of the surgery to the exclusion of the other two areas. However, by considering all these areas, you help increase the probability of a successful outcome.

Medical preparations for surgery include:

- ✔ **Consulting with your internist or other physician before surgery:** Your family doctor can help ensure that you can safely undergo the procedure.

- ✔ **Reviewing the medications you're taking:** Stop taking aspirin, compounds that contain aspirin, non-steriodal anti-inflammatories, and blood thinning medications for at least three to ten days (depending on the medicine) prior to your surgery. These medicines can increase bleeding, leading to complications during or following the surgical procedure. Your physician should direct and monitor this process.

Smokers and fusions

If you smoke, you face an important risk for fusion. Studies show that smokers have significantly less chance of a successful fusion (as low as 60 percent compared with 85 percent in the nonsmoking population). In these cases, the fusion fails, and the bones of your back do not grow together as they should.

We recommend that you stop smoking for a minimum of four to six weeks before surgery. You should make every effort not to smoke until you have a solid fusion post-operatively as well. And if you make it that long, you may as well never start smoking again, right?

Psychological screening and preparation for surgery can be important, especially if you have prior unsuccessful surgeries or are having an extensive operation. In these cases, we recommend that you undergo a preoperative psychological evaluation with a psychologist skilled in the evaluation and management of chronic pain problems. Your doctor may recommend that you undergo a brief, psychological preparation program. Such a program gives you the opportunity to discuss any anxiety or fears, your expectations about the experience, and the predicted course of treatment. Make sure that you have accurate information about what to expect before and after your hospital stay. You may also want to look into relaxation training or more effective pain and anxiety control (see the sidebar on preparing for surgery).

Psychosocial preparation for surgery includes making arrangements and explanations at work and at home: You need to arrange for time off of work, prepare your household for the postoperative recovery phase, and educate your family members as to what to expect.

You can, and should, engage in normal activities until the time of surgery and use the time to address any predictable problems before your surgery.

Preoperative plans can include:

- ✔ Resolving insurance and financial issues
- ✔ Planning for your absence, and your return, to work
- ✔ Anticipating your return to a more active lifestyle including exercise
- ✔ Helping your family prepare for your postoperative rehabilitation

If you are older, you may need to arrange for a transition to an extended care facility after the surgery before you return to your home environment.

The Future of Spine Surgery

The last decade has seen dramatic changes in the field of spine surgery, and these are likely to continue. For instance, if you had lower back surgery for a disc herniation several years ago, your surgery involved an incision three to five inches long and a hospital stay of four days to one week. You could then expect a two to three month period before returning to your normal activity.

With the advent of microsurgical techniques, an entire surgery is now done through a 1 to 1½-inch incision and requires only a one night hospital stay (or perhaps less). You can then return to normal light duty activities within two to three weeks.

Mind-body preparation for surgery improves outcome

Surgery, whether inpatient or outpatient, can be one of the most stressful events in your life. Recent advances in mind-body approaches yield many benefits including:

- Less post-operative pain

- Reduced need for pain medicines

- Fewer complications

- Decreased distress before and after surgery

- Return to health more quickly

- Improved satisfaction with the surgery overall

Drs. William Deardorff (one of the authors of this fine book) and John Reeves II designed a clinically tested program that improves response to spine surgery and other stressful medical procedures. We produced a ground-breaking workbook which incorporates the findings of more than 200 research studies and provides a number of mind-body exercises.

The workbook program is based on a review of over 200 research studies done with thousands of patients over the past 30 years. These studies were primarily done in university settings with materials developed specifically for each research project. The interactive workbook we developed distills the important components of this clinical research into a supportive, step-by-step guide that allows you to successfully:

- Create an individualized surgery preparation program

- Learn cognitive restructuring techniques

- Develop coping strategies

- Draw upon spiritual resources

- Communicate effectively

- Maintain control of your situation

- Use relaxation and imagery skills

- Prepare family and friends

- Deal with the hospital environment

You can order the workbook by calling New Harbinger Publications at 800-748-6273 (in the U.S.) or 510-652-0215. You can also obtain more information at www.surgeryprep.com (which includes surgery links to help you find valuable information about your spine surgery).

The developments for lower back surgery have a bright future. Dr. Patrick Johnson, a neurosurgeon at UCLA Medical Center and co-director of the UCLA Comprehensive Spine Center, predicts there will be further miniaturization of incisions as well as the use of more advanced instruments, which will help spine surgeons to work even more accurately within the small confined space of your spine.

Another exciting development may be the ability to perform these surgical procedures within a MRI scanner. This would give your spine surgeon a continuous update on how the surgery is going by high-definition body scanning. MRI technology may also allow your surgeon to revise the procedure during the operation as necessary.

Part III

Complementary Approaches: Are They for You?

The 5th Wave — By Rich Tennant

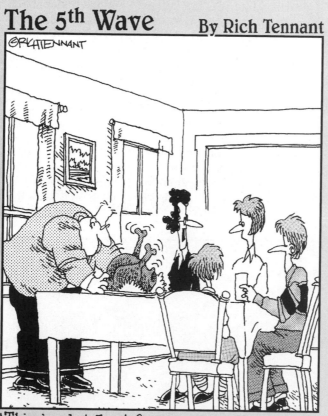

"This is what I get for marrying a chiropractor. Every Thanksgiving he's got to align the turkey's spine before he'll carve it."

In this part . . .

You may find yourself drawn to non-traditional back pain treatments. We believe that these complementary approaches can work very well under the right circumstances — especially when you combine them with the traditional options that we discuss in Part II of this book.

Complementary approaches sometimes get a bad rap. Although they're not a panacea, they may help you, and you are the important one here. This part takes a look at some of the common complementary methods, including chiropractics and yoga, among others. Finding a qualified professional to administer and/or teach you these methods can be difficult, so we also spend a good deal of time telling you how to separate the wheat from the chaff.

Chapter 9

Ancient Eastern Wisdom and Contemporary Ideas

*I*ndividuals suffering from any of a variety of health problems (including back pain) are looking more and more toward alternative medicine approaches for relief. These patients are either abandoning treatment prescribed by their regular doctors or supplementing traditional medical treatment with alternative measures. We can safely say that people are flocking to alternative approaches in record numbers.

In response to this public interest, many health centers and insurance companies across the country are now including alternative approaches in their programs. For example, many medical centers now have departments of complementary medicine, and more health insurance plans are including some type of coverage for alternative care approaches. In addition, the National Institutes of Health has formed a special Office of Alternative Medicine and various other agencies to evaluate these treatment approaches.

Throughout this book, we use the terms *alternative medicine, complementary medicine,* and *holistic medicine* interchangeably. In working with back pain, we prefer the term *complementary medicine* because this term connotes the idea of traditional medical approaches to back pain working in concert with complementary medical interventions. We don't like to think of alternative medicine approaches as being alternative to standard medical treatment. In our opinion (and in the way we practice), the most powerful approach is to combine the two orientations in an appropriate manner. In this chapter, and those following in this part, we present information that can help you pursue complementary medicine treatments in a safe manner while avoiding any treatments that may injure you.

We first discuss the general issue of selecting a complementary medicine practitioner. This practitioner may be in any of the complementary medicine fields (such as chiropractic, acupuncture, herbal therapy, and magnetic therapy, to name just a few). Then we focus on complementary medicine approaches commonly used for back pain. We also discuss issues relevant to any complementary medicine approach you may choose to pursue.

Selecting an Alternative Medicine Practitioner

When you seek out an expert in complementary medicine, you can use many of the same criteria you use to select a traditional doctor. The following sections offer basic guidelines for choosing a practitioner.

- ✔ **Choose a generalist with a diverse background:** If you're selecting a general practitioner of complementary medicine, choose someone who has a diverse background and expertise in a wide variety of areas. We often recommend finding someone who can use both complementary medicine approaches and traditional medicine treatments. This person is more likely to be able to balance her approach in a rational manner.

  If you're looking for a practitioner to treat a specific ailment, such as back pain, this advice to seek a generalist may not apply. If you're seeking treatment with an alternative medicine practitioner who specializes in one approach, be sure the treatment is coordinated with your conventional physician.

- ✔ **Find a practitioner with whom you can establish a good rapport:** As with any doctor, you want to find a complementary medicine practitioner with whom you feel comfortable. A good relationship with your health practitioner includes such elements as open communication and an overall sense of trust in that person's abilities.

- ✔ **Rely on a referral source that you trust:** One of the best (and most common) ways to find a good practitioner is through a referral, either from your doctor or from someone who has been treated by the individual. Because most mainstream physicians are not involved in complementary medicine approaches, the referral probably will be from another source. Talking to someone who has been treated by the practitioner can give you a good idea about that person's bedside manner, conduct, and practices.

✔ **Select a practitioner who is sensitive to your needs:** Find a practitioner who has experience treating back pain and attending to any requirements specific to your case, such as associated symptoms.

✔ **Beware of a practitioner who isn't willing to work with your doctor:** Successful treatment of conditions such as chronic back pain is often a collaborative effort by a variety of different healthcare professionals. If any practitioner is unwilling to work with other disciplines you have found helpful, this refusal can be a warning sign of a problem.

This advice includes not only complementary medicine practitioners, but also your physician. Your doctor should be willing to discuss complementary medicine approaches with you in a nonjudgmental and open fashion. Your doctor may not agree with certain complementary medicine approaches; in these cases, she should help you make an informed decision about pursuing this type of treatment.

✔ **Don't depend on credentials alone:** A medical degree (or other degrees for that matter) is not an automatic guarantee that a complementary medicine practitioner's recommendation is safe. Investigate recommended treatments yourself, in addition to developing a trusting relationship with the practitioner.

Choosing the Best Complementary Medicine Approach for You

In complementary medicine, the mental and emotional aspects of healing must be dealt with in conjunction with the physical. Even when the complementary medicine approach you choose seems to focus primarily on the physical, you still need to be mentally and emotionally comfortable and confident in the treatment. This section helps you evaluate complementary treatment methods.

Asking the right questions

After you decide to try some type of complementary treatment approach (based on the preceding guidelines), you can identify a practitioner or two with whom you may be interested in working. Asking the practitioner (or the practitioner's office staff) the following questions can help you get the information you need in order to wisely decide among complementary treatments for back pain:

✔ How long has this treatment been available?

✔ How commonly is this treatment used for back pain, and in what percentage of back-pain cases has this treatment been documented to be successful?

✔ What risks or potential side effects are associated with this treatment?

✔ Are any other treatments better or more effective, and would they achieve the same result?

✔ At what point in the treatment will you and your practitioner know whether the treatment is working?

✔ What is a reasonable *treatment trial* (for example, how many sessions)?

Avoiding quackery

When you choose a complementary medicine method, avoiding quackery is important. Given the popularity of alternative medicine approaches today and the overall lack of regulation, the area is ripe for patient rip-offs.

For you to have a positive experience with complementary medicine, you must be sure to avoid being treated by a *quack* (someone who performs a treatment or service without having the necessary knowledge, skills, or qualifications).

The following guidelines can help you identify quackery:

✔ **Beware of quick fixes:** Quacks often claim that their treatments or remedies can produce immediate cures. If you have chronic back pain, you may be more susceptible to claims for a quick fix due to your frustration over the ongoing pain and your longing for relief.

✔ **Beware of anecdotal evidence:** Testimonials and case histories are often used to support claims for a particular treatment that allegedly cures a condition such as back pain. These testimonials often target conditions that traditional medicine has found difficult to treat. Chronic back pain falls into this category. Even if the testimonials are given sincerely by patients, any such dramatic improvement could be explained by a number of factors other than the complementary medicine approach. These factors include the natural improvement or fluctuation of the back pain over time or the *placebo effect* (getting better because you expect to improve).

✔ **Beware of secret formulas:** The active ingredients of any medicine or other medicinal substance should be disclosed on the label. Pharmaceutical companies patent medications, and those companies must publish reports listing the ingredients of their drugs and explaining how they work. You should expect the same labeling approach from any product that claims to have a medicinal benefit. Avoid any product that doesn't list its contents.

✔ **Beware of treatment approaches supposedly condemned by the medical establishment:** A common but unscrupulous practice of marketing certain alternative approaches is to claim that the treatment has been censored or condemned by mainstream medicine or some governmental agency (such as the Federal Drug Administration). The advertisements often claim that the products possess curative powers that the medical establishment doesn't want you to find out about (usually because this disclosure would somehow rob doctors of their income). No mechanism exists within the medical profession for this type of censorship or condemnation. The only condemnation or warning that may occur is if a product is found to be a health hazard to the public. (See the section, "How can you use herbs safely?" later in this chapter for more information.)

Considering Specific Alternative Treatment Methods

Alternative medicine offers many treatment options for back-pain sufferers. The following sections introduce some of those treatments and provide information about their effectiveness.

Acupuncture: Needling your way to a better back

Acupuncture is one of the more common complementary medicine approaches in the treatment of back pain. The following sections offer the basics on the theory and practice of acupuncture.

Acupuncture has been practiced in China for more than 5,000 years. It is a complete system of healing that is based on the ancient Chinese theory of *qi* (also referred to as *chi* and pronounced "chee").

The traditional Chinese theory on acupuncture

Qi is thought to be the vital life energy that is present in all living organisms. According to traditional Chinese acupuncture theory, qi circulates in the body along 12 to 14 major energy pathways called *meridians*. These meridians are on each side of the body and crisscross along the arms, legs, torso, and head, as well as deep within tissues. Each meridian is believed to be linked to a specific internal organ and organ system.

CLINICAL INFO

A contemporary Western take on acupuncture

Not surprisingly, the ancient Chinese explanation of the reason acupuncture works differs markedly from the theory proposed by Western medical researchers.

Western researchers typically dispute the existence of qi and provide different explanations for the effects of acupuncture. They believe that stimulating an acupuncture point causes the release of endorphins in the brain as well as other biochemicals in the body. *Endorphins* are substances that naturally occur in the brain and cause a decreased perception of pain. This theory about the way acupuncture works is supported by research showing that when animals or humans are given a chemical that blocks the action of endorphins (Naloxone), the effect of the acupuncture is stopped.

In addition to rejecting the concept of qi, many Western scientists don't accept the existence of a separate independent system of meridians. Instead, they point to studies demonstrating that acupuncture points, when viewed under a microscope, show a greater concentration of nerve endings than other skin locations. According to this view, acupoints are part of the nervous system instead of being an independent system.

Many Western physicians are critical of acupuncture and believe that its effects are simply a placebo response (meaning that acupuncture doesn't actually provide any active treatment). These physicians feel that accounts of acupuncture responses can be attributed simply to the patient's belief that it will work.

The meridians surface at different locations on the body, and these are called *acupuncture points* or *acupoints*. Traditional acupuncture theorists and researchers believe that hundreds to thousands of these acupoints exist within the meridian system, and they can be stimulated to enhance the flow of qi. This stimulation, in turn, causes healing. Special needles that are placed just under the skin at specific acupoints provide the necessary stimulation to correct and rebalance the flow of energy. Opposing forces within the body, called *yin* and *yang,* must be in balance before the qi can get your vital functions (spiritual, mental, physical, and emotional) to work normally. This stimulation of the acupuncture points provides pain relief and acupuncture's healing properties.

What is a typical acupuncture treatment program like?

Acupuncture treatments differ from conventional Western treatment programs. The following sections outline the acupuncture treatment process.

The initial evaluation

As with a traditional medical office, if you're a first-time acupuncture patient, you most likely will complete a questionnaire regarding your medical history and the condition for which you're seeking treatment. The acupuncturist then interviews you and investigates symptoms not typically addressed by Western medicine.

For example, the practitioner may take a very close look at your tongue, which is considered to be a primary source of diagnostic information. Other areas that the practitioner may assess include the tone of your voice, your body language, the color of your urine, your menstrual cycle, any sensitivity to temperatures and seasons, digestive problems, your pulse, your eating and sleeping habits, as well as your emotional status.

A treatment session

After the initial evaluation is complete, the acupuncturist places special acupuncture needles in the appropriate acupoints, as she determines. Acupuncture needles are extremely thin ($\frac{1}{17,000}$ to $\frac{1}{18,000}$ of an inch in diameter) and vary in length from a fraction of an inch to several inches. These needles are made of stainless steel over copper but can also be composed of gold, silver, bamboo, and wood.

Although using disposable needles is a common modern practice, checking to make sure that the acupuncture needles are sterile and disposable is still extremely important.

Depending on your condition, an acupuncture treatment involves using up to 10 or 12 needles placed at specific locations. As the needles are placed, the practitioner may gently twirl or twist them by hand for approximately 15 to 20 minutes.

The placement of the needles is generally painless. Patients tell us that they experience a slight pricking sensation when the needles are inserted. The competence and experience of the acupuncturist certainly relates to the amount of physical sensation that you may notice.

Be sure to tell the acupuncturist if you feel any discomfort as a result of needle placement. Sometimes, the acupuncturist needs to slightly change the needle position or pressure, which can eliminate the discomfort you're experiencing.

You may notice that the needle placement doesn't necessarily correlate with the location of your pain or symptoms. This discrepancy is based on the theory of meridians. (See the earlier section "The traditional Chinese theory on acupuncture.") The practitioner may place needles in your ears, head, face, legs, arms, or torso, all of which may be nowhere near the place where you're experiencing symptoms.

The needles are generally left in 15 to 30 minutes, but in certain instances they are left in for longer periods of time. Many of our patients report a temporary feeling of "heaviness" or a slight ache at the location of needle treatment, but this reaction is by no means universal.

The number and frequency of sessions depends greatly on the condition being treated, as well as the competency and orientation of the practitioner. We have had back pain patients respond to as few as two sessions of

Other approaches to stimulation of acupoints

Acupuncturists use other means of stimulating acupoints in addition to using the acupuncture needles. One common technique is to apply heat by burning an herb called *moxa* (mugwort) above the acupoint to be treated. Chinese studies suggest that this herb is unique in its ability to stimulate the acupoints and facilitate your body's self-healing abilities. The acupuncturist burns a very small amount of moxa on a slice of ginger that is placed on top of an acupoint. In some cases, the moxa is placed and burned directly on the acupoint and then removed when the patient reports it is too warm to tolerate further.

Another traditional treatment for areas of large muscle pain is *cupping,* which utilizes a glass or a bamboo cup. The cup creates a suction on the skin over the painful area. Acupuncturists may also use other techniques in place of the needles. This may include such things as ultrasound waves, electrical stimulation, lasers, or heat.

acupuncture. Other patients start off at a higher frequency of twice per week and gradually taper their frequency of visits to a maintenance regimen of two to four times per month. This schedule is a highly individual response, and you should work closely with your acupuncturist regarding these treatment issues.

How effective is acupuncture on back pain?

We believe that acupuncture is most effective when provided as part of a comprehensive medical treatment approach. Your acupuncture plan may be complementary to a traditional medical intervention and/or in conjunction with other alternative medicine approaches, such as herbal therapies, appropriate exercise, and healthy lifestyle changes.

The effectiveness of acupuncture continues to be controversial in scientific communities as does its mechanism of action. Scientists have difficulty teasing out the mechanical effectiveness of acupuncture from the patient's belief that it will work. Not surprisingly, this is a problem with many other medical approaches as well. In our clinical practice, we don't see this issue as particularly important, because the reason doesn't really matter as long as you have a positive response to the treatment with little risk.

Pain control is one of the more common areas that acupuncture is used for. Physicians who specialize in pain management (such as neurologists, physiatrists, anesthesiologists, and internists) often use acupuncture as a treatment in addition to other approaches such as exercise and medications. In our experience, patients who receive acupuncture treatment for painful conditions have a highly individual response. Some patients respond in a few sessions with long-lasting benefits, some have a good initial response but require periodic maintenance treatments, and some experience no benefit at all. Acupuncture is best offered as part of a package of treatments, but if you don't notice any benefit after the first 6 to 12 sessions, it is unlikely that you will benefit from further treatment.

For more information about acupuncture, check out the resources listed in Appendix B.

Herbal medicine

Herbs have always been a key part of the practice of medicine. Before modern medicines, doctors treated their patients with plants and herbs. In fact, herbal medicine is the most ancient form of health care known to humankind. Unfortunately, your physician is not likely to recommend an herbal medicine approach. Therefore, if you choose to pursue herbal medicine approaches to your back pain, an herbal medicine practitioner will likely perform the treatment.

What is an herb?

An *herb,* as the term is used in herbal medicine, is a plant or part of a plant that is used to make medicine, spices, or aromatic oils for soaps and fragrances. An herb can be a leaf, flower, stem, seed, root, fruit, bark, or any other plant part that is used for its medicinal, food-flavoring, or fragrant properties.

An estimated 250,000 to 500,000 plants exist on the earth today, and only about 5,000 of these have been investigated extensively for their use in medicine. Currently, about 25 percent of all prescription medications are still derived from trees, shrubs, or herbs. Some of these medicines are derived directly from the plant, and others are synthesized to mimic the plant substance. In fact, 120 commonly prescribed medicines are extracted from 90 species of plants. Almost half of the world's drug companies are working with locals on every continent to analyze the medicinal properties of plants that previously had been ignored by the medical establishment. Eighty percent of the world's population continues to depend on herbal medicine for treatment.

Herbal medicines work in much the same way as conventional pharmaceutical drugs (by their chemical action in the body). Herbs come in many forms, including:

- **Whole:** Whole herbs are plants or parts of plants that are dried and then cut or powdered. They are then used to make teas, or used in some other form.

- **Teas:** When steeped in hot or boiling water, an herb's medicinal properties are released into a tea which a person then consumes.

✔ **Capsules and tablets:** Herbs are often prepared in the form of capsules and tablets. Tablets and capsules are made by removing the liquid from an herbal extract, powdering the remaining herb, and shaping it into pill form. The sale of capsules and tablets is one of the fastest growing markets in herbal medicine over the past 15 years. Capsules and tablets have become popular with consumers because they are convenient and, in many cases, mask the unpleasant taste of the herb.

✔ **Extracts and tinctures:** If an herb is soaked in alcohol or glycerin and the resulting solution is strained off it forms a *tincture*. If you filter or distill out some of the alcohol from a tincture, you have an *extract* (which is usually more potent than a tincture of the same herb). The alcohol helps to extract various non-water-soluble compounds from an herb and to function as a preservative to maintain shelf life. Extracts and tinctures have the advantage of a high concentration in a low weight and space. They are also absorbed in the body faster than tablets or capsules.

✔ **Essential oils:** Essential oils are usually distilled from various parts of medicinal and aromatic plants. Essential oils are very concentrated (usually the dosage is as low as one or two drops). Because these oils are so concentrated, they must be used carefully and sparingly when ingested. Also, you may need to dilute them before applying them topically (rubbed on the skin) in order to avoid irritation.

✔ **Salves, balms, and ointments:** Humans have used plants to treat conditions such as skin irritation, wounds, and bites for thousands of years. Today, a number of ointments are available that contain herbal extracts.

What is herbal medicine?

The practice of herbal medicine is extremely varied. It can be as simple as going to your family doctor for an herbal prescription or as comprehensive as going to a Chinese medicine practitioner who ascribes to a completely different philosophy than Western counterparts. Because of this diversity and the vast number of herbal substances available on the market, discussing an exact herbal treatment for back pain is beyond the scope of this chapter. The herbal medicine practitioner generally uses a variety of approaches to treat a specific ailment (for example, back pain) and for overall health.

For example, a Chinese medicine practitioner may use herbs, acupuncture, and exercises to treat back pain. An *Ayurvedic* medicine practitioner may focus on the mind, body, and spirit equally, and use treatments such as herbs, diet, exercise, meditation, massage, and breathing techniques. However, the use of herbs in Western medicine generally follows a pharmaceutical model in which the herb is simply used as a medicine to induce a physical change in the body. Given this complexity, in this section, we limit our discussion to the right questions you should ask to get good herbal medicine treatment.

How can you use herbs safely?

Don't equate *natural* with *safe*. Herbal medicinal products have been generally unregulated and unmonitored by the Food and Drug Administration. People often assume that using herbs isn't harmful. Nothing can be further from the truth. Therefore, you must be cautious in their use — not only due to the effect (and possible side-effects) of the herb itself, but also because several serious incidences of contamination have occurred.

To safely pursue herbal therapy, consider the following guidelines for using herbal compounds:

- ✔ **Interactions:** Notifying your physician prior to taking any herb is extremely important, especially if you are on other medications. Herbs are medicines, and they can interact dangerously with other prescribed medicines.

- ✔ **Potency:** The potency of an herbal preparation can vary from brand to brand. Unless the label says *standardized,* you can't know the potency of the preparation. Look for the words *standard* or *standardized extract* on the label. Those terms indicate that the herbal product meets an international standard of quality.

- ✔ **Dosage:** Herbal preparations also vary greatly in the amount of active ingredient they contain. Some products have too little of the active ingredient to produce any effect, and others contain more than is necessary, making you vulnerable to side effects. When you start taking an herb, begin with a small dose and increase slowly.

- ✔ **Form:** Choose an herbal preparation that can be effectively utilized by your body. The forms available can vary by manufacturer, depending on the way the herb is produced and packaged (for example, capsule, tablet, tea, or oil).

- ✔ **Contaminants:** Some herbs have been found to be contaminated with substances such as arsenic, mercury, and lead. Purchase herbal products from a reputable manufacturer and distributor who uses appropriate quality control measures.

- ✔ **Other ingredients:** Some herbal compounds contain other ingredients that may or may not be listed on the label. These other ingredients may have side effects or interactions with other medications you are taking. In some cases, herbal compounds are fortified with substances that are not safe.

- ✔ **Cultivation:** Try to find out where the herbs come from, especially if you suspect that the point of origin is Asia or South America. Without knowing the location, you can't be sure that safe insecticides or pesticides were used in the production of these herbs.

Don't simply rely on the advice of the clerk at the health food store regarding the safety of these compounds. Following the preceding guidelines will help you get high quality herbs and assure that you know what you are getting. And remember, don't take any herb if you are pregnant or nursing, unless you discuss the herb with your primary care doctor.

For more information about herbal remedies, take a look at the resources listed in Appendix B.

Magnetic therapy

The idea that magnets may have healing properties has been around for quite some time. Until recently, no actual scientific evidence showed their medicinal properties, although anecdotal evidence continued to mount. For example, many athletes (especially professional golfers) swear that magnets help them control pain and heal injuries faster.

Advertisements for magnets are prevalent, including products such as magnetic back belts, biomagnetic bracelets, and magnetic beds. Mainstream medicines criticism of magnets for medicinal reasons may now be changing as mounting scientific evidence indicates that magnets may provide certain treatment benefits. You should be aware that some magnet manufacturers claim their products treat a variety of conditions but, in this section, we focus only on the effects of magnets on pain — particularly back pain.

What is magnetic therapy?

Magnetic therapy as a complementary medicine approach involves exposing the body, or certain body parts, to a magnetic field. Magnetic therapy can be applied in many ways ranging from small, simple magnets placed on the skin to large machines capable of generating high levels of field strength. In this section, we focus on the use of simple magnets that are commonly purchased over the counter.

The use of magnets and electrical devices to generate magnetic fields already has many accepted applications in mainstream medicine. For example, magnetic resonance imaging relies on the creation of a powerful magnetic field in order to obtain tissue pictures that are more accurate than X rays. Also, magnetic therapy has been found to be useful for accelerating the healing of bone fractures. Beyond these applications, most physicians have been skeptical of complementary medicine uses of magnetic therapy for pain control and healing.

Magnetic therapy for back pain involves the placement of magnets at various points on the back. Treatment variations include placing the magnets (either individually or in clusters) over the painful or injured area or at various acupressure sites, depending on one's condition. The strength of the magnets and the length of time they are applied can also vary.

What are the basic principles of magnetic therapy?

All magnets have two poles: One is called positive, and the other is negative. Researchers in the field of magnetic therapy claim that the negative pole generally has a calming effect and helps normalize the body's functioning. In contrast, the positive pole has a stress effect, and prolonged exposure can interfere with various bodily processes in an unhealthy way.

The strength of a magnet is measured in units of *gauss* or *Telsa* (one Telsa equals 10,000 gauss). Every magnetic device has a manufacturer's gauss rating. However, the actual strength of the magnets at the surface of the skin is often much less than this number. For example, a 4,000 gauss magnet transmits only about 1,200 gauss to the patient. Magnets used in pillows or mattresses deliver an even lower amount of field strength at the skin surface because a magnet's strength quickly decreases the further away it is from the patient.

How does magnetic therapy affect the body?

Although a magnetic field's mechanism of action on the body is not entirely clear, the following are leading theories:

- **Blood flow:** Many experts agree that magnets probably help increase the blood flow to a painful area of the body. Increased blood flow helps carry more oxygen to the region, decreases inflammation, and relieves pain.

- **Pain perception:** Researchers suggest that a magnetic field may affect pain receptors in the painful area. The magnets seem to provide pain relief, but the mechanism of action is unknown. The magnetic field may disrupt the pain signal going to the brain, causing the release of the body's natural pain-relieving substance (endorphins), or some other as yet undiscovered action.

How can you safely get magnetic treatment?

Magnetic therapy for back pain is quite popular even though the scientific research is just now being conducted. Treatment generally involves using a back belt or elastic wrap that has magnets imbedded in it and fits around your waist. Other back pain sufferers also sleep on magnetic mattress pads.

Although magnetic devices for pain relief are marketed over-the-counter and don't require any type of medical prescription, some experts recommend that these products should be used under the supervision of a qualified professional. However, no serious side effects have been clearly documented. The following are some other cautions:

✔ Get clearance from your physician before trying any type of treatment, including magnetic therapy. If you wear any type of implanted electronic device such as a pacemaker, be sure to ask your doctor about trying magnetic therapy before starting and don't place a magnet directly over the device.

✔ Don't use magnets on the abdomen during pregnancy.

✔ Don't use a magnetic bed for more than 8 to 10 hours at a time.

How effective is magnetic therapy in treating back pain?

We believe that the potential benefits of magnetic therapy for back pain relief, along with the relative lack of side effects and relatively low cost, make this treatment approach worth a try if you're interested. As with all the complementary medicine approaches, keeping your physician aware that you're pursuing this treatment is important.

Until recently, not one speck of scientific evidence showed that magnets provided any pain relief. That situation has now changed with the recent publication — in *The Archives of Physical Medicine and Rehabilitation* (November, 1997) — of a well-controlled research study. This study investigated the effects of magnets on 50 patients suffering from pain associated with post-polio syndrome. Half the patients were given actual magnets, and the other half received inactive magnets. Both groups believed that they were getting active magnets. The patients were instructed to hold the magnets on the points where they felt the most intense pain and keep them in place for 45 minutes.

After the magnets were removed, 75 percent of the patients who had used the active magnets reported a significant reduction in pain. Only 19 percent of the patients who used the inactive magnets reported pain relief, and they reported only a *small* decrease in pain. No side effects to the magnets were reported. Patients reported pain relief lasting from as short as a few hours to as long as several months. As a result of these types of findings, the Food and Drug Administration (FDA) has approved several independent review boards to track current research in magnetic therapy. The use of magnets to treat pain is not currently approved by the FDA.

For more information on magnetic therapy, check out the resources listed in Appendix B.

Bodywork

The therapeutic use of touch has been used for centuries to heal the body and reduce tension. *Bodywork* refers to therapies such as massage, deep tissue manipulation, movement awareness, and energy balancing. Bodywork is used to reduce pain, soothe injured muscles, stimulate blood and lymphatic circulation, and promote deep relaxation. Patients often seek some type of bodywork for help with their back pain problems. Hundreds of types of bodywork treatments are available. In this section, we review several well-established bodywork systems.

This section deals with *professional* bodywork and massage techniques. It doesn't tell you how to give massages. This section can help you find a style of bodywork or special practitioner focus, that may be effective for your back pain problem.

Some common elements of bodywork treatments include:

- ✔ **Pressure or deep friction** to alter muscles, connective tissues, and other body structures
- ✔ **Patient education and awareness** of posture and movement to improve physical functioning and pain
- ✔ **Stretching, muscle balance, and relaxation** to affect physical functioning and pain
- ✔ **Breathing and emotional expression** to eliminate tension and enhance physical abilities

Bodywork treatment for back pain is highly variable in terms of the actual approach to treatment, the length and frequency of treatment recommended by the practitioner, and the cost per session. As you investigate bodywork treatment, use the same list of questions presented earlier in this chapter for selecting a complementary treatment and practitioner. As with all complementary treatment approaches, we recommend that you clear your bodywork treatment choices with your doctor.

For additional information about various types of bodywork, check out the resources listed in Appendix B.

Pilates

The next time you're at a fine Italian restaurant, be sure to order Pilates, they're delicious (just kidding!). Actually, Pilates is a system of physical conditioning developed by Joseph Pilates almost a century ago. Determined to overcome his childhood illnesses, Pilates studied Eastern and Western forms of exercise in addition to developing special machines to help with his rehabilitation.

The *Pilates Method* (or just *Pilates* as people in the know say) has a strong emphasis on proper body alignment, injury prevention, and correct breathing, as well as muscle stretching and strengthening. Although originally made popular by professional dancers, Pilates is appropriate for people of all ages, abilities, and lifestyles, including those suffering from back pain.

Pilates emphasizes muscle stretching and its goal is to promote muscle elongation, rather than building bulk. (You don't have to worry about turning into the "Hulk.") Pilates attempts to develop your abdomen and lower back into a firm *core* of support for your whole body. The program promotes alignment, balance, and stabilization of your spine which, in turn, makes it easier to safely work other parts of your body.

Along with specific floor exercises, Pilates training takes place on a *universal reformer,* which sounds like a Star Trek device but is actually a low bench-like piece of exercise equipment that uses springs and ropes for resistance. You lie, sit, stand, or kneel on the movable platform and control a sliding carriage by pushing or pulling with your feet or hands on straps, bars, or pulleys. Your abdominal muscles are the main focal point for each movement, and each movement is performed with breath, ease of motion, and relaxation.

Risa Sheppard, founder of The Sheppard Method Fitness Program in Los Angeles, warns that Pilates is unique from other exercise approaches; therefore, you should make sure that you are treated by a professional Pilates instructor. Also, before committing to any one training facility, find out the trainer's background and credentials by using the questions at the beginning of this chapter.

Therapeutic massage

Massage is one of the most frequently used therapies for musculoskeletal problems, particularly for controlling pain. Research indicates that therapeutic massage can have several beneficial effects on back pain including

- ✔ Relaxing the nervous system and muscles
- ✔ Breaking down scar tissue and lessening fibrosis and adhesions that develop as a result of injury
- ✔ Helping to reduce swelling
- ✔ Improving blood flow through the muscles

Therapeutic massage releases muscle tension and promotes relaxation. Muscle tension (either from activity, injury, or stress) may contribute to muscle fatigue and pain by pushing on nerve fibers in the muscle. Muscle *contraction* (tightening) for an extended period of time interferes with the elimination of chemical waste products in the muscles and surrounding tissues. The longer a muscle is tense, the more these chemical waste products build up and irritate the nerves and muscles in the area, causing more pain. Therapeutic massage can help break up these muscular waste deposits and stimulate more blood flow to the painful areas.

The Alexander Technique

Around the turn of the century, Frederick Matthias Alexander was one of the first to notice that faulty posture (sitting, standing, and moving) during daily activities relates to physical and emotional problems. The *Alexander Technique* seeks to rebalance the body by using awareness, movement, and touch. The technique focuses on developing the correct relationship between the patient's head, neck, and back while engaging in proper (or natural) movements.

The Feldenkrais Method

Moshe Feldenkrais was a physicist who suffered a personal trauma in the form of a sports-related injury. Rather than submitting to surgery, he searched for another solution through the study of the nervous system and human behavior. He applied his experience with martial arts, physiology, anatomy, psychology, and neurology to develop his own treatment program. Feldenkrais was able to reverse his impairment and walk without pain.

The *Feldenkrais Method* focuses on improving your self image, changing negative habitual patterns of movement, and teaching healthy breathing. You are taught to function with greater ease, fluidity, and motion. This effort, in turn, is said to improve your self-image and increases awareness. The approach encourages you to explore and experiment in order to find your own optimal style of movement. In addition, the practitioner actively directs your movements by using touch.

Rolfing

Ida Rolf, Ph.D., was a biochemist who was first exposed to therapeutic manipulation when she was successfully treated by an osteopath for a respiratory condition. As a result of this treatment, Dr. Rolf began to develop the primary tenet of her treatment approach: The structure of the body affects all physical and psychological processes. Dr. Rolf was also influenced by her exposure to yoga. She established the Rolf Institute in 1970.

Rolfing is based on the idea that human function improves when the body is properly aligned. Dr. Rolf believed that if your body is out of alignment, your muscles are overly contracted and stressed. After maintaining this unhealthy posture for months or years, other tissues in your body have to compensate to hold everything in this out-of-balance position. Movement becomes impaired and this, in turn, reduces your mental clarity and increases emotional stress.

During Rolfing, the practitioner re-establishes balance by manually manipulating and stretching your body's fascial tissues. The *fascia* is a thin, elastic, membrane that surrounds every muscle, bone, blood vessel, nerve, and organ. The practitioner applies pressure to the fascia using her fingers, knuckles, and elbows. This treatment can cause mild to significant pain depending on the amount of pressure applied. In addition to the physical manipulations, Rolfing includes education about movement.

Rolfing (and many other forms of bodywork) often include an approach developed originally by Dr. William Reich. Dr. Reich, a psychoanalyst and student of Dr. Sigmund Freud, was one of the first to purport that your body posture and behavior reflect your feelings and emotions. He developed a system of bodywork and breathing techniques that he believed could bring buried emotions to the surface. Reich felt that bodywork could decrease chronic physical tensions and release unconscious feelings and memories. Many practitioners of bodywork, as well as psychotherapists, have incorporated his techniques in order to address physical and emotional issues simultaneously.

Other popular systems of bodywork include Aston-Patterning, Hellerwork, The Trager Approach, Myotherapy, Therapeutic Touch, and Reflexology. All systems of bodywork focus on either physical manipulation of body structures, energy fields, or both. Practitioners often incorporate bodywork into other treatment approaches, such as acupuncture, herbal therapies, and traditional Western medicine.

Chapter 10

A Chiropractic Solution to Back Pain

● ●

In This Chapter

▶ Understanding the chiropractic approach

▶ Deciding when to use chiropractic

▶ Getting a grip on diagnosis and treatment methods

▶ Boning up on the possible side effects

▶ Knowing when to end chiropractic treatment

● ●

*Y*ou probably know the adage, "Never discuss religion or politics at cocktail parties." For a long time, chiropractors were on the same list of no-no's. Some people swear by their chiropractor, often seeking help from him or her before going a more traditional route. Other people are very suspicious, wondering whether a chiropractor is even a "real" doctor. Some people get great relief from the treatment that their chiropractors give, while others say they can't bear the thought of someone "cracking their bones."

Up to 40 percent of back-pain sufferers seek relief from a doctor of chiropractic each year. Another 25 percent see a chiropractor after having tried to get relief from an MD. If you've never considered consulting a chiropractor for your back or neck pain problem, you may want to know more about these health care professionals and their methods. In this chapter, John J. Triano, DC, Ph.D., of the Texas Back Institute, helped us put together some guidelines that you can use to determine when a chiropractor may be the doctor for your back pain problem, when a chiropractor is probably not your best option, and how to find a qualified chiropractor.

More than 70 nations legally recognize chiropractic health care. As a result, some controversy exists as to whether this healthcare approach is complementary or mainstream. Many of the early controversies between political medicine and chiropractic have been resolved. Beginning with research in 1975, the evidence now shows that chiropractic holds some benefits for back pain sufferers.

The chiropractic profession has made considerable strides in education, training, and quality control to warrant public trust over the past 25 years. Most insurers, employers, and managed-care organizations provide insurance benefits for chiropractic.

In this chapter, we look at chiropractic as a legitimate form of treatment for back pain.

How Chiropractors Think about Back Problems

The core philosophy of the chiropractic approach is the belief that your body has the inherent capacity to heal itself. In the chiropractic approach, the doctor of chiropractic is a facilitator who helps you achieve health naturally. That philosophy isn't a bad one to follow!

Chiropractors attempt to help your body resolve problems by using a mechanical treatment (known as *manipulation* or *adjustment)* to correct or offset the original mechanical injury, thus allowing your body to heal.

Sometimes, however, the damage done by trauma or degenerative disease may be too severe for chiropractic medicine to help completely. If that is the case, additional help may be necessary from a medical doctor for medical or surgical intervention. The result of any treatment may not always be expected to help you recover to full health.

Chiropractors agree with the modern traditional medicine idea that most back problems begin with some type of injury to your spine or surrounding muscles. They have promoted that notion since the late 19th century! Injury can occur from a single event (a car accident) or from repeatedly using bad posture. Scientifically, the injury leads to a series of events thereafter that determines how you experience the back symptoms. For instance, you may experience symptoms that are close to the injury site, such as local back pain and spasm. Alternatively, you may also have symptoms that are remote from the injury site, like radiating pain to your arm or leg.

Similar to traditional medical practice, chiropractors vary greatly on their attention to possible emotional and psychological contributions to back pain. Some focus only on structural explanations for your back symptoms and plan their treatment accordingly. Others focus on both mind and body influences on your symptoms.

The good news is that most back or neck problems get better, without treatment. They usually get better faster with treatment!

When to Choose Chiropractic

Typically, pain medications and a day or two of bed rest are enough to improve your back pain situation. If you do nothing but continue with your normal routine as best you can (for acute back pain), your situation is likely to improve. If your pain persists or becomes severe — or if you just can't afford to take time off and want to get better faster than just waiting — then seeing a chiropractor is for you. Appropriate chiropractic treatment may speed the rate of improvement and reduce your overall costs, including the expense of lost work time!

An unbiased review of chiropractic shows that chiropractic is a safe and effective method for dealing with various types of pain. For example,

- **Acute back pain** is most likely to benefit from chiropractic.

- **Radiating pain,** traveling through your legs, may be more difficult to help, but chiropractic is still worth a try.

- **Chronic pain** may benefit from chiropractic care, but don't expect your pain to go away totally — even with lots of treatment.

Sometimes, the tissue injury from trauma or degenerative disease may be too severe for chiropractic to help. If your pain is not relieved in a reasonable time, your chiropractor should suggest you consult with a medical doctor for medical or surgical intervention.

Before you choose to undergo chiropractic treatment for your back pain, ask your chiropractor a few questions:

- What is the problem that I'm being treated for?

  Your doctor should be able to tell you what he believes is causing your pain. He or she should also explain the activities of daily living that you need to avoid since they may slow your improvement. Certain activities may be helpful.

- How long should it take before I feel an improvement?

  Most patients (about eight of ten) feel some temporary improvement right away. A few people have some local soreness the first time that may last a day or less. Ice usually helps relieve that soreness. Lasting improvement should occur within two weeks for most and four weeks for the tougher cases.

- What other treatments are available to me?

  The treatment options depend on what is causing the pain and whether it is a recent onset or long-standing problem. Depending on the problem, alternate treatments may include watchful-waiting, medication, massage and physical therapy, rehabilitation exercise, or various types of injection procedures.

✔ If the planned treatment doesn't work as expected, what next?

During the first four weeks of treatment, if your pain lasts that long, the chiropractor modifies the plan of care and customizes it for you. If there is no improvement in that time, other appropriate steps may include special diagnostic tests to clarify the cause of pain or a consultation with a medial doctor. Your pain may respond best from treatment that includes chiropractic and medical teamwork.

✔ What can I do for myself to improve the pace of my recovery?

Mostly, you can help yourself by recognizing that back pain problems are an inconvenience (sometimes major) and usually not going to seriously alter your enjoyment of life. Following recommendations on restrictions and being consistent with exercises that a doctor assigns is very useful. In general, walking, swimming, or bicycling may be helpful.

✔ Will you speak to my family doctor (or specialist) about your findings and recommendations?

Absolutely! Open communication and cooperation between your doctors is the very best way for you to get the treatment that you need.

What to Expect — Diagnosis and Treatment

Your first visit is the time for you and your Doctor of Chiropractic to get acquainted. The doctor's office staff has you complete some forms giving personal information for billing and insurance. Other forms are used to help shorten the time needed to find out what is wrong with you. They ask about your health history and how your current pain began and affects you. When you get into the room you may need to remove some of your clothing in the area of the pain so that the doctor can properly examine you. Gowns are available as you need or want them. Many of the doctor's tools should be familiar to you. There are also a few special instruments that may be unfamiliar to you. These instruments help the doctor find out what is wrong and what to do about it.

After the doctor makes a diagnosis, he explains what he believes is wrong and recommends a treatment plan. What he suggests depends on what your problem is. If you agree with the plan, the treatment begins. As you leave, you may receive various health aids designed to speed your relief including braces or corsets, and nutritional supplements, as well as exercises for you to do at home.

Diagnostic methods

Chiropractors rely heavily on examining you in order to determine the site of the problem and the best method of treatment. Like their medical colleagues, chiropractors should question you about how, when, and where your pain or symptoms occur. Your chiropractor then performs a physical examination and asks you to perform simple tasks such as bending your back, legs, and arms in different directions; contracting your muscles against resistance; responding to light touch on the skin; and testing your reflexes.

Your chiropractor also feels the muscles and bones of your back, neck, or extremities to determine any tight muscles and tender areas. The chiropractor may apply special maneuvers that test the integrity of your joint ligaments and other tissues. These take the form of putting the area of pain through specific motions and applying light pressure to detect if it makes the symptoms worse.

Depending on the combined picture from your history and physical examination, the chiropractor may ask for special tests. Your doctor should be able to explain the following:

- Why you need the test
- What differences the test will make in your treatment
- What risks are associated with the test

The special tests can include:

- **X rays** to examine the bony structure of your back are the most frequently used test
- **MRI scans** to look for disc, nerve, or other soft tissue problems
- **Blood tests** to help check for internal medical disorders that may cause your pain including infection, cancer, and systemic diseases affecting the spine

Occasionally, your chiropractor may refer you to other specialists for invasive procedures to study suspected nerve damage or injection procedures to numb specific structures (similar to when a dentist uses novocaine to numb your jaw) and further define the source of your pain. These invasive procedures are the same ones used in traditional medical practice such as nerve studies and nerve blocks or epidurals.

Chiropractic terms: Say what?

As you find in most areas of health care, chiropractic has many insider terms that may make you feel as if you're listening to another language. Never fear! The following hit list can help you become a fluent speaker of *chiropracticese:*

✔ **Active care:** Treatment that asks you to take responsibility for your own recovery through exercise, ergonomics, and lifestyle changes.

✔ **Diversified technique:** The most widely used system of manipulation procedures in use today. Most scientific studies on the effectiveness of manipulation involve this method. Manipulations using this technique are quickly performed and may result in a popping sound similar to what you hear when someone "cracks their knuckles."

✔ **Ergonomics:** Literally, the term means "the study of work." This is the science that chiropractors use in making recommendations on proper spinal mechanics and posture, and on reducing work stress on your back.

✔ **Maintenance care:** In this theory of chiropractic care, your chiropractor performs regular maintenance spinal treatments to prevent or reduce the frequency of repeated problems — similar to periodically visiting your dentist for a check-up. Maintenance care is an elective form of treatment that insurance or managed-care programs usually don't cover. The effectiveness of this approach has never been tested and we aren't big advocates of it.

✔ **Manipulation (adjustment):** The application of controlled, directed forces and torques to the spine in order to relieve physical stresses and to increase movement.

✔ **Passive care:** Treatment administered by a doctor where you take no active role or responsibility for your own improvement. Contrast with **active care.**

✔ **Subluxation:** The term chiropractors use to describe poorly functioning joints that are associated with the pain and symptoms. Subluxations are found by themselves or along with other problems like disc degeneration or herniation.

Although some chiropractors recommend that all patients have X rays, as a precaution, many patients don't need X rays or more extensive imaging testing. X rays are necessary only when your pain was brought on by injury, your examination suggests the possibility of serious pathology (tumor, infection, systemic or severe degenerative disease) as the source of your pain, or when you haven't healed as expected. MRIs are specifically useful when your doctor suspects a disc herniation. Check out Chapter 6 for more on testing.

Most back pain problems don't require special testing! Always ask how the result of a special test may possibly change your treatment.

Treatment methods

The most common type of chiropractic treatment for back problems is *spinal manipulative therapy* (SMT). Chiropractors have more experience with this form of treatment than any other type of healthcare provider. Chiropractors are responsible for more than 94 percent of manipulation treatments given in the United States — see *Spinal manipulation for low-back pain.* Shekelle P.G., Adams A.H., Chassin M.R., Hurwitz E.L., Brook R.H. Ann Intern Med, 1992 117(7), 590-8.

Manual treatment procedures are part of the training that all chiropractors undergo; and most chiropractors focus on joint manipulation of the spine and extremities. Less well-known is the fact that chiropractors can often offer a wide variety of complementary, conservative (non-surgical) treatments to relieve your back or neck pain. Training in these complementary treatments usually is an elective part of regular chiropractic training or part of post-graduate education and advanced residency programs.

Other treatment methods that your chiropractor may recommend include a number of additional manual techniques (massage, stretching, and other methods) to help relieve symptoms, self-help recommendations for home exercise programs, ergonomic modifications for home and office, supervised exercise therapy to rehabilitate your spine, nutritional counseling to promote healing, and various other supportive procedures.

If you're getting appropriate treatment, you should see some type of improvement fairly quickly. If your problem has been going on for quite some time (over three months), the improvement may begin slowly, and be gradual. In addition, you may not see improvement in all of your symptoms simultaneously.

It's always a good idea to keep in mind the "three steps forward, one step back" rule (no, it's not a new dance for curing back pain). In treatment of back pain problems we often see patients move forward nicely in terms of feeling better and becoming more active, only to have an occasional set-back. Remember, if you move three steps forward and one step backward in your treatment, you are still two steps ahead (and that's done without using the "new math"). Keeping this rule in mind prevents you from getting discouraged when set-backs or flare-ups occur.

Possible Side Effects

Any effective treatment has some possible side effects. Fortunately, chiropractic care is generally very safe, and the likely potential complications are minor. The most common side effect (about 12 percent of the time) is some local soreness after the first treatment. Other temporary symptoms include feelings of fatigue or warmth in your extremities. These complications are short-lived and leave no permanent effect.

Straights and Mixers

Early this century, as chiropractors expanded their training and practice to include treatment beyond spinal manipulation (Mixers), a small group of dissenters (Straights) disavowed the need for integrating additional methods. The descriptive terms are no longer used much. However, the usual modern practice follows the precedent of expanded expertise. These practitioners are more likely to work closely with other health professionals. A small proportion of practitioners today (Straights) continues to rely almost solely on spinal manipulation to treat back problems.

Much less common are nerve damage or stroke; these complications occur so infrequently that most chiropractors never see one in their entire careers. The risk of having these complications is much smaller than the chance of having stomach ulcers from use of some over-the-counter pain medication.

Stopping Chiropractic Treatment

Modern chiropractors look for measurable improvement in your pain and function. Treatment should stop when your symptoms are no longer improving or, if for any reason, they are getting worse. You should seriously consider discontinuing treatment if your chiropractor offers only passive care on a prolonged basis.

No one (including your doctor) knows exactly how long effective treatment will take. On average, uncomplicated cases should take less than eight weeks. We recommend trying 6–12 sessions and stopping if there is no lasting improvement at that point.

Factors that may make recovery take longer include:

- Symptoms that have been present longer than eight days
- Severe symptoms that are not getting better on their own
- A history of more than three prior episodes of the same problem
- Presence of another problem in your bones or joints (arthritis, disc degeneration, or herniation)

We don't recommend spinal manipulation for a disk herniation with nerve compression as it may worsen the condition!

Chapter 11

All in Knots: Yoga for Your Back Problem

Yoga is one of the oldest known systems of health practiced in the world. The breathing exercises, physical postures, and meditation practices of yoga can help you with reducing stress, regulating heart rate, lowering blood pressure, and relieving pain (yes, even back pain).

Technically, the meaning of the word yoga is *union*. Yoga is the integration of physical, mental, and spiritual energies that come together to enhance your overall health and well being. In the 2nd century BC, Patanjali was the first to describe yoga systematically in writing in *The Yoga Sutras*. One of the ideas of yoga is that if your mind is chronically agitated and restless, then that anxiety will negatively affect the health of your body. Alternatively, if your body is in poor health, your mental strength will be drained.

Yoga actually extends beyond the practice of a few exercises and includes a complete system of lifestyle changes, hygiene, and detoxification methods. It includes both physical and psychological practices. Volumes have been written about yoga, and it is beyond the scope of this chapter to present an actual yoga approach. (That effort would take at least an entire book, such as *Yoga For Dummies* by Georg Feuerstein, Ph.D. and Larry Payne, Ph.D., published by IDG Books Worldwide, Inc.)

This chapter offers advice on using yoga to relieve your back pain. Appendix B can lead you to more information.

Beginning Hatha Yoga

One of the most widely used yoga practices is called the *Hatha yoga.* In Hatha yoga, you complete a series of body positions and movements (asanas) that involve stretching and holding, in addition to breathing exercises (pranayama). These exercises can create almost immediate positive changes in your body that can help with your back pain. The asanas and pranayama prepare you for meditation (which is called *samadhi* at its most advanced state), which is another aspect of yoga.

- ✔ **Asanas** bring the spine and head into alignment to promote proper blood flow throughout your body, and then bring your mind into a state of relaxation. Also, asanas help energize your glands, lungs, and heart. Asanas are also commonly prescribed for back, neck, and joint-pain problems.

- ✔ **Pranayama** focuses on regulating your breath, thereby promoting physical relaxation, calming your restless mind, and creating mental focus and increased energy.

- ✔ **Samadhi** is an advanced level of meditation that comes from practicing the asanas and pranayama. We discuss the nature of samadhi later in the chapter.

Practicing yoga postures: Asana

Asana literally means "ease" in Sanskrit. Even though many of the yoga postures, or asanas, involve little movement, the mind is actively involved in the performance of every asana. Thus, by practicing yoga postures, you discover how to regulate automatic nervous system functions (such as your heartbeat and breath) while allowing physical tensions to relax. This process, in turn, can help teach you to prevent or relieve back pain.

The asanas are designed to help you balance opposites such as forward with backward, stillness with movement, and inhaling with exhaling. One of the most well-known asanas is the *lotus position* (you know, the pretzel sitting position). In the lotus position, your left ankle is on top of your right thigh, and your right ankle is on top of your left thigh with the backs of your hands resting on your knees. (Don't try this on your own. You need to work up to this level of flexibility under the guidance of a qualified yoga instructor.)

Controlling your breath: Pranayama

Breath control or *pranayama* focuses on the way you regulate your breath. Pranayama literally means the regulation or control of *prana,* which is the life force. An interruption in the flow of prana (due to factors such as stress, improper diet, or toxins) damages your physical, emotional, and mental health. The pranayama exercises promote the proper flow of prana throughout your body.

The pranayama exercises guide you to focus your mind while bringing your breathing into a steady and rhythmic state. For a simple pranayama exercise, see the sidebar titled, "The alternate nostril breathing exercise." The breathing exercises are very useful to relax your mind and body. As we discuss in Chapter 12, these breathing exercises induce the *relaxation response,* which can provide you with benefits such as decreased heart rate, lowered blood pressure, reduced muscle tension, and lowered levels of pain. The pranayama or breath exercises are often performed as a preparation for meditation.

The alternate nostril breathing exercise

Alternate nostril breathing is a simple pranayama exercise that can help promote the flow of prana (the life force) and promote relaxation.

Begin by sitting upright on a cushion or firm chair with your head, neck, and body aligned. Take three complete breaths focusing on breathing from your diaphragm. (We cover this breathing technique in Chapter 12. This way of breathing primarily involves filling your lungs from the bottom up rather than chest breathing.) Your inhaling and exhaling should be of equal length as well as being slow, controlled, and smooth.

After taking the three complete breaths, you can begin the alternate nostril breathing technique. First, close your right nostril with the thumb of your right hand and exhale completely through your left nostril. After you have exhaled completely, close your left nostril with your right index finger and inhale completely through your right nostril.

Repeat this cycle of exhaling through your left nostril and inhaling through your right nostril two more times. Be sure that you maintain an equal length of time for inhaling and exhaling. At the end of inhaling the third time through the right nostril, exhale completely through the same nostril while keeping the left nostril closed. At the end of this exhalation, close your right nostril and inhale through your left nostril.

Repeat this cycle of exhaling through your right nostril and inhaling through your left nostril two more times. Then place your hands on your knees while exhaling and inhaling through both nostrils evenly for three complete breaths. At this point, you have completed one cycle of the alternate nostril breathing exercise. The following is a summary of the entire exercise:

Complete breaths, both nostrils	Three times
Exhale left and inhale right	Three times
Exhale right and inhale left	Three times
Complete breaths, both nostrils	Three times

As you practice this technique, gradually lengthen the duration of your inhales and exhales. We recommend that you practice the alternate nostril breathing exercise at least twice per day, once in the morning and once in the evening.

Meditating toward samadhi

The asanas and pranayama can lead to a state of meditation in which your physical body is extremely relaxed and your mind is highly focused. The most advanced practice of meditation leads to spiritual realization, or *samadhi,* which is the culmination of lengthy, dedicated, and disciplined practice. Those in the know describe samadhi as a different state of consciousness beyond states of waking, sleeping, or dreaming.

Rest assured that the meditative state can be very beneficial even if you never get to samadhi. When you're in a meditative state, you may notice a heightened sense of awareness and overall well-being. The state of meditation has been shown to reduce muscle tension, slow heart rate, lower blood pressure, slow brain wave patterns, improve oxygen consumption in the body, improve immune function, and reduce pain.

Using Yoga to Treat Back Pain

Yoga can be very effective for your back pain problem because it addresses several factors that may be making your condition worse. Yoga can help with your posture, strength, flexibility, weight or diet, and overall mind and body relaxation. Given yoga's positive effects on your body, it is not surprising that one national survey of patients showed that 98 percent of the people found yoga to be beneficial for their back pain problem. See the Burton Goldberg Group, *Alternative Medicine: The Definitive Guide* (Fife, Washington: Future Medicine Publishing, Inc., 1994) and K. Nespor, "Pain Management and Yoga," *International Journal of Psychosomatics* 38 (1991): 76–81.

One of the common causes of back problems may be prolonged overstretching of the back ligaments and muscles due to poor posture during sitting and standing, but probably mostly sitting. (For more information about posture, see Chapter 13.)

If you're like most people, you bend forward too much throughout your day. Improving your everyday posture (whether sitting, standing, walking, lifting, or sleeping) can help with your back pain problem or even prevent pain from occurring. Poor posture takes a toll on your body — especially your back — after days, weeks, and years of repetition. Poor posture can cause people even in their 30s and 40s to be beset by chronic physical problems.

Think about your average day: You wake up in the morning, sit on the edge of the bed and bend forward. You walk into the bathroom, sit on the commode and bend forward. As you prepare for the day, you stand in front of the mirror and bend forward, perhaps shaving or putting on makeup. You may then get into a car and bend forward while driving to and from work. After arriving at work, you may sit in a chair and bend forward at your desk. Finally, if you are connected to the Internet, you may find yourself spending more and more time at home sitting and bending forward in front of your computer. That's a lot of bending forward, and it may be too much for your body.

A simple way to experience the effects of bending forward too much is to turn both palms up with your fingers extended. Push the tip of your left index finger down with the tip of your right index finger (right palm above left palm) while keeping the left palm and forearm parallel to the floor. At first you will notice pressure at the end of your left finger; after a short while, however, you will feel radiating pressure going first down the entire finger, then your hand, and eventually your entire arm. This process is exactly what happens to the back ligaments and muscles during prolonged periods of slouched sitting or standing. Tension in one part of your body (for example, your back) causes pain and tension in other areas as well.

At first, maintaining a healthy back may seem to you like a full-time job. Be assured that after you practice the techniques (such as posture and exercise) we discuss throughout this book, they will become second nature. When that happens, promoting a healthy back becomes a lifestyle rather than an ordeal you have to think about all the time. A session or two of yoga or exercise therapy during your week won't help much if you misuse and abuse your back the rest of the time.

Yoga therapy can be an excellent approach either by itself or as part of an overall treatment plan for your back problem. In fact, yoga can not only help improve your posture and back pain, but it can enhance your entire lifestyle.

As with any alternative medicine treatment, check with your doctor before proceeding with yoga practice.

Yoga and back exercise

If you have a serious back problem that significantly interferes with your activities or limits your ability to exercise, you should consider initially work-ing one-on-one with a competent yoga therapist. Be sure that the yoga therapist has experience in working with people who have back pain prob-lems. Some of the yoga movements may have to be altered in order to accommodate your back. In addition, the yoga therapist may have you move through the exercises at a slower pace in order to keep your pain under con-trol while you are learning the techniques.

Often, yoga is offered in classes where general techniques are taught. Although you may eventually progress toward group classes, starting out with an individual yoga therapist is probably the wisest choice. A group yoga class can be very risky when you have a back problem, especially if the class is large. Of course, always check with your medical doctor before starting a program, to ensure that it is safe for you to proceed. To find a yoga instruc-tor, start with the resources in Appendix B. Other good places to start are local community centers and health clubs. You may also be able to find a dedicated yoga center in your area (some may even specialize in back patients), given yoga's current popularity.

Because no national standards or certifications exist for yoga instructions, getting a recommendation for an instructor from family, friends, or your healthcare professional can be helpful. As you check out an instructor, consider asking to talk to one or two satisfied clients.

One main goal of any good yoga or exercise program for the back is to restore the normal range of motion to your spine, including flexion (bending forward), extension (bending backward), and rotation. The challenge is to determine which type of program your back problem requires and to inspire you to complete a daily exercise routine that fits your lifestyle and allows for progress at the proper speed. This goal is often accomplished by having your yoga therapist and medical doctor work together (or at least communicate periodically) to design a safe yoga program that will be maximally effective.

The key to yoga exercises for your back problem is knowing what to do, when, and how much. Every case is a little different, and your back problem is unique. As such, prescribing a particular yoga posture or program for your unique back problem is beyond the scope of this chapter.

In general, if you are like many people, you suffer from weak abdominal muscles, tight hamstrings, and strained or sprained ligaments and muscles that support the curves in your spine. Additionally, if you have had injuries to or surgeries on your spine, you may have built up scar tissue that needs to be stretched out in order for your spine to become functional again. A specific yoga exercise program can help achieve these goals for your back problem and bring your body into balance.

Daily journal

As we discuss in Chapter 7, you can make yourself accountable for exercising by getting an exercise buddy. Another method (either in addition to the exercise buddy or on its own) is to keep a daily back journal. Your journal can be long and complicated, or it can be very simple. In most cases, the simpler the better because you will tend to shy away from anything that takes too much time. On a piece of paper or on a calendar, keep track of the following information on a daily basis:

✔ Did you do your yoga or back exercises today? Yes or No.

✔ Did you feel pain and at what time of the day? If so, give the degree of pain a rating from 0 to 10, with 0 being no pain and 10 being the worst pain possible.

✔ Keep track of the amount of water you drink. The goal is to drink from six to eight 8-ounce glasses per day.

On another piece of journal paper, take a few minutes to record the activities during your normal day that cause pain in your back. For example, "My lower back hurts on the right side when I take out the trash," or "My back hurts when I sit too long." After a week or two of writing in the journal, review your entries and look for patterns. With this information you can better tailor your activities and yoga exercise program to keep the pain under control.

For example, you may find that taking short breaks throughout the day helps prevent a buildup of back pain. You may also discover that doing a few yoga movements and breathing/meditation exercises throughout the day helps you break up the pain cycle. In addition, if you are having a particularly bad day, you'll feel a lot better if you look back on your calendar and notice how many good days you've had. An occasional bad day is part of the normal healing curve (we always tell our patients to expect three steps forward, one step back), so don't let it get you down.

Rest and relaxation

Let's face it: If you don't get a good night's sleep, you are inviting more back pain problems and other poor health conditions. Many people don't understand that the mind as well as the body needs a rest. In our fast-moving society, getting your thoughts off of work or other stress-related matters is very difficult. Just because you physically lie in a bed for eight hours doesn't mean that you are getting the rest you need.

Reducing back pain requires good sleep hygiene. Yoga breathing and meditation exercises can be an integral part of this program. Sleep hygiene means that you take steps to ensure that you obtain a restful night's sleep. Examples include not doing stressful activities in bed (such as working on your checkbook or watching the news), getting up after a half hour if you are unable to fall asleep, and not doing any energizing activities (such as exercise) just prior to going to bed.

What goes into your mind just before going to bed and while you are trying to fall asleep can affect your entire night's sleep pattern. Thus, even though you may be physically asleep, your mind can remain quite stressed. This anxiety results in a restless night's sleep that doesn't restore your energy for the following day. Symptoms of a stressful night's sleep can include clenching your teeth, awakening during the night and not being able to readily fall back to sleep, and feeling tired the following day. Yoga breathing and meditative exercises can help you get a good night's sleep, which in turn, helps your body and mind effectively fight off the back pain during the day.

Rope yoga

Fear not! *Rope yoga* does not involve getting tied up (or whips and chains, for that matter!). Rope yoga is a new, innovative conditioning program developed by Gudni Gunnarsson. Rope Yoga integrates many of the principles of traditional yoga, which we discuss in this chapter, with an additional special piece of equipment that increases the efficiency of the exercises. The equipment is a rope and pulley system that helps coordinate the movement of your arms and legs. Specific exercises with the rope and pulley system provide a total body workout, with a special emphasis on your abdominal and back muscles.

An instructional video and manual leads you through a four-stage workout including: strength and posture alignment exercise, mobility and directed exercises at the abdomen and back, breathing exercises, and stretching and stress reduction. For more information about this program contact: Rope Yoga, c/o RHL Group, 1640 S. Sepulveda Blvd, Suite 500, Los Angeles, CA; phone 310-444-8801, extension 401.

Chapter 12

Using the Power of the Mind-Body Connection

In This Chapter

▶ Changing your thoughts to decrease pain

▶ Relaxing: Not just "mellowing out"

▶ Using cue-controlled relaxation

▶ Practicing relaxation and imagery

▶ Beginning biofeedback training

▶ Using self-hypnosis

Many factors — physical, mental, and emotional — influence your back pain. As we state elsewhere in this book, you can have severe pain with minimal physical findings and minimal pain with horrendous physical findings. Your mind can influence your body in significant ways including

✔ Whether you experience certain types of back pain, such as stress-related back pain

✔ How quickly you heal from a back injury or pain problem

✔ Whether you experience depression and anxiety as part of your back pain

Both thoughts and emotions have a significant influence over your pain level and suffering. Given this fact, you can use your thoughts and emotions to help make the back pain better.

The *mind-body connection* refers to how your mental and emotional states ("the mind") affect your physical being or "body," and vice versa. Even though the connection goes both ways (mind affecting body and body affecting mind), the focus is generally on the mind's influences on the body. The mind-body connection can work *against you,* making your pain and suffering worse, or it can work *for you,* becoming a powerful connection you can use to overcome your pain problem.

Mind-body techniques are gaining in popularity and are useful for the management of many medical conditions, including back pain. This chapter reviews the mind-body techniques of changing your thoughts and emotions, as well as using various types of relaxation and imagery exercises, biofeedback, and hypnosis.

You may notice that the mind-body techniques we feature in this chapter differ from most medical approaches in that you must practice mind-body techniques on a regular basis in order for them to be effective. Keeping yourself motivated is the most important component of successfully using mind-body approaches to improve your back health. Motivation and practice can reward you with positive results such as improved health and less pain. You can help yourself stay motivated by giving yourself rewards along the way. For instance, you may buy yourself that special something you've been wanting after you practice a mind-body technique for a certain amount of time.

Taking Control of Your Thoughts and Emotions

You constantly evaluate the world around you. You constantly evaluate the sensations going on inside of your body as well.

These constant thoughts are *automatic thoughts* because they occur almost automatically, outside of your awareness. Automatic thoughts tend to be very fast, *unconscious* (out of your awareness), and highly believable. How can a thought be unconscious *and* believable. Actually, it happens all the time. For instance, when you play golf and are facing a challenging shot, you may have the unconscious thought that you can't make the shot because you've missed it a few time before (even though consciously you are trying to tell yourself that you can). The unconscious thought can be highly believable even though it is unconscious. The evidence that you believe the unconscious thought is your emotional and physical sensations such as self-doubt, anxiety, and trembling.

Because of the characteristics of automatic thoughts, they have a great influence over your emotions, behaviors, and pain. As we discuss later in this chapter, the good news is that you can change automatic thoughts from negative to positive.

Recognizing automatic thoughts

Research shows that human beings under stress have a tendency to engage in irrational *negative* automatic thoughts. Negative automatic thoughts, as the term implies, tend to produce negative emotions such as depression, anxiety, and fear as well as create increased pain sensations. Identifying when you're experiencing negative automatic thoughts and understanding how negative automatic thoughts work can put you on the road to changing them.

Experiencing back pain is often a stressful situation — one that can result in a variety of negative automatic thoughts, including some, or all of the following:

- ✔ I'll never get better.
- ✔ My back is getting worse and worse.
- ✔ I'm going to end up a cripple.
- ✔ Why is this happening to me?

This type of thinking is not only negative, but (more important) these statements are also often inaccurate if you explore them carefully.

Almost all the back pain patients we work with acknowledge having the preceding types of thoughts at one time or another. Patients also admit that these thoughts are highly believable at the time they occur.

You can probably guess the consequences of having and believing negative thoughts. Try reading the thoughts in the preceding list out loud. Research shows that by simply reviewing a list of negative statements, most people begin to feel somewhat sad and nervous. In fact, if you have back pain, you may notice your pain worsening as you review and think about these statements.

Using automatic thoughts to your advantage

Coping, or rational, thoughts are directly opposed to negative automatic thoughts. *Coping thoughts* reflect the true reality of the situation and help you focus on the range of options available to help solve a problem like back pain. Coping thoughts may be similar to the following:

- ✔ Because no one can predict the future, I benefit more by being optimistic than pessimistic.
- ✔ This pain doesn't mean that I'm getting worse. I'm showing improvement in the following ways. . . .
- ✔ I have no evidence that this back pain is going to make me a cripple.
- ✔ I'm going to think about what can I do to better my situation instead of spending my time asking why this happened to me.

Notice that each of the preceding coping thoughts directly disputes an associated negative automatic thought we list in the previous section. Try reading the coping thoughts in the preceding list out loud. You will find that by simply reviewing these coping statements, you may begin to feel a little more hopeful and optimistic. We sometimes have patients make a list of coping thoughts to carry around in their purses or billfolds and review throughout the day.

You do not have to be a victim of negative automatic thoughts. You can learn how to identify negative automatic thoughts as they occur and replace them with coping or nurturing thoughts.

Changing your thoughts

Negative automatic thoughts can cause negative emotions such as depression, anxiety, fear, and anger, which can in turn worsen your back pain. Then, in a vicious cycle, the back pain causes more stress, resulting in a cascade of more negative automatic thoughts.

A useful model for understanding how your thoughts, emotions, and behaviors interact has been developed by Drs. Aaron Beck, Albert Ellis, and others. The *ABCDE model* can be a useful tool in changing your thoughts and dealing with your back pain. In the ABCDE model:

> **A** is the **activating event** or **antecedent event,** which is simply the event to which you're responding. This can be an outside event such as sitting in a traffic jam or an internal event such as a severe back spasm.

> **B** is your **belief** or automatic thought about the activating event. For instance, your belief about your back pain may be "I'll never get better. My back is getting worse and worse. I'll end up a cripple." On the other hand, your thoughts about the back pain may be "This pain doesn't mean I'm getting worse. This is usually a temporary thing. I am getting better overall. This pain is nothing to be frightened of."

> **C** is the **consequent** emotion resulting from your automatic thoughts. Most people think that the activating event causes this consequent emotion, but in reality, your belief causes your emotion. A person's emotional response to a situation is caused by his or her beliefs about the situation and not the situation itself.

> **D** is the **disputing thought** that you can use to change negative automatic thoughts. Disputing thoughts can help change the way you think about a stressful situation (such as back pain) from a negative standpoint to a coping standpoint. We like to call this process "the power of realistic thinking" when working with our patients.

E is the **evaluation** part of using the disputing thoughts to challenge the negative automatic thoughts. In the evaluation part, you assess how well disputing thoughts are working to challenge your negative automatic thoughts and replace them with coping thoughts. We discuss this process later in the chapter.

Table 12-1 takes you through two examples of how the ABCDE model operates.

Table 12-1	The ABCDE Model in Action	
Event	*Scenario 1*	*Scenario 2*
Activating event	You experience a mild increase in your heart rate and feel "uncomfortable and jittery."	You experience back or neck pain.
Belief	I'm having a heart attack!	Something is seriously wrong with my spine. My spine is weak and fragile. Nobody really understands my pain.
Consequent emotions	Fear, anxiety, panic	Hopelessness, helplessness, anxiety, depression, anger
Resulting behavior	Call doctor or go to the emergency room.	Slow, robotic movements; social isolation; irritability; use of pain medicines

In Scenario 1, the symptoms are interpreted as a heart attack. Subsequent emotions and behavior follow from this belief. Given the same activating event, an alternative belief is: "I just drank four cups of coffee and I'm on a caffeine jag." With this explanation, the emotions and resulting behavior would be entirely different — even though the situation prompting the beliefs is exactly the same.

In Scenario 2 the back pain symptoms trigger a number of negative automatic thoughts that are likely to make you feel worse. Negative emotions and other behaviors then follow from these negative thoughts. Alternative coping beliefs are "My spine is a strong structure," "I am finding ways to manage this increase in back pain," and "I can choose to not allow the pain to control my life." Again, you can analyze the same situation using different thoughts. Using coping thoughts results in more positive emotions and less pain.

Your beliefs are what cause your emotional response and behavior, not the situation itself.

Using the three- and five-column techniques

The examples in Table 12-1 illustrate how your thoughts and beliefs influence your emotions and behavior. But, how can you use this information to help with back pain? You use the *three-* and *five-column* techniques. By using both of these techniques, you can change your negative automatic thoughts to realistic, coping, and nurturing thoughts.

A three-column worksheet utilizes the ABC parts of the ABCDE model. Filling out the three columns on the worksheet enables you to run through your automatic negative thoughts in slow motion. Figure 12-1 shows an example of a three column worksheet.

Antecendent	Beliefs	Consequent Emotions
Sitting at work. Supervisor gave me too much to do. I'm noticing worse pain in my back as well as my neck.	There is something seriously wrong with my back.	Fear
	My spine is weak and fragile.	
	If I move the wrong way, I'll do myself in.	
	I'll never lead a normal life.	Helpless
	I can't cope with this pain.	
	There is nothing I can do about this pain.	Hopeless
	My back pain is all their fault.	Anger and Entitlement
	My boss doesn't understand my pain.	
	My boss expects too much from me.	
	I should be better by now.	Guilt
	I should never have let myself get injured in the first place.	
	This pain is ruining my family.	

Figure 12-1: Example of a three-column worksheet.

At first, you may have a difficult time fleshing out your beliefs (the B column) or automatic negative thoughts (the C column) about a situation. Automatic negative thoughts often contain such words like *should, ought, must, never,* and *always*. Examples may be something like "I should be able to handle this pain better," "I ought to be better by now," and "I must be a terrible person with this pain."

Often, it is easier to first identify your emotional reactions and then work backward to identify the negative automatic thoughts or beliefs.

When you have become adept at identifying the ABC components of stress and pain, you can expand the three-column technique to a five-column technique: Simply add the columns for disputing thoughts and evaluation to your worksheet. (Refer to Figure 12-2.)

The disputing thoughts (in column D) are constructed to directly attack and counter the negative automatic thoughts you wrote in column B. You use the evaluation column (column E) to record how your disputing thoughts affect your original negative thoughts, emotions, and overall stress.

Antecendent	Beliefs	Consequent Emotions	Disputing Thoughts	Evaluation
Sitting at work. Supervisor gave me too much to do.	There is something seriously wrong with my back.	Fear	Hurt does not equal harm! This pain does not mean injury.	Much less fear
I'm noticing worse pain in my back as well as my neck.	My spine is weak and fragile.		The spine is a strong structure.	
	If I move the wrong way, I'll do myself in.		I am not at risk for injury.	
	I'll never lead a normal life.	Helpless	No one can predict the future.	More feeling of control
	I can't cope with this pain.		I'm learning ways to cope. I've made it through before.	
	There is nothing I can do about this pain.	Hopeless	There are things I can do. They are	Somewhat better
	My back pain is all their fault.	Anger and Entitlement	Blaming does not help me get better.	Mild decrease in anger
	My boss doesn't understand my pain.		My boss acts that way to everyone.	
	My boss expects too much from me.		I can get a lot done if I work steady and pace myself.	
	I should be better by now.	Guilt	I am trying to get better and working hard at it.	Guilt improved
	I should never have let myself get injured in the first place.		It was not my fault.	
	This pain is ruining my family.		There are things I can do to lead a quality of life regardless of the pain.	

Figure 12-2: Expansion of the three-column worksheet to five columns.

What is stress?

Stress generally can be defined as a mental or physical demand made upon the body. Your body responds to stress by increasing your blood pressure and heart rate, causing rapid breathing, tensing your muscles, and reducing blood flow to your head, stomach, skin, hands, and feet.

When you're tense, your body also produces stress hormones to give you an energy burst. If you're in danger, these hormones help your body perform at maximum efficiency for survival reasons. But, when these hormones are released inappropriately over a long time, they damage your body. It's like running your car's engine beyond the design capabilities: It's okay for a quick get-away, but will blow up the engine if done extensively.

Scientific studies suggest that up to 85 percent of all medical problems are caused by stress. This is not to say physical problems are all "in your head." Rather, prolonged stress causes physical changes in your body that result in various medical conditions. For example, stress-related problems can include such things as headaches, back pain, sleep problems, digestive disorders, and high-blood pressure. Stress can make virtually any medical problem worse, and can make a surgical procedure more difficult at every stage — before, during, and after. See D. Coleman J. Gurin, *Mind-Body Medicine: How to Use Your Mind for Better Health* (Yonkers, New York: Consumer Reports Books, 1993) and D.S. Sobel and R. Ornstein, *The Healthy Mind, Healthy Body Handbook* (Los Altos, CA: DRX Publishing, 1996).

The Relaxation Response: More Than Just Relaxing

Distinguishing between the "relaxation response" and simply "relaxing" is important. When we discuss relaxation training, our patients often ask us if they can simply do something they enjoy, such as listening to music or sitting out in the backyard. Although these types of activities are certainly "relaxing" they do not elicit the "relaxation response."

The relaxation response, first described by Dr. Herbert Benson and his colleagues at Harvard Medical School in the early 1970s, involves a number of physical changes, including:

- Decrease in heart rate
- Decrease in respiration rate
- Decrease in blood pressure
- Decrease in muscle tension
- Decrease in metabolism rate and oxygen consumption

Practice makes perfect

Just like learning any new skill, you need to practice the relaxation exercises we feature in this chapter in order for them to be effective. The following guidelines can help you establish a regular practice regimen and get the most out of each session.

- **Practice once or twice a day.** Practicing at least once a day is necessary in order to elicit the relaxation response. Initially, your relaxation sessions may take more time. As you practice regularly, you may find that the amount of time required to elicit the relaxation response decreases.

- **Find a quiet location.** Practice your exercises in a location where you will not be disturbed or distracted. For instance, try turning off your phone's ringer or using a fan or air conditioner to block out outside noise while you're practicing.

- **Give a five-minute warning.** Give yourself and other family members a five-minute warning before you begin your exercises. This can help you and other family members take care of loose ends prior to practicing your relaxation techniques.

- **Practice at regular times.** Setting up regular practice times increases the likelihood that you will follow through on your relaxation exercises. Choose a time when you are most likely to follow through on completing the exercises. Your regular practice times should not be when you are so tired that you are likely to fall asleep (right after a big meal or just prior to bed, for example).

- **Assume a comfortable position.** A common position is lying flat on your back with your legs extended and your arms comfortably at your sides. Depending upon your back pain, you may want to flex your knees, or support them with a pillow. If even this position causes pain, you can complete relaxation exercises while sitting or standing.

- **Loosen your clothing.** Loosen any tight clothing and take off such things as your shoes, belt, watch, glasses, jewelry, and other constrictive apparel. Again, the objective is to be as comfortable as possible while you practice the exercises.

- **Set your worries aside.** Try writing down all the things on your mind, and then physically putting that paper aside prior to practicing. You can focus better on the relaxation exercise if your other concerns are documented for your attention after you finish with your relaxation exercise.

- **Assume a passive attitude.** You need to *allow the relaxation response to happen.* You should not *try* to relax or *control* your body. Don't judge your performance. Focusing on your breathing is all you need to do. Relaxation occurs on its own.

You can only achieve the relaxation response by regularly practicing a relaxation technique. After you learn to elicit the relaxation response, you notice feeling more relaxed in other areas of your life, even when not directly practicing the relaxation technique. Achieving the relaxation response

- ✔ Reduces generalized anxiety.
- ✔ Prevents stress from building up over time.
- ✔ Increases energy levels and productivity.
- ✔ Improves concentration, memory, and ability to focus.
- ✔ Induces deeper, more restorative sleep and a reduction of insomnia and fatigue.
- ✔ Increases awareness of your actual emotional state and feelings (being "stressed out" tends to make you unaware of your actual feelings).

You can use a variety of techniques and exercises to bring about the relaxation response, including breathing techniques, cue controlled relaxation, imagery, biofeedback, and hypnosis, among others. The following sections cover these techniques in greater detail.

Different Types of Breathing

It may seem strange to even be discussing learning how to breathe properly. Breathing is essential for life, and we all take for granted that we know how to do it properly. In reality, very few people actually breathe in the most healthy fashion.

In our experience, breathing exercises are the easiest way to learn to elicit the relaxation response. The exercises in this section are straightforward and require minimal body movement.

You have two basic ways of breathing:

- ✔ **Chest Breathing.** Chest breathing, or *shallow breathing,* occurs when you expand your chest with each in-breath, raise your shoulders, and tuck in your abdomen. The breaths tend to be shallow and short. They can also be quite irregular and rapid. Chest breathing tends to cause excess tension in your neck and shoulders.

  Chest breathing is often associated with high anxiety states in which you may hold your breath and experience hyperventilation, shortness of breath, constricted breathing, or feeling like you are going to pass out. You are more prone to chest breathe when you are under stress, which in turn decreases your ability to cope with stress.

- ✔ **Abdominal Breathing.** Abdominal, or *diaphragmatic breathing,* is how newborn infants breathe. Adults also breathe abdominally when they sleep. Unfortunately, most of us learn to be chest breathers over the years.

Learning how to breathe diaphragmatically is a key component to learning how to elicit the relaxation response. By regularly practicing proper breathing techniques, you can elicit the relaxation response.

Breathing awareness

Before you begin doing any breathing exercises, follow these steps to discover how you normally breathe.

1. **Lie down on your back in a comfortable place.**

   You may want to raise your knees because this position can help reduce back pain (see Figure 12-3). If for some reason, lying on your back is just not comfortable, you can try sitting in a chair.

2. **Close your eyes and place one hand on your breastbone and the other hand over your belly button.**

3. **Without trying to change how you normally breathe, become aware of which part of your body is moving as you inhale and exhale.**

   The hand on your breastbone monitors chest breathing, and the hand over your belly button monitors abdominal breathing.

4. **Pay attention to which hand rises when you inhale — the one on your abdomen or the one on your chest.**

   If your abdomen moves up and down with each breath, you're breathing diaphragmatically. If your chest moves up and down with each breath, then you may be more of a chest breather.

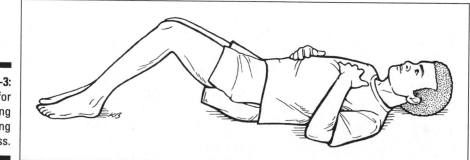

Figure 12-3:
Position for practicing breathing awareness.

Diaphragmatic or abdominal breathing

The following exercise helps you develop your abdominal breathing skills. Practice it until you can breathe abdominally for five to ten minutes.

1. **Lie down in a comfortable position on your back with your legs straight and slightly apart.**

   Allow your toes to point comfortably outward and let your arms rest at your sides without touching your body. Place your palms up and close your eyes.

2. **Focus your attention on your breathing and place your hand on the spot that seems to rise and fall the most as you inhale and exhale.**

   Notice the position of your hand. It may be on your chest, abdomen, or somewhere in between.

3. **Gently place both of your hands (or a book) on your abdomen and again focus on your breathing.**

   Pay attention to how your abdomen rises as you inhale and falls as you exhale. Try to make your hands rise and fall as you inhale and exhale.

   Breathe through your nose during this exercise. You may need to clear your nasal passages prior to doing your breathing exercises.

   If you have difficulty breathing into your abdomen, press your hand down on your abdomen as you exhale and allow your abdomen to push your hand back up as you inhale deeply. The pressure from your hand helps you become more aware of the action of your abdomen during breathing.

4. **Take a few minutes and let your chest follow the movement of your abdomen.**

   Notice whether your chest is moving in harmony with your abdomen, or if it appears rigid. Continue to focus on making your abdomen move up and down as you breathe and allow your chest to follow your abdomen's motion naturally.

   If you have difficulty breathing abdominally, try lying on your stomach with your head resting on your folded hands. Take deep abdominal breaths so that you can feel your abdomen pushing against the floor as you breathe.

5. **As you practice abdominal breathing for five or ten minutes, scan your body for tension.**

   Start at the top of your head and mentally scan your body down to your toes looking for any left-over tension. Tension "hot spots" that you may feel as you scan over your body include your neck, shoulders, and back. If you find any tension, try and relax that part of your body more and more as you continue the breathing exercise.

Relaxed breathing

After you master abdominal breathing, a relaxed breathing exercise can be helpful to begin to elicit the relaxation response:

1. **Lie down on your back.**

   Bend your knees and move your feet about eight inches apart with your toes turned slightly outward. This position helps straighten your spine and keep you comfortable. If you have back problems, you may want to place a pillow under your knees for extra support.

2. **Mentally scan your body for any tension as we discuss in the preceding section.**

   You can often notice tension by feelings of tightness or aching in a particular part of your body. If you notice any tension, make a mental note of it ("My shoulders and back feel a little tight"). You can re-scan your body after the relaxed breathing exercise to see whether these tense spots have loosened up.

3. **Place one hand on your abdomen and one hand on your chest.**

4. **Inhale slowly and deeply through your nose into your abdomen, so that your hand rises.**

   Your chest should move only a little and should "follow" your abdomen.

5. **When you feel at ease with Step 4, try the deep breathing cycle: Inhale through your nose while smiling slightly.**

6. **Exhale through your mouth, gently blowing the air out of your lungs and making a "whooshing" sound.**

7. **Take long slow deep breathes that raise and lower your abdomen.**

   Focus on the sound and feeling of breathing as you become more and more relaxed.

   Continue the relaxed breathing pattern for five or ten minutes at a time, once or twice a day. After you do this exercise daily for a week, try extending your relaxed breathing exercise period to 15 or 20 minutes.

8. **At the end of each relaxed breathing session, take time to once again scan your body for tension.**

   Compare the tension you feel at the conclusion of the exercise with that you were feeling at the beginning of the exercise. This will give you some idea as to how the relaxed breathing exercise is working. The more you practice, the better it works.

As you become more proficient at relaxed breathing, you can practice it anytime during the day, in addition to your regularly scheduled sessions.

Cue-Controlled Relaxation

Cue-controlled relaxation is an effective technique you can use either in conjunction with relaxed breathing or alone. In *cue-controlled relaxation,* you use a cue to signal the relaxation response. Although the cue can be anything, it is usually a verbal signal such as a word that you say quietly to yourself such as *relax, breathe,* or *one;* a phrase, such as *I am calm* or *My back and neck are relaxed;* or a line from a prayer.

Before trying to learn cue-controlled relaxation, you need to have a basic mastery of relaxed breathing and eliciting the relaxation response. (See the section "Different Types of Breathing" for more information.) Practice relaxed breathing for at least a week prior to beginning cue-controlled relaxation.

To begin using cue-controlled relaxation:

1. **Choose a verbal cue.**

2. **Condition yourself to the cue.**

    Conditioning yourself to the cue means saying the cue (the word *relax*) or seeing the cue (a spot) to cause your body to almost automatically relax. For conditioning to occur, you need to associate the cue with the relaxation response. Whenever you practice the relaxed breathing exercise, use the last several deep breaths at the end of your sessions for cue-controlled relaxation. If you choose a word cue such as *relax,* stretch out the sound of the word while you exhale and say "Reeelaax." With practice, simply saying *relax* to yourself in any situation can help you relax.

You can use cue-controlled relaxation in many situations where it is either difficult or impossible to actually engage in relaxed breathing, or when you need to slow things down and decrease your pain or anxiety. Use cue-controlled relaxation:

- ✔ **To signal the relaxation response in any situation:** Especially when you can't actually do relaxed breathing, you can use your cue to help you stay calm and relaxed.

- ✔ **To stop negative thoughts:** Cue-controlled relaxation is a powerful technique for stopping or disrupting negative and unproductive thinking. If you find yourself carried away by anxiety, distress, or negative thinking, use your cue to disrupt or stop these thoughts and redirect your thinking towards positive, coping statements.

- ✔ **To prepare yourself for an uncomfortable medical procedure:** Cue-controlled relaxation is an excellent way to prepare yourself for any medical procedure, particularly those related to your back pain — a nerve block injection or to help you hold still during an MRI.

- ✔ **To manage an acute back pain flare-up:** Use your cue as soon as you experience increased pain to help you get you through these episodes.

Cue-controlled relaxation is a very useful skill that you can call upon in a variety of situations. As with any skill, *it is important to take time to practice.* The cue will work for you, but only if you practice it and give it a chance to become associated with your relaxation response.

You can obtain more information about relaxation techniques from the resources listed in Appendix B.

Using Imagery Techniques

Imagery, or *visualization* — for example, picturing a pleasant situation or scene — is a great technique that can help you manage your back pain successfully. In this section, we use the terms *imagery* and *visualization* interchangeably.

Imagery is nothing magical. In fact, you engage in imagery every day: When you daydream or dream while sleeping, you are actually engaging in imagery. Imagery is also used in athletic activities. You may imagine in your mind's eye the golf ball landing on the green before hitting the shot, or the basketball going through the hoop before making the free throw.

Day-to-day life offers ample evidence of the truth of this phenomenon. Think about what happens when you watch a scary movie. During the course of the movie, your heartbeat may increase, your palms become sweaty, and your breathing may accelerate. All these very real physical reactions occur in response to something that is not real. The movie simply activates your imagination, and your brain responds, not knowing whether the monster is in the room or on the screen.

Practicing imagery

As you develop your imagery exercises, you need to decide which imagery approach works best for you. Remember that imagery is a natural process and that you are always in complete control. Think of imagery as if you are the director of a movie — you can project whatever image you want onto your mental screen.

As you develop your own imagery exercises, keep the following in mind:

- **Prerecord your imagery exercise:** Prerecording your imagery exercise on audiotape can help a great deal in terms of your regular practice and making the imagery experience as robust as possible.

TIP

Your first task is to write out your imagery script, including the places where you'll pause. Consider recording the breathing techniques from earlier in this chapter before the imagery exercise. Then record the script onto a tape for use in regular practice. When making an audiotape of this type, read through the script very slowly and pause often. Speak in a calm, comforting, and steady voice. Let your voice flow in a smooth and somewhat monotonous manner, without whispering.

✔ **Use a familiar image:** Our clinical experience, as well as a number of research studies, suggests that patients who use images which are quite familiar to them have more success with this technique. Generally, people have an easier time of conjuring up all aspects of the image if it is something that they have actually experienced. So, choose a beach or forest you actually visited (and, of course, a place with pleasant associations). This way, you can have a better experience with all the elements of the image.

The benefits of imagery

Your natural ability to imagine can be used for many beneficial health purposes:

✔ **To enhance physical healing:** Many imagery exercises are designed to activate your body's natural ability to heal itself. Some imagery techniques include thinking about such images as white blood cells attacking germs or injured tissues receiving valuable nutrients from increased blood flow. Imagery exercises can be especially useful in healing a back injury and back pain management. For instance, you cam imagine the muscle around your spine as a bunch of tied up knots that you slowly loosen and undo as a way to decrease muscle tension.

✔ **To provide a method for pain relief:** Imagery can help you actually remove yourself from the experience of pain. Using imagery techniques, you can mentally put yourself in another place to decrease your perception of pain and discomfort.

✔ **To improve sleep:** Sleep disturbances are not uncommon when you're experiencing

back pain. Imagery can promote sleep. Often sleeping imagery involves *passive* techniques in which you imagine your body feeling the physical sensation of relaxing (for example, feeling "warm and heavy").

✔ **To promote muscle relaxation:** This type of imagery involves activities such as imagining your muscles "unwinding" like the knots in a twisted rope, seeing a "ball of tension" in your body dissipate each time you exhale, or feeling your muscles become more "smooth" and loose.

✔ **To provide a distraction from a stressful medical procedure:** Imagery can be effective when you are undergoing an unpleasant medical procedure that causes discomfort or pain. Imagery, in which you "guide" your imagination through a sequence of events such as walking on the beach or down a forest path, is particularly effective for this purpose.

Images developed from your own memories and experiences do not have to contain the entire memory. You can draw from bits and pieces of different memories in order to form a complete image.

✔ **Use all five of your senses in developing the image:** For instance, if you are imagining a beach scene, be sure to notice the view of the ocean and beach, the smell of the salty water, the sounds of the sea gulls and the waves crashing, the salty taste of the ocean air, and the feel of your bare feet walking on the warm sand.

✔ **Use an image that is pleasing to you:** The old adage that "one person's feast is another person's poison" applies to imagery as well. Imagery is a personal and individualized experience. Be sure that your imagery is pleasing to you.

✔ **Sneak up on the image:** Sometimes immediately focusing on an entire image at one time can be difficult. Research by Margo McCaffrey, R.N. suggests that "sneaking up on the image" can be a helpful technique.

"Sneaking up on the image" simply involves constructing it slowly in order to avoid becoming frustrated in creating the scene. For example, if you are using a forest scene as your image, you can begin by imagining that you are at home preparing to go to the forest, or that you are on the way to the forest. You can imagine driving to the trail head, getting out of the car, and slowly walking into the beautiful mountain scene which is your final goal image. Using this technique helps ensure that the imagery is relaxing and that you adopt an attitude of letting it happen, rather than trying too hard. See M. McCaffrey and A. Beebe, *Pain: Clinical Manual for Nursing Practice* (St. Louis: C.V. Mosby, 1989).

✔ **Use one image at a time:** Trying to maintain several images at once is stressful and usually does not accomplish the goal of imagery.

✔ **Precede the imagery with a relaxation exercise:** Although not required, using a relaxation exercise — such as those we discuss throughout this chapter — can greatly improve your use of imagery.

✔ **Each session of relaxation and imagery should total about ten to twenty minutes:** Depending upon your back pain situation, you may have trouble sitting or lying down longer than 10 to 20 minutes, so keep the total time limited in order to stay comfortable. However, a session shorter than 10 minutes doesn't allow you enough time to relax and develop the image. Also, trying to do imagery quickly can cause you to rush and defeat the purpose. As you practice, you may want to go longer than 20 minutes, which is fine.

✔ **Practice the image:** The ability to create a mental image utilizing all five senses may be difficult at first but it does improve with practice. If your images aren't vivid initially, don't worry. As you practice, more details will come into focus, and you'll feel more and more as if you are actually in the image.

The attraction of distraction

Distraction is literally defined as causing a person to turn away from an original focus or attention. Clinical experience and research studies show that distraction can be a powerful technique for managing stressful medical procedures and controlling pain. Distraction techniques involve helping your mind focus on something other than the stressful event. The imagery exercises we discuss in this section may be used as one method of distraction because they serve to keep your mind busy and turn your attention away from pain or a particular situation.

You may have already discovered your own distraction techniques for coping with medical stressors. One study interviewed patients after undergoing an uncomfortable, stressful medical procedure (such as an MRI with back pain) and found that patients employed such distraction methods as counting the holes in ceiling tiles, repeating words or poems, singing and humming, engaging in conversation, and whistling.

Other distraction techniques include staring at a stationary object or a spot on the wall (a focal point), tapping the rhythm to a song with your finger or foot, listening to music, and humor.

✔ **Develop a technique to end your image gradually rather than stopping it abruptly:** One of the most common side effects of using imagery is a slight sense of drowsiness afterwards. You can avoid this by using a technique for ending the image. One of the most common methods is to count silently from one to five. Then, on the last count, you inhale deeply, open your eyes, and say to yourself, "I feel alert and relaxed."

Standard imagery exercises

You can use the following imagery example if you like or develop more individualized and personal ones. In the following example, the series of dots represent places where you pause in order to develop a nice, slow pace to the exercise.

✔ **Passive Muscle Relaxation.** As you feel ready, allow your eyes to slowly close.... Take in a full, deep breath through your nose, allowing your lungs to fill completely. Let the air go all the way in, breathing down into the bottom of your lungs. Notice the cool sensation in your nose as the air rushes in.... Then, breathe out through your mouth while slightly pursing your lips.... Notice that the air you exhale is warm and moist.... Release all of the air in your lungs as you exhale completely.... Slowly repeat this cycle several times.

Allow yourself to relax more and more fully. Begin to focus your attention on your fingers and hands.... Notice the sensations that are coming from that part of your body.... Imagine what it would feel like for your hands and fingers to become more and more relaxed.... Let go of any excess tension you may feel in your fingers or hands.

As you continue to relax and breath peacefully, slowly move your mental attention to the sensations coming from your forearms and upper arms.... As your fingers and hands continue to relax, allow that feeling of relaxation to move into your forearms and upper arms.... You may notice your hands or arms feeling warm or heavy as they relax. Or you may notice them feeling cool and light.... Simply focus on what the relaxation response feels like for you. As your arms continue to relax with every breath, allow the feeling of relaxation to move into your head, neck, and shoulders.... Let your forehead relax completely.... Allow the muscles around your eyes to relax.... As you relax the muscles of your jaw you may notice that your lips separate slightly.... Allow your shoulders to relax completely....

When you are ready, focus your attention on the sensations coming from your stomach and back. Imagine what it would be like for all of the muscles in your stomach and back to unwind and loosen up completely.... It is as if you are inhaling relaxation and exhaling tension with every breath.... As you continue to enjoy this feeling of relaxation, imagine the pleasurable sensation moving into your upper legs.... Notice how the relaxation spreads throughout all the muscles of your legs and feet.... Again, you may notice your entire body becoming heavier and heavier, or lighter and lighter. You may also notice a tingling sensation as part of the relaxation response. These are all normal feelings as part of relaxing.... Simply focus on what the relaxation sensation feels like for you....

The preceding passive muscle relaxation exercise can lead to other imagery scenes such as a beach scene or a pain reduction scene. The following are parts of these types of images that you can expand upon:

- **The Beach Scene:** It is about five in the afternoon on a midsummer day. You're walking along a shady path that opens up to a beautiful and expansive beach. As you walk from the path onto the sandy beach, you notice that it is virtually deserted. The deep and golden sun has not yet begun to set, but it is getting very low on the horizon. The sand is warm and comfortable on your toes, and you notice the taste and smell of the salt in the ocean air. You settle deeply into the comfortable sand dune as you enjoy the sun's reflection off the water.

- **Breathing Out Pain:** Imagine that your breath goes to that part of your body in which you are experiencing pain or discomfort. Each time you breath in, imagine the healthy air flowing to that area of your pain and discomfort. Each breath brings with it a sensation of health and comfort. Each time you breathe out the air, notice the area of pain and discomfort becoming smaller and smaller. As you breathe out, you are exhaling discomfort and pain. Continue to breathe in the relaxation and breathe out the pain.

You can obtain more information about imagery training from the resources listed in Appendix B.

Biofeedback Training

Biofeedback training measures a physical process (your heart rate or brain waves) and immediately reports the information back to you so that you can learn to consciously influence that physical state. Biofeedback can measure a variety of things including:

- **Skin temperature,** which is influenced by blood flow beneath the skin
- **Galvanic skin response (GSR),** which is the electrical action of the skin due to sweat gland activity
- **Muscle tension**
- **Heart rate**
- **Brain wave activity**

The purpose of monitoring the preceding physical states is to develop the ability to control them. For instance, if muscle tension is contributing to your back pain, monitoring tension and learning how to decrease it can help relieve your pain. If anxiety is a problem, then monitoring heart rate and galvanic skin response can help you decrease anxiety. Monitoring any of these systems can help you achieve a general state of relaxation.

Humor, health, and back pain

"A cheerful heart is good medicine." Proverbs 17:22

Laughter and humor are not only fun but can improve your mood, reduce emotional tension, exercise your cardiovascular system, and promote social interactions. Beyond these obvious benefits, research shows that there may be a physiological basis for the conclusion that laughter is good medicine. Studies demonstrate that laughter can provide such health benefits as decreasing pain sensitivity, improving sleep, and boosting your immune system.

As suggested by Drs. David Sobel and Robert Ornstein, you can use humor for health as follows — see D.S. Sobel and R. Ornstein, *The*

Healthy Mind, Healthy Body Handbook (DRx Publishing, 1996).

- Expose yourself to humor through such things as films, joke books, and television.
- Keep a humor journal in which you record funny thoughts or experiences.
- Tell a joke and be able to laugh at yourself.
- Look for the funny side of a stressful situation. Sometimes laughing about a stressful situation is the only control you can exert; so, you may as well have fun with it.
- Spend time around happy, optimistic people.

Biofeedback training is a painless, noninvasive procedure involving placing electrodes on the skin to monitor the muscle to be retrained. This may be an area of soreness, spasm, or suspected muscle imbalance. The computer connected to the electrodes then measures the amount of electrical activity, related to tension, present in the muscle, as shown in Figure 12-4. You can see the amount of "tension" on the monitor and begin to learn to decrease it. Your brain learns how to decrease the muscle tension simply by having the feedback available.

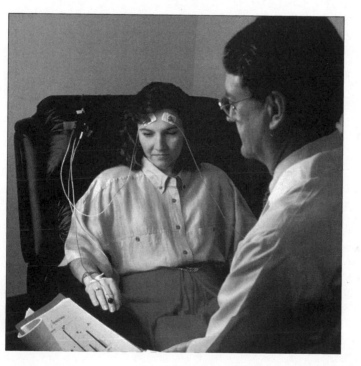

Figure 12-4:
Not a crazy science experiment, but rather a patient undergoing biofeedback training.

Despite the wide use of biofeedback training for back pain relief, there are very few well-controlled scientific studies on the effectiveness of this treatment. It is unclear whether the positive results often seen are due to actual treatment effects of decreased muscle tension, giving the patient a sense of increased control over the pain, or some other reason. Increasing the difficulties of gathering definitive evidence is the fact that patients often report a reduction in their tension and pain levels even when the computer doesn't measure any changes. Regardless of these technical issues, many patients report benefits from biofeedback in terms of improved control of their back pain. We think that makes it worth a try.

We recommend a short trial of biofeedback (5 to 15 sessions) if muscle tension appears to be part of your back pain problem or if you're anxious about your symptoms.

Train your brain

Just like the rest of your nervous system, messages get transmitted through your brain by tiny electrical signals. Special electrodes can measure the activity of millions of nerve cells in your brain all at once. The result of this recording is called an electoencephalogram (or EEG). The EEG looks like a series of waves going up and down depending upon your brain's activity. The pattern of brain wave activity indicates different states (anxious, agitated, relaxed, and so on).

Dr. Stephen Sideroff of the UCLA School of Medicine explains that neurofeedback helps you attain control over your brain waves and that, in turn, can help you be more relaxed and decrease your sensitivity to pain. The training uses a computer monitor that gives you both visual and auditory feedback. Similar to other forms of biofeedback, you can learn to change the frequencies of various wave patterns through this feedback. Using this training, brain activity can be normalized, you can become more relaxed, and your pain sensitivity can be reduced. See Appendix B for more information.

The essential feature of biofeedback training is rapidly teaching the patient to relax without needing the equipment. This is most often done through relaxation training and the use of practice with relaxation audio tapes at home. You can obtain more information about biofeedback training from the resources listed in Appendix B.

Biofeedback can be abused by practitioners who require too many sessions and keep patients dependent on the biofeedback machines. Some research even indicates that the biofeedback machine itself may not be necessary and that the same result can be achieved through relaxation training. Even so, we find a significant effect for the patient of being able to "see" the changes occur as learning takes place.

Here's a Suggestion: Hypnosis

Hypnosis is a natural state of focused concentration that can make relaxing and controlling your mind and body easier. This fascinating technique has seen cycles of acceptance and rejection since the time it was discovered by Franz Anton Mesmer, considered the father of hypnosis, more than 200 years ago. Currently, hypnosis is widely used to treat many psychological and medical conditions, including back pain. It can also be a useful tool to help patients manage stressful medical procedures such as nerve blocks and MRIs, and as a preparation for spinal surgery.

Hypnosis for spinal problems is best performed by a licensed healthcare professional such as a psychologist or physician. After you pick up the hypnotic skills from a professional, you can use self-hypnosis to duplicate the effects.

The hypnotic process involves the following:

- ✔ **Relaxation:** In hypnosis, relaxation is first induced. This usually includes relaxed breathing similar to the exercises we discuss earlier in this chapter.

- ✔ **Imagery:** Relaxation exercises and healing imagery help to deepen the level of hypnosis. Often, the hypnosis professional uses special imagery to help deepen your level of relaxation. Examples include having you imagine going down some steps, an escalator, or an elevator.

- ✔ **Suggestion:** The hypnosis professional presents *hypnotic suggestions* that address specific needs. Suggestions may include such things as control of the back pain or control of the stressful medical procedure. Examples of possible suggestions include the following:

  - Breathing comfortably and deeply makes you stronger.

  - You feel calm and relaxed. You have nothing to worry about. You can set your troubles aside until you heal.

  - You will sleep soundly.

You can make specific suggestions a part of your back pain management program by repeating the suggestions when you practice during your relaxed breathing and imagery exercises. If you choose to give yourself hypnotic suggestions, a process known as *self-hypnosis,* be sure to make the suggestions realistic. Realistic suggestions can be something like "When I tell myself to relax, I will notice less back pain," "I will feel more and more confident throughout the day," and "Each time I hear the phone ring I will feel more relaxed."

You may notice there is an overlap among the relaxation response, cue-controlled relaxation, and hypnosis. They all have similar features that you can combine into an effective pain management program.

We know of no reported cases of harm resulting from hypnosis. If you're interested in using hypnosis as part of your back pain management program, we recommend that you seek professional help from a licensed healthcare professional such as a psychologist or physician. This person should have special training in hypnosis dealing with medical problems, such as back pain or managing stressful medical procedures. The World Health Organization (WHO) suggests that hypnosis should not be performed in certain cases such as with patients with psychosis or other psychiatric conditions.

You can obtain more information about hypnosis from the resources listed in Appendix B.

Seven hypno-myths

Widespread misconceptions about hypnosis (particularly perpetuated by stories in the media and movies) have limited its use in clinical and professional settings. Seven of the most common misconceptions include (based on G.J. Pratt, et al., in *A Clinical Hypnosis Primer* [La Jolla, CA: Psychology and Consulting Associates Press, 1984]):

✔ **Hypnosis is a state of deep sleep or unconsciousness:** Hypnosis is actually a state of relaxed attention in which you can hear, speak, move around, and think independently. Your brain waves in a hypnotic state are similar to those when you're awake. Reflexes, such as the knee reflex, which are absent when sleeping are present when you're hypnotized.

✔ **You must be gullible, weak-willed, or passive to be hypnotized:** In actuality, the opposite is true. Because their powers of concentration are better, individuals most responsive to hypnosis tend to be more intelligent, creative, and strong-willed. The primary factor in benefiting from hypnosis is a strong motivation to participate.

✔ **Hypnosis allows someone else to control your mind:** This is probably not only the biggest misconception about hypnosis but also the one that keeps people from pursuing and benefiting from hypnosis. You cannot be hypnotized against your will. Once hypnotized, you cannot be forced to do something you find objectionable.

✔ **You may not be able to come out of a trance:** Actually, becoming hypnotized is more difficult than coming out of hypnosis. If left alone and hypnotized, you will become alert and awake naturally in a short period of time.

✔ **Under hypnosis, you will give away secrets:** When hypnotized, you're aware of everything that happens both during and after hypnosis; unless you want to accept and follow specific suggestions for amnesia. Thus, you can't be forced to express secrets that you would be unwilling to divulge if not under hypnosis.

✔ **You probably cannot be hypnotized:** Although some people are more responsive than others, almost everyone can achieve some level of hypnosis and can benefit from it with practice. Challenges to hypnosis include such things as trying too hard, fears or misconceptions about hypnosis, and unconscious desires to hang on to troublesome symptoms. A licensed practitioner can help you overcome these stumbling blocks.

✔ **Hypnosis is a quick, easy cure-all:** This misconception is due to extravagant and inaccurate claims regarding hypnosis. Such claims are detrimental and result in a loss of credibility for the overall practice.

Part IV
Rehabilitation

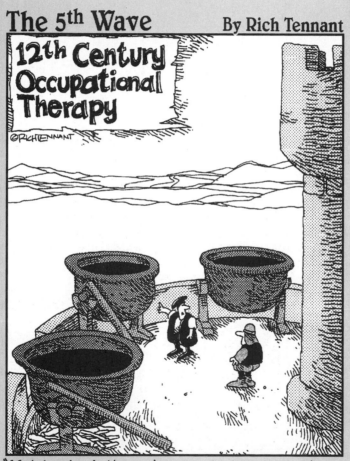

The 5th Wave   By Rich Tennant

12th Century Occupational Therapy

©RICHTENNANT

"Well, here's what's causing your back problem. It's having to tip these vats of boiling oil onto the storming hordes. Is there a lighter substance you could be using?"

In this part . . .

Even if you never pinpoint the exact cause of your back pain, your doctor (or other healthcare professional) will devise a treatment program for you. By following your doctor's recommendations, you can manage your pain and return to all your normal activities. However, carrying out the treatment plan is up to you.

This part is hands-on. We tell you what things your doctor is likely to ask you to do, we help you design a solid back exercise program, and we give you tip after tip of things that you can do on your own. We also throw in a few nifty back products that can help alleviate pain, or at least make you more comfortable.

Chapter 13

The Importance of Posture

*W*hen we talk about *posture,* your first thought may be remembering being told as a child to "Stand up straight," or "Don't slouch." Your parents knew that good posture keeps your back healthy, but a healthy spine involves more than standing at attention.

Posture can be divided into two categories:

✔ **Static posture** is the position of your body when you're stationary. Examples of static posture are standing and sitting.

✔ **Dynamic posture** is the position of your body as it moves. Examples of dynamic posture are walking, bending, and lifting.

Understanding what healthy static and dynamic postures look and feel like may help you prevent back pain episodes from occurring as well as manage your back pain when it does occur. Throughout this chapter, we help you identify when your posture is unhealthy, and we tell you what you can do to make it better.

Sizing Up Static Postures

Even though you're not moving, static postures can place unnecessary pressures on your spine if you assume an unhealthy position. Without a doubt, you spend a great deal of time standing, sitting, and lying down during a typical day. Understanding how to be in these positions comfortably may play an important role in your total back health.

Standing up for yourself

As an individual, you have a unique standing position that is efficient, comfortable, and healthy for your back. The ideal standing posture supports your body in a balanced, upright alignment with minimal use of muscle energy and no perception of strain.

Examining your standing position

A good way to assess your current standing posture is to stand sidewise in front of a full-length mirror.

If you have another mirror available, you can place the two mirrors at an angle so that you can look straight ahead into one while getting a side view of yourself from the other. Using two mirrors helps you avoid having to turn your neck to the side to observe your posture.

As you look in the mirror, allow yourself to assume a posture that is an exaggeration of your normal standing posture. For instance, if you tend to slump your shoulders, slump them more. Or, if your stomach tends to stick out, push it out more. Although your exaggerated posture is not your everyday posture, it can help you identify problems as you go through the following list. As you assume your exaggerated posture, ask yourself these questions:

- **Are my knees locked or bent?** Your knees should be relatively straight, but not entirely locked.

- **What's going on with my lower back, pelvis, and abdomen?** Ideally, your waistline (representing your pelvis) is fairly level: Your lower back exhibits only a mild curve and your abdomen is "tucked in." This is a position of a *pelvic tilt,* as we describe in Chapter 14. We give you more tips on how to achieve this position later in this chapter.

- **Are my shoulders slumped over?** Ideally, your shoulders are not rounded forward and slumped over. Generally, your shoulders should be in a straight line with your torso.

- **Are my head and neck tilted forward from my shoulders?** Your head should be fairly centered over the top of your chest and in a level position. Your neck should appear fairly straight, with a slight forward curve.

As you check yourself out in the mirror, you may notice some unhealthy aspects of your standing position. See whether your stance has any of these features:

- **The military stance:** This is the stance that you probably assumed as a child when you were told to "Stand up straight." In this position, you stand as straight, tall, and rigid as you can (refer to the first example in Figure 13-1). Even though the military stance may look good, it is not

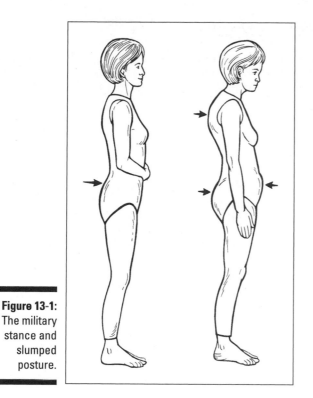

Figure 13-1:
The military
stance and
slumped
posture.

healthy for your back. It can actually cause your lower back to curve more (causing your stomach to stick out) and your head to tip backwards over your neck, which strains the ligaments and muscles of your upper back.

✔ **Slumped posture:** In the slumped posture, your head is tilted forward, your shoulders are slumped forward and down, and your stomach sticks out, increasing the curve of your lower back (refer to the second example in Figure 13-1). Slumped posture may irritate and put excessive strain on structures in your lower back. The tilted head and curve of your spine can also cause neck pain.

Adopting healthy standing habits

After assessing your posture using the mirror technique we describe earlier in this chapter, you can adopt a healthy standing posture, as shown in Figure 13-2.

A healthy standing position may feel uncomfortable at first, especially if you've been "practicing" an unhealthy standing posture for 30 or 40 years (or more). Rest assured that you can develop a better standing posture and that doing so can help you feel better.

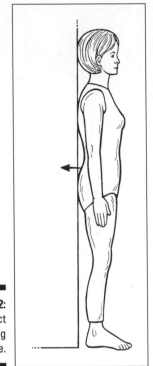

Figure 13-2:
Correct
standing
posture.

To practice a healthy standing position, stand against a wall with your heels approximately two inches away from it. (Standing slightly away from the wall allows room for your buttocks.) Do a *pelvic tilt* — move the small of your back toward the wall by tilting your pelvis. Keep your knees slightly bent and making sure not to lock them in a straight position.

The *pelvic tilt* is a healthy standing posture. Practicing the pelvic tilt exercise, as demonstrated in Chapter 14, can help strengthen your abdominal muscles, which help you maintain a healthy posture while standing.

The following guidelines can help you develop a healthy standing posture:

✔ If you must stand for an extended length of time, be sure to use a footrest. Most people are likely to stand with both feet on the ground as the "incorrect standing posture" in Figure 13-3 shows. The second part of Figure 13-3 shows how simply placing one foot up on a short stool or stack of books gives you a healthier standing posture. Be sure to alternate your feet every once in a while. This position reduces the curve in your lower back and decreases the strain on the facet joints in your lower spine.

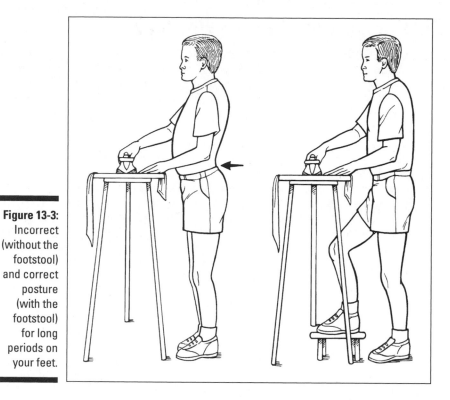

Figure 13-3:
Incorrect
(without the
footstool)
and correct
posture
(with the
footstool)
for long
periods on
your feet.

✔ When you are standing for an extended period of time, try to avoid bending or leaning over. For instance, bending over a counter while working in the kitchen places quite a bit of strain on your lower back. If you must maintain a bent or leaning posture for an extended period of time, bend your knees slightly to absorb some of the strain on your lower back.

✔ Wearing high heels increases the curve of your lower back, possibly placing more strain on it.

✔ You can decrease strain on your back simply by placing commonly used household items at eye level. Doing so helps you avoid bending and leaning throughout the day as you use these items.

✔ If you are standing for a long period of time, try to move about and alternate your position frequently. You can change positions to keep your muscles and spine relaxed.

As you become more aware of your unhealthy habits, you can begin to substitute them with healthy habits and decrease your back pain problem.

Sitting on the dock of the bay

If you're like many people, your job and daily activities involve a great deal of sitting. Some studies of United States workers indicate that more than half of today's workforce is made up of people who sit during most of the workday. Unfortunately, research has only recently paid attention to the types of stress that extended sitting places on your spine.

Sitting, especially in the same position for an extended time, is thought to be more stressful on your back than standing, lying down, and, in some cases, lifting. Sitting is stressful on your back because your muscles have to work harder to keep you upright and stable. If your back is not well supported while sitting, your muscles tire quickly. When this happens, you tend to slouch in order to give your muscles a break. Slouching causes your center of gravity to shift forward and your pelvis to rotate backward, which puts your lower spine in an unnatural position. This unnatural position means that the discs of your lumbar spine must bear the weight of your entire upper body unevenly. Studies have shown that pressure between discs increases with sitting. Although certain well-designed chairs can help decrease distress on your spine, people often sit on the edge of their chairs out of habit, which defeats the design of the chair.

Assessing your sitting posture

As with standing, it's important to assess your own sitting posture so that you can determine whether it is unhealthy and what to do to change it. First, sit in a chair and allow yourself to exaggerate your normal, comfortable sitting posture. To help you exaggerate your posture, try moving yourself away from the backrest and allowing your entire upper body to "let go" and relax. You can either imagine a side view of your posture in this position, or you can look at yourself in a mirror as described in the section "Examining your standing position."

While you are in an exaggerated posture, assess it for the following characteristics:

- **Slumped posture:** If your sitting posture is slumped, then your lower back tends to be rounded out, your chest is depressed inward, your upper back is rounded forward, and your neck is arched backward in order to keep your head level. Your head probably feels like it is projecting out in front of your chest rather than being balanced above your torso.

  Slumped sitting greatly increases the pressure on your lower back. In this position, the middle and upper joints of your neck tend to be crammed together because of the increased backward arching. The muscles of your neck and shoulders are also overworked in this position. After sitting in this position for an extended period of time, you may also notice difficulties straightening up into a standing position.

✔ **Tense sitting:** In this type of sitting, you sustain a certain level of tension in your muscles due to your back being unsupported, being in a stressful situation, or simply by habit. We find that people who engage in tense sitting are often not even aware that their bodies are tense until we monitor their muscle tension through biofeedback (see Chapter 12).

Tense sitting can occur either in conjunction with unhealthy posture or even with healthy posture for sitting. For example, you may maintain a healthy posture while having virtually all the muscles in your body in a state of low-level tension. Becoming aware of muscle tension and practicing relaxation, as we describe in Chapter 12, can help reduce this muscle tension.

✔ **Sitting too long:** If you're like most people, your most common posture in the course of a day is sitting. The problem is that your body is not designed to be in this position for an extended period of time without any movement. Even when you are sitting correctly, it's important for your body to move about regularly. Sitting for long periods of time puts strain on the structures of your back, including the muscles.

✔ **Crossing your legs:** Another common posture is to cross your legs while sitting. For short periods of time, this posture is comfortable and allows your muscles to relax. Staying in this position for an extended period of time, however, causes some of the same problems as sitting too long. Also, crossing your legs while sitting in a chair that does not provide support causes you to hold a slumped or tense sitting posture.

First, become aware of whether you tend to cross one leg over the other consistently. If you do, pay attention to switching legs regularly to help cancel out the imbalance in your posture it causes. Also, pay attention to keeping your legs uncrossed as an alternate position, when you can.

Sitting pretty (and healthfully)

The first rule of healthy sitting is to become aware of whether you experience any of the unhealthy patterns we describe in the preceding section. The following healthy sitting guidelines can help you sit more comfortably and reduce the stress on your lower back:

✔ **Position your pelvis:** Healthy sitting involves paying attention to the position of your pelvis — it affects the position of your lower back and your entire upper body. To position your pelvis properly, move your tail bone back as far as possible in the chair with your upper body tilting forward (imagine tucking your buttocks into the back of the chair). After you tuck your pelvis into the back of the chair, bring your body into the upright position. This move repositions your pelvis into a healthy posture. You may need to adjust this position slightly (for example, rolling your pelvis slightly forward or backward) until it feels good for you. Figure 13-4 shows the entire process.

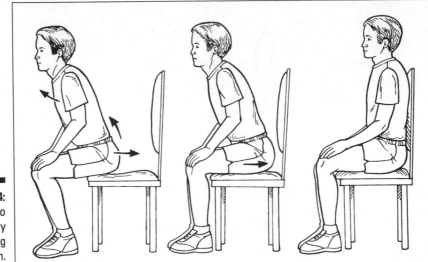

Figure 13-4:
Getting into
a healthy
sitting
position.

✔ **Keep your pelvis, chest, and head aligned:** As you become familiar with a healthy sitting position, you can change your position frequently and keep stressful forces on your lower back to a minimum. The primary goal is to keep your pelvis, chest, and head aligned whether you are sitting back, up, or forward. Thus, as your upper torso leans backwards, your lower body should tilt upward to maintain the proper posture or angle between your upper and lower body. A healthy sitting posture at a workstation (including angles for the elbows and knees) is shown in Figure 13-5.

- If you're sitting with your pelvis back in the chair (and your upper body slightly backward), you may want to place a small footstool (these are often designed with a slant to fit your feet) or telephone book under your feet (see Figure 13-5). Using a footstool helps raise your knees slightly above hip level, which puts your pelvis in a healthy position.

- If you're sitting on the edge of a chair, you should keep your knees lower than your hips, move your legs wider apart than normally, and position one foot forward and the other foot farther back on the floor.

✔ **Use a good chair for sitting:** Getting a chair designed for healthy sitting is very important, especially if the chair is one you sit in for extended periods of time on a regular basis, such as in the office. The more you sit, the more your body takes on the shape of the particular chair you use (although changing positions frequently does help). The sidebar "Buying a chair" talks about how to shop for a good chair.

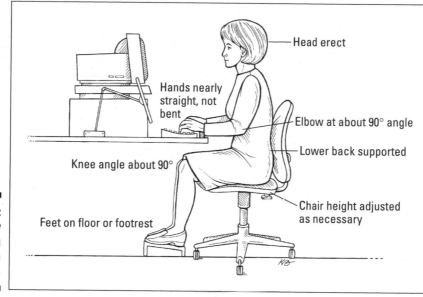

Figure 13-5:
Healthy
sitting
position at a
workstation.

In figure: Head erect · Hands nearly straight, not bent · Elbow at about 90° angle · Lower back supported · Knee angle about 90° · Chair height adjusted as necessary · Feet on floor or footrest

✔ **Use proper supports in unsupported chairs:** If you must use a chair that does not provide proper support, you can take steps to improve your sitting position. First, if the chair does not provide support for your lower back, you can put a rolled-up towel or small pillow across the small of your back to help keep the natural curve of your lower back while sitting. Many lumbar support pillows are available commercially. Second, if you tend to sink down in the chair (as often happens in worn-out restaurant booths or soft couches), you can put a folded towel or even a book under your buttocks to fill in part of the seat you are sinking into.

✔ **Take breaks and move around:** One of the best ways to keep your back healthy while sitting is to take frequent breaks and move around. Taking breaks is sometimes quite a challenge, though, especially when you become engrossed in a task and don't realize that you have been sitting in the same position for two or three hours.

If you're prone to sitting too long, try setting a timer for about every 30 minutes to remind you to get up and take a break. When you do, try such activities as walking around or doing some of the back stretching exercises as we describe in Chapter 14.

Buying a chair

When you go shopping for a chair that will be kind to your back, you're confronted with an overwhelming number of choices. Gathering information about the various types of chairs available is important. Choosing the best chair for you depends upon such factors as your body shape and the type of work you'll be doing while sitting in the chair. You can gather valuable information from a physical therapist or a well-trained salesperson at some of the stores that specialize in these products.

The following are some general guidelines related to getting a proper chair:

- A good chair supports and maintains your spine in its natural shape as you sit in it. Particularly, the curve in the small of your back should not be either excessive or reduced, but rather maintained in its natural form. If you're not using a chair at a desk, try one that tilts back slightly with a footrest to support your feet.

- The height of a desk chair should be easy to adjust. If the seat of your chair is too high, the curve of your lower back increases to a unhealthy position, your feet almost dangle, and the muscles of your upper and lower back strain. Most good chairs have a hydraulic mechanism for changing height.

- Most high-quality (another word for *expensive*) office chairs provide specific lumbar support for your lower back — something you want to be sure you get. When the muscles of your lower back are not properly supported, they contract. This low-level muscle contraction, when sustained for many hours, causes muscle fatigue and spasm, which may lead to pain.

- Avoid a chair that you "sink into. "A soft chair actually causes the muscles in your lower back to be more tense as they attempt to provide your spine with the support that the chair lacks.

- The chair should have a curved front edge. A sharp edge that puts undue pressure on your upper legs can decrease blood flow to your thighs and lower legs.

- The chair should transfer the majority of your weight to your buttocks rather than your thighs while you are sitting. Some chairs are so straight-backed that they "push" your upper body forward, causing pressure on your thighs.

- If possible, choose a chair with armrests. Armrests can help decrease the tension and fatigue on your neck and shoulders. Armrests can also help you stabilize the chair when making the transition from sitting to standing and vice versa.

Lying down on the job — and anywhere else

One of the first areas to assess for healthy lying down is your mattress. If your bed is too soft, your spine must rely on your muscles and ligaments to keep its natural shape, which may increase your muscle tension and the stress on your spine.

Simply putting a piece of plywood between the box spring and a soft mattress is not a reasonable solution for a soft mattress. Doing so simply creates a situation in which your soft mattress sags into the hard surface of the board. Also, if you place a board between a good mattress and a good box spring, you can cause the mattress to wear out sooner than it normally would. Using a board under a mattress can help if you have a good mattress on a sagging metal frame that provides inadequate support for the mattress. The sidebar "Choosing a mattress" covers how to shop for a mattress that is kind to your back and comfortable to you.

Assuming that you have a decent mattress, you can still cause more back problems by lying down in an unhealthy position. Although a great deal of advice is available on proper sleeping positions, the research is not all that clear on whether different sleeping positions impact your back pain. It appears that sleeping positions may be an individual thing: For you, it may be important, and for others, it doesn't matter.

The important thing is for you to be comfortable. You can try some of the following tips while keeping in mind that your overall comfort is the most important thing while sleeping:

The following healthy sleeping guidelines can help you sleep more comfortably:

- **Solving the "sleeping on your stomach" problem:** Lying on your stomach increases the curve of your lower back. If sleeping on your stomach is a difficult position for you to give up, you can try to straighten out your spine by placing a pillow or towel under your pelvis.

- **Solving the "lying flat on your back" problem:** Lying flat on your back with your legs outstretched increases the curve in your lower back and may cause stress to that area. If you prefer to sleep on your back, you can support your hips by bending your knees and placing a pillow underneath them. Doing so places your lower back in a natural, comfortable position.

- **Using the fetal position:** Like many other people with back pain, you may find that the fetal position is the most comfortable. In this position, you lie on your side with both hips and knees bent equally. Placing a small pillow between your knees may make you even more comfortable. Also, you can put a small pillow under your head and neck to fill the space between your head and shoulders.

- **Being aware of the couch:** Your couch can be thought of as a small-size soft bed. Therefore, lying down on the couch (to sleep, watch TV, or read) may cause the same stresses as lying on a soft bed. Instead, you may want to lie on your back on the floor with your knees bent over some pillows or a chair. You can place a small pillow under your neck to support your head.

Choosing a mattress

As with chairs, you have a great many choices when it comes to buying a mattress. Mattresses and box springs are designed to work together to provide support for your body. The following are some bed tips that can help you make a good choice:

- ✔ A well-made mattress and box spring set should last between 7 and 15 years, depending upon the quality and how you take care of the bed.

- ✔ Part of proper bed maintenance includes turning the mattress end to end and upside down every month for the first few months so that it adjusts evenly to your body weight. After that time, you should turn the mattress every couple of months. Of course, if you have a back pain problem, get help to turn your mattress and use proper lifting techniques (see "Opting for healthy lifting and bending" later in this chapter).

- ✔ Because you spend about one-third of your life in bed, you should invest wisely.

Unfortunately, it is not possible to "try out" a bed for a few weeks to decide whether you like it. Even so, you should spend five or ten minutes seeing how it feels in the showroom.

- ✔ Most mattresses use a spring coil construction. Mattresses can vary greatly in terms of the number and thickness of the coil springs. Other mattresses use things like "baffles" and other design features in conjunction with the coil springs. Finding a bed that is comfortable for you is a highly individual choice. Just like Goldilocks (remember her?), you want a mattress and box spring set that is neither too firm nor too soft but provides enough support to keep your back in its natural curves.

You can get specific information about different features available in beds from your specialty mattress store. You can even review this information with your physical therapist or other healthcare professional.

Dealing with Dynamic Postures

Dynamic postures involve the position that your body takes while it is in motion. Movement requires that your muscles, ligaments, and bones all work together in a coordinated fashion. Proper dynamic posture is moving in such a way that places the least amount of stress on your body to complete the required motion, and using the posture most likely to prevent injury to your spine.

Paying attention to proper dynamic posture is a little more difficult than static posture because you may not have as much time to plan ahead. In the following sections we review healthy dynamic postures.

Walking tall

If you're like most people, you spend a great deal of time walking. Not only is walking your most basic form of transportation, it is also good exercise.

Checking out your walk

As with standing and sitting, you need to evaluate your walking posture for unhealthy habits. A good way to assess your walking is to watch yourself walk from the side either in a mirror or in the reflection from a store window as you head down the sidewalk. As with assessing your sitting and standing postures, exaggerate your movements. If you tend to walk with your head forward or your stomach out, do it more. If you walk fairly loose and casually, loosen up even more. And, if you walk in a fast and more rigid manner, exaggerate those qualities. Understanding what type of unhealthy patterns of walking you are likely to engage in helps you correct them and adapt the healthy walking patterns we describe later in this chapter. The following walking patterns may put more stress and strain on your lower back:

- ✔ **Stomach-out walking:** Increasing the forward arch of your lower back, along with stretching out your lower stomach, causes your pelvis to tilt forward as you walk. This alignment can aggravate low-back pain. In this unhealthy walking posture, you tend to walk with your abdomen leading far out in front of the rest of your body.

- ✔ **Head-forward walking:** Head-forward walking is generally caused by looking down at the ground directly in front of you while you walk. When you do so, you also put your chest in a depressed position, which puts stress on your neck, shoulders, and lower back due to unhealthy alignment. It also results in poor breathing and overall endurance.

- ✔ **Loose walking:** Loose walking is characterized by a tendency to be wobbly and engage in extraneous movements of the joints of your legs, arms, neck, and back. You may be prone to this type of walking if you have a tendency toward joint instability and muscle weakness.

- ✔ **Stiff walking:** The opposite of loose walking, stiff walking can be due to such things as being tense and uptight, having a fear of falling or re-injury, or a concern about making your back pain worse. People who stiff-walk look like they have a corset or brace from their neck to their lower back (or, in more severe cases, from their head to their toes). This type of walking looks very robotic. Stiff walking causes your muscles to work too hard as they try to prevent any motion from occurring around your neck and back. This muscle overactivity tends to pull all the joints of your body together in a state of total body contraction. Stiff walking causes you to tire rapidly due to the amount of energy you expend to maintain rigidity. Stiff walking actually increases the probability of injury and pain flare-ups in your back.

- ✔ **Heel-pounding walking:** This type of walking pattern is characterized by a heavy heel- or foot-strike each time you take a step. It is as if you are pounding out a beat as you walk. This type of walking sends shock waves from your foot to your leg and up to your pelvic and spinal joints. The shock waves create extra stress throughout these body parts. This type of walking is usually developed through habit and is more exaggerated when you are in a hurry, emotionally upset, barefoot, or wearing heels that are either hard or spiked.

✔ **Stress walking:** Stress walking is characterized by taking fast, choppy steps with your upper body held forward and your head down. Similar to the heel-pounding walk, stress walking transmits shock waves from your lower body to your pelvis and spine. Stress walking also includes total body muscle tension, especially around areas of pain such as your lower back. You may stress-walk as a matter of habit, and it gets worse when you are under emotional pressure.

Becoming a healthy walker

Before attempting to adopt healthy walking, identify whether you are exhibiting any of the unhealthy patterns we describe in the preceding list. Doing so helps you focus your practice of the healthy walking techniques. The following are some tips for healthy walking:

✔ **Make your pelvis level:** Keep your hips and lower back in a stable position as you walk. This tip involves doing a slight pelvic tilt as you walk. Imagine a straight line coming directly out of the center of your stomach or bellybutton as you walk. Generally, that line points at a downward angle. In order to get a slight pelvic tilt, imagine shifting the line up slightly. Doing this slight shift while you walk results in a tilt that brings your pelvis to a more level position and makes walking easier on your spine.

✔ **Release tension as you walk:** Use breathing techniques (we describe some in Chapter 12) while you walk to keep the muscles of your body, including your back, in a fairly relaxed state. Each time you slowly exhale while you walk, think about releasing any tightness that is holding your body rigid. This technique can help prevent stiff walking, stress walking, and heel pounding.

✔ **Keep your head light:** This one may sound funny, but thinking in terms of keeping your head and neck light on your shoulders as you walk can help you walk better. You should allow your head and neck to relax and simply "ride," centered and at ease, on top of your shoulders. This helps decrease any tension you may be carrying in your shoulders or neck.

✔ **Use a soft landing:** As you walk, think about your legs moving smoothly and your feet landing softly as they touch the ground with each step. The most important thing is to reduce the amount of pounding and theshock waves generated throughout your lower body. Simply focus on landing each foot more quietly, softly, and smoothly. As you practice smooth walking, you can do it efficiently while walking as fast as you desire. The type of shoes you wear can also help you walk more smoothly and decrease heel pounding. Especially good shoes are running shoes with a snug heel, room for the front of your foot, proper support, and excellent cushioning.

✔ **Walk smoothly:** As you walk, allow your head and trunk to be relatively upright in order to maintain a healthy posture and improve breathing. Limit any extra movement of your hips, and keep your head from tipping forward, backward, or off to either side. There should not be much twisting between your various body parts, such as your upper and lower body. Visualize your face, shoulders, chest, and hips being in a relatively stable position and facing forward while you walk. Healthy walking involves a smooth motion of the muscles of your legs and feet. An excellent resource for walking is *Walking Yourself Healthy* by S. Brourman (Hyperion Books, 1994).

Buying a pair of shoes

The type of shoes that you wear might impact how your back feels while standing and walking. Your shoes determine how your lower body interacts with the ground in two ways: positioning and transmission of shock waves. No matter what type of shoe you wear, from athletic to dressy, pay attention to some basics of healthy footwear:

- The part of the shoe that surrounds your heel (the *heel counter*) should be stable enough to hold your heel upright while you stand and walk. The heel counter should be made of reinforced and durable material. If the heel counter is weak, it allows your heel to move either inward or outward, increasing strain on your legs and your lower back.

- The *heel* of the shoe is the platform under the bones of your heel. The heel should be well padded to absorb shock and be elevated slightly above the ball of your foot. The width of the heel should be equal to the width of the heel counter in order to help distribute the shock from walking. Hard and dense heels increase the amount of shock transmitted from your legs to your back. Spiked heels can cause an unstable effect on the legs that may increase muscle tension in the lower back.

Beware of heels that have worn unevenly, because they can cause you to walk and stand unevenly and increase the stress on your spine.

- A shoe should have a reasonable amount of flexibility at the ball of the foot to provide a smooth motion while walking. If the sole of the shoe is too rigid, it doesn't "give" when you try to bend it. A stiff sole is not only uncomfortable but causes you to walk in an unnatural and unhealthy way. On the other hand, a sole that is too flexible and soft does not give your feet the proper support that they need (especially in the arches).

- The *insole* is the inside, flat part of the shoe and extends from the toes to the heel. The insole of your shoe should provide comfortable support to the heel and arch of your foot. As you look inside one of your shoes, you should see a contour that matches the shape of the bottom of your foot. A good insole has a buildup of material to support the arch. If this buildup is not there, your feet tend to fall inward and flatten out, putting your lower body into a state of misalignment that increases pressure on your lower spine.

- The *toe box* is that part of the shoe that surrounds your toes. The toe box should allow enough room for your toes to move around while providing adequate support on either side of your foot. The side support should prevent your toes from moving excessively from side to side. The toe box should not in any way cramp or crunch your toes. You should not feel the top of your toes hitting the roof of the toe box.

Lift and bend, one-two-three

Lifting and bending are among the movements most commonly associated with the onset of back pain problems. Think about your typical day: On any given day, you probably bend over and lift items multiple times. If you use unhealthy bending and lifting techniques, you place a significant amount of pressure and strain on your spine each time you perform these motions. Repeated bending and lifting can cause a back pain problem even when the things you lift are very light. Using good, healthy lifting and bending techniques is one of the most effective ways to reduce stress on your lower spine.

Identifying unhealthy bending and lifting

As you read through the following characteristics of unhealthy bending and lifting, identify the ones that you commonly engage in. Identifying your bad habits helps you be aware of them and helps you more readily adapt the healthy techniques:

 ✔ **Feet too close together:** One of the most common unhealthy moves in bending and lifting is keeping your feet too close together. If your feet are closer than shoulder-width apart, you have poor leverage, you are unstable, and you tend to round out your back as you bend and lift.

 ✔ **Bending at the waist:** Another unhealthy move is to bend at the waist while keeping your knees and hips straight and arching your lower back forward. An example of this move is shown in Figure 13-6. Bending at the waist is probably the most common and stressful lifting. It's even worse if you do this move while twisting at the same time.

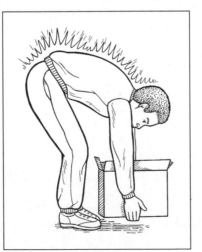

Figure 13-6:
Incorrect
lifting
posture.

- ✔ **Lifting and carrying an imbalanced load:** Examples of this common, unhealthy manner of bending and lifting include carrying a heavy suitcase in one hand with nothing in your other hand or carrying a heavy purse on one shoulder.

- ✔ **Lifting objects that are too heavy for you:** Lifting, or trying to lift something that is really too heavy for you places strain on your back. One tip-off that this problem is occurring is when you attempt to lift something in one big "strained" move.

- ✔ **Lifting and bending repetitively:** This common problem in work injuries involves repetitive bending and lifting within a short period of time without taking breaks. If you are getting tired from repetitive bending and lifting, you tend not to use a good technique, which increases your chances for injury.

- ✔ **Lifting objects away from your body:** Another common mistake is attempting to lift an object away from your body. It may surprise you to know that lifting a 10-pound weight that is 14 inches from your body rather than being close to it is equivalent to lifting approximately 150 pounds as far as your spine is concerned. Lifting even a light object that is extended from your body causes a great deal more pressure on your spine than lifting close to your body.

Opting for healthy bending and lifting

If you follow healthy bending and lifting guidelines, you can avoid a back injury and help prevent any future flare-ups of back pain. Most of these tips involve using common sense and not taking any shortcuts:

- ✔ **Place your feet at proper width:** When bending and lifting, your feet and knees should be at least shoulder-width apart if side by side. If your feet are front to back, you should be in a wide step position. Positioning your feet in this manner helps you bend at the hips and keeps your back relatively straight and unstressed.

- ✔ **Use your legs when lifting:** When bending and lifting, you should bend your knees so that your legs take on most of the stress. Squat with your chest sticking out forward and your buttocks protruding out backward. This position helps keep your lower back straight and subjects it to a minimal amount of pressure from lifting (see Figure 13-7).

- ✔ **Keep the weight of the object close to you as you lift:** When you lift and carry an object, keep it as close to your body as possible. When lifting a heavy object from a full squat, keep your elbows and forearms in contact with the insides of your thighs. Doing so helps you to be more stable and transfers more weight off your spine and onto your legs — a proper *squat lift.*

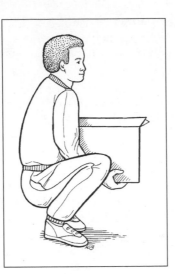

Figure 13-7:
Preparing to lift properly.

Another good lifting technique is the *half-kneeling lift,* as shown in Figure 13-8. This technique is good for lifting such items as suitcases or groceries. Simply go down into a half-kneeling position and then push up with both legs to a standing position. Keep your upper torso straight as you lift. If the object is heavy and doesn't have handles, you can use the half-kneeling position to roll it onto your raised thigh. From this position, you can hold the item close to your chest and push up with your legs from the half-kneeling position to standing. Be sure to keep your back straight throughout this maneuver.

✔ **Carry a balanced load:** If doing so is an option, balance your load on both sides of your body. For instance, rather than carrying a heavy bag of groceries on one side, divide it into two lighter bags that you can carry on either side. If that isn't an option, switch sides frequently so that you balance the stress on your body across both sides. If it is a very heavy load, avoid carrying it on one side or the other altogether. Instead, choose some other option, such as using a cart or getting help from another person. Remember, it may take a little more time to do it right, but helping to prevent a back injury is well worth a few extra minutes.

✔ **Avoid lifting objects above waist-level:** If possible, avoid lifting objects above your waist and certainly above your shoulders. Both of these postures increases the curve of your lower back, placing unnecessary strain on the muscles, ligaments, and joints in that area. You are much more vulnerable to a low-back injury when you lift an object above waist- or shoulder-level.

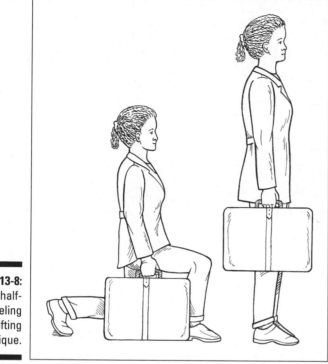

Figure 13-8:
The half-
kneeling
lifting
technique.

✔ **Avoid twisting when lifting:** One of the worse things you can do is twist while you are lifting an object. Twisting and lifting places a great deal of pressure on the structures of your lower back and can result in a disc herniation or other injury (see Chapter 3). Instead, pick up the object using one of the healthy techniques we describe earlier in this chapter, and then turn your entire body to face the place where you want to put the object you're lifting. Doing so avoids putting any twisting motion on your back.

✔ **Push rather than pull:** In most cases, pushing a heavy object is easier than pulling it. Pushing a heavy object along the floor places less stress and strain on your lower back.

✔ **Pay attention to maximum lifting guidelines:** In very general terms, the maximum lifting load for women is 30 to 35 pounds, and for men, it is about 50 to 60 pounds. If you are attempting to lift an object that is much heavier than these guidelines, consider getting help or using some other technique to avoid lifting, such as a cart or dolly.

Tips for safe lifting

If you are like most people, you simply go up to the object you need to lift, bend over, grab it, and pick it up. You do so without thinking or planning ahead because, in most cases, you can get away with it and not injure your back — underscoring that your spine is a strong and amazing structure. Unfortunately, the one time you don't get away with it and sustain a back injury can be the start of an ongoing back pain problem. The following safety tips (in addition to the ones discussed in this section) can help you avoid a back injury:

✔ **Keep your arms straight:** If possible, keep your arms as straight as possible when lifting an object while using your legs. Your arms should be straight down, not straight out. With your arms straight down, your leg muscles (which are much stronger) do most of the work.

✔ **Lowering objects is also stressful:** It may seem easier to lower an object rather than lift it, but lowering objects can also cause stress and strain on your lower back. Many people injure their backs when they lose control of a heavy item while lowering it then grab for it in an effort to prevent it from hitting the floor.

✔ **Lift at a moderate speed:** Lifting an object at a moderate speed, neither too fast nor too slowly, is best. Lifting too fast can cause you to use unsafe techniques and lose control of the object. On the other hand, lifting too slowly can also make you unstable and increase the time that your lower back is under stress. You should lift at a moderate speed using a smooth motion.

✔ **Beware of odd-shaped objects:** The most difficult type of object to lift is one that is oddly shaped, heavy, and has no handles. If you are faced with lifting such an object, be very careful. If possible, either get help from someone else or find a way to avoid lifting the object altogether.

✔ **Plan ahead:** Before doing any type of lifting, your most important safety technique is to plan ahead. Unfortunately, this is also the step that is most often skipped. Planning ahead helps ensure that you use proper lifting techniques or avoid lifting an object that is more likely to cause a back injury altogether.

Chapter 14

Exercising Your Way to a Healthy Back

. . . .

In This Chapter

▶ Combining aerobic and back exercises for the best workout

▶ Understanding the do's and don'ts of exercise

▶ Getting on your way to a better back: The exercise program

. . . .

A regular back exercise program helps keep the muscles of your back and abdomen strong and flexible, giving your back support and decreasing the chances of a back pain attack. Even if you have never had a significant back pain problem, back exercises can help prevent future back pain attacks. Exercising can also ease a chronic back pain problem.

This chapter presents a comprehensive back exercise program, which you should combine with some type of aerobic conditioning such as walking, bicycling, or swimming. A good way to be sure that you get both is to alternate your back exercise program and aerobic conditioning every other day.

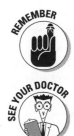

General aerobic conditioning is important not only for your back, but also to improve muscle tone, relieve stress, and improve sleep habits, along with other benefits as we discuss in Chapter 7.

Consult with your physician prior to starting any type of exercise program, including a back conditioning program. Doing so is especially relevant if you haven't been exercising for quite sometime or if you have risk factors that need to be monitored. General medical risk factors requiring evaluation prior to beginning an exercise course include heart disease and high blood pressure.

Exercise Tips

To make your exercise program safe, beneficial, and effective, heed the following tips and warnings:

✔ **Set aside time to exercise:** Plan ahead. Make sure you can be private and undisturbed during your exercise time. The exercises in this chapter take anywhere from 15 to 30 minutes to complete and do you the most good when you do them three to five times per week.

If you choose to exercise in the morning, it's a good idea to walk around a little bit after getting up before doing your back exercises.

✔ **Exercise on a firm but comfortable surface and wear loose-fitting clothing:** Carpeting or an exercise pad provide a good exercise surface. It is not a good idea to do your exercises on a very soft surface such as a bed or couch. Soft surfaces do not provide your body or your back with adequate support to do the exercises safely.

✔ **Move slowly and smoothly:** Especially when you're just starting this type of exercise program, concentrate on making your movements easy and graceful. Take a brief rest between each exercise if you find that helps you complete the program.

✔ **Progress at your own pace:** When beginning an exercise regimen, do the number of repetitions that cause you little, if any, discomfort. Increase your repetitions using the quota system (see Chapter 7). For example, start out with two or three repetitions of a particular exercise and add one repetition per week until you reach your goal.

At no point during your back exercise program should you feel that you are straining beyond what you feel are your physical capabilities or to the point of significantly increasing your pain.

✔ **Make a public commitment:** Tell as many people as possible about your exercise program. Making a public commitment to exercising helps ensure that you follow through with this healthy idea.

✔ **Get an exercise buddy:** An *exercise buddy* is someone with whom you make a commitment to exercise. Setting up a regular exercise time and regimen with a buddy makes you accountable to someone else, and therefore less likely that you will cancel or drop your exercise program.

✔ **Focus on your breathing:** As you progress through your back exercises, focus on healthy breathing as we discuss in Chapter 12. Try to breathe evenly and deeply. Avoid holding your breath or taking shallow breaths.

A good technique to ensure healthy breathing is to inhale slowly through your nose and exhale slowly through your mouth.

Exercise Warnings

Just as there are specific tips to enhance your exercise program, there are also specific warnings:

✔ **See a physician if you experience numbness in the genital area, sexual problems, or muscle weakness in your legs:** If you experience any of these symptoms contact your doctor immediately. Refer to Chapters 5 and 21 for in-depth information on these, and other, warning signs.

✔ **Do not start your exercise program in the middle of an acute attack:** Wait until any acute back pain calms down before starting on the exercises (unless your doctor recommends exercise). This waiting period may be anywhere from one day to three weeks after onset of the pain.

✔ **Expect some soreness and discomfort:** If you haven't stretched or strengthened your back muscles for some time, those muscles will naturally be sore after you start exercising them. For this reason, start your exercise program at a very low level such as two or three repetitions of each exercise. Your exercise routine will become more enjoyable and less painful as you do it regularly.

If at any time you experience a dramatic increase in pain, any of the warning signs discussed previously, or any new type of pain, see your physician. If at any time you have difficulty doing the exercises due to an increase in your back pain, stop that exercise for a few days then return to it at a lower level of repetitions.

✔ **Don't bounce:** Bouncing is fine if you are Tigger in *Winnie-the-Pooh* but there is no place for it when doing back stretching exercises. Stretch using a gradual, smooth, and slow motion. Do not stretch beyond what is comfortable for you. Using a bouncy or jerky motion puts you at risk for muscle and ligament injury.

Your Back Exercise Program

Our back exercise program is excellent for strengthening and stretching the muscles of your lower back and abdominal area. The exercise routine takes 15 to 30 minutes depending on how many repetitions of each exercise you do. Begin the program slowly and gradually work up to higher repetitions as you become stronger.

The following sections outline a general back conditioning program. Your doctor or healthcare advisor may recommend a slightly different program, depending on your symptoms. The first part of the exercise program is done while you lie on your back. After that, you move to lie on your stomach, then a position on your hands and knees. You do the exercises in the last portion while standing.

Exercise 1: Pelvic tilt

This exercise not only stretches your abdominal and back muscles and increases the flexibility of your pelvis (hips), it also really lets you "get down" — on the floor, that is (see Figure 14-1).

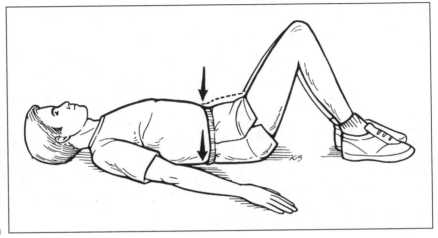

Figure 14-1:
Pelvic tilt to stretch abdominal and back muscles while increasing flexibility.

1. **Lie on your back with your knees bent, your feet flat on the floor, and your arms at your sides. Your feet should be about hip width apart with your knees slightly closer together than your feet.**

2. **Flatten the small of your back against the floor.**

   This causes your hips to tilt upward.

3. **Hold this position for a few seconds and then relax.**

   Breathe in as you do the pelvic tilt and breathe out as you relax.

Begin with two or three repetitions as you are able and gradually work your way up to between five and ten repetitions.

Exercise 2: Single leg pull

This exercise stretches the muscles of your hips, lower back, and buttocks.

1. **Lie on your back with one leg bent, one foot flat on the floor, and your other leg extended straight out (see Figure 14-2).**

2. **Use the arm on the same side to pull the bent knee to your chest in a continuous motion while keeping your lower back and other knee pressed against the floor.**

3. **Hold this position for a count of five seconds.**

4. **Lower your leg to the starting position.**

   Repeat this movement two to five times with the same leg.

5. **Switch legs and repeat Steps 2, 3, and 4.**

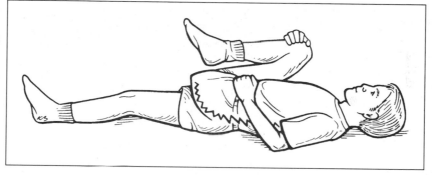

Figure 14-2:
Single leg pull to stretch your hip, lower back, and buttocks.

Exercise 3: Double knee to chest

This exercise stretches the muscle of your hip area, buttocks, and lower back.

1. **Lie on your back with your knees bent, your feet flat on the floor, and arms at your sides. Your knees should be enough distance apart to be comfortable for you (usually fairly close together for this exercise).**

2. **Raise both knees, either one at a time or together, to your chest. You can use your arms to help pull your knees to this position.**

   Use your arms to gently pull your knee(s) to your chest, as shown in Figure 14-3.

3. **Hold for a count of five ("one rhinoceros, two rhinoceros"...).**

4. **Lower your legs one at a time to the floor and rest briefly between each repetition.**

Begin with two or three repetitions and work your way up to between 10 and 20 repetitions.

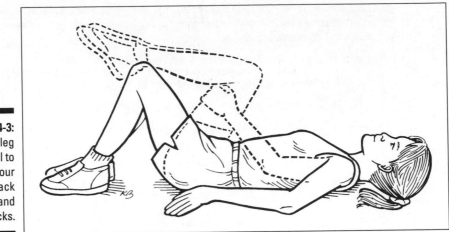

Figure 14-3:
Double leg
pull to
stretch your
lower back
and
buttocks.

Exercise 4: The pretzel

This exercise is great stretch for your inner leg and hips.

1. **Lie on your back with your knees bent.**

2. **Cross one leg over the other at the knee.**

3. **Take hold of your bent leg and pull both legs toward your chest (see Figure 14-4).**

4. **Hold the stretch for five seconds.**

5. **Release and uncross your legs. Repeat this stretch using your other leg.**

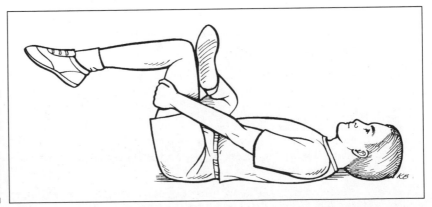

Figure 14-4:
You won't
get tied in
knots with
the pretzel
stretch.

Exercise 5: Pelvic lift

This exercise is designed to strengthen the muscles of your buttocks.

1. **Lie on your back with your knees bent, your feet flat on the floor at about shoulder width, and arms at your sides.**

2. **Raise your hips bit by bit as shown in Figure 14-5.**

   It is important that you raise your hips without arching your back. Focusing on not sticking your stomach out can help you keep from arching your back. Try to keep a straight line from your shoulders to your knees.

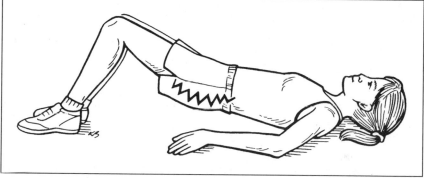

Figure 14-5:
Pelvic lift to strengthen buttock muscles.

3. **Hold for a count of five (you know how it goes).**

4. **Slowly lower your hips to the starting position.**

Begin with two or three repetitions and gradually work up to five.

Exercise 6: Partial sit-up

Strengthen your abdominal muscles with this sit-up.

1. **Lie on your back with your knees bent, your feet flat on the floor, arms at your sides.**

2. **Cross your arms over your chest and, keeping your middle and lower back flat on the floor, raise your head and shoulders off the floor slightly, as shown in Figure 14-6.**

   Raise up only far enough to get your shoulder blades just off the floor. It's okay if you can't go up too far at first.

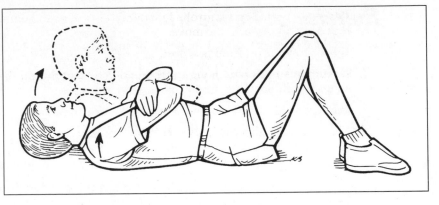

Figure 14-6:
Partial
sit-up to
strengthen
the
abdominal
muscles.

3. **Hold this position for just a few seconds.**

   As you get stronger, you can work up to holding the position for five to ten seconds.

4. **Gently return your upper body to a relaxed position on the floor.**

Start out with two or three repetitions and gradually increase to between five and ten repetitions.

Exercise 7: The oblique sit-up

This variation of the sit-up works your obliques.

1. **Lie on your back with your knees bent and your feet flat the floor. Place your hands behind your neck.**

2. **Lift one side of your upper back off the ground and rotate your elbow toward your opposite knee (see Figure 14-7).**

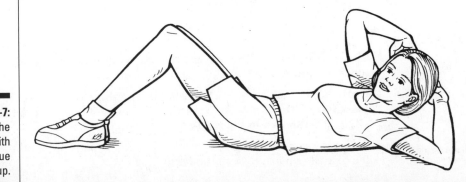

Figure 14-7:
Doing the
twist with
the oblique
sit-up.

Move slowly and in a controlled manner. Don't use momentum from your arms to perform the move.

3. **Return to your original position.**

4. **Repeat this motion with your other arm leading the way.**

Exercise 8: Hamstring stretch

The backs of your thighs are worked in this stretch.

1. **Lie on your back with one leg bent, one foot flat on the floor, and your other leg extended straight out.**

2. **Lift your straight leg (the one flat on the floor) upward until you feel a slight stretch along the back your leg.**

   Use your hands to grasp behind your knee and help raise and hold your leg, as shown in Figure 14-8. If you have difficulty reaching your knee with your hands, place a towel under your knee or thigh and pull up on that. It's okay to have a slight bend at the knee in the leg that's being stretched — keeping it perfectly straight is a feat reserved for Olympic gymnasts.

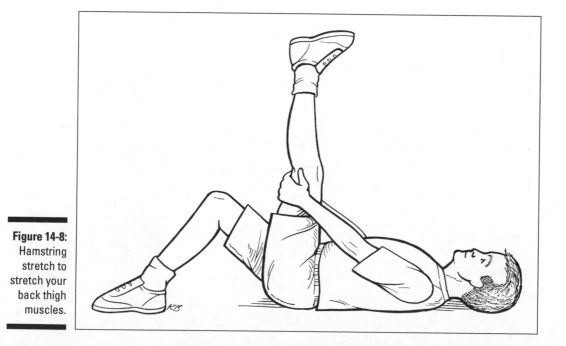

Figure 14-8:
Hamstring
stretch to
stretch your
back thigh
muscles.

3. **Hold that position for 20 seconds.**

4. **Let your leg relax unhurriedly down to the floor.**

5. **Switch legs and repeat Steps 2, 3, and 4.**

Begin by doing two or three repetitions on each leg and work your way up to about five repetitions.

Exercise 9: Press-up

This exercise stretches the muscles of your abdominal area and provides some upper body strengthening.

1. **Lie on your stomach with your feet slightly apart, place your face near the floor or rest your forehead on the floor, and your hands palm-down at face level, as shown in the first image in Figure 14-9.**

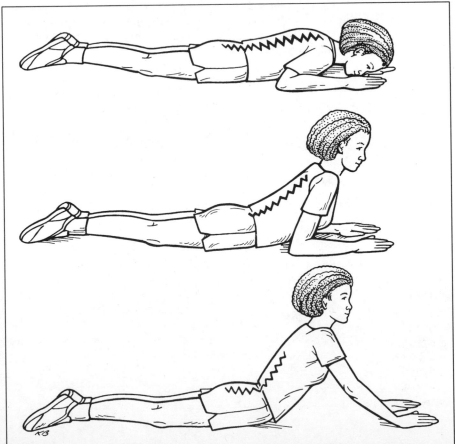

Figure 14-9: This press-up exercise stretches and maintains your lower back curve.

2. **Use your arms to gradually push the top half of your body to a resting position on your elbows (as the second image in Figure 14-9 shows).**

   You may feel tightness in your lower back or abdomen. Try to hold this position for 20 seconds or more until you feel comfortable.

3. **Push up with your arms (with your hands on the floor) as high as possible while keeping your hips and legs flat on the floor (as demonstrated in the third image in Figure 14-9).**

   Remember to keep your back relaxed.

4. **Hold the position for 20 to 30 seconds.**

5. **Slowly lower yourself back to the floor.**

Initially, do two or three repetitions, and work your way up to about five repetitions.

Exercise 10: Cat and camel

As the first image of Figure 14-10 shows, this exercise also begins a new starting position. This exercise is designed to strengthen your back and abdominal muscles.

1. **Start on your hands and knees with your weight evenly distributed and your neck parallel to the floor, as shown in the first image of Figure 14-10.**

2. **Arch your back upward by tightening your abdominal and buttock muscles, letting your head drop slightly, as shown in the second image in Figure 14-10.**

3. **Hold for a count of five.**

4. **Let your back sag gently toward the floor while keeping your arms straight, as shown in the third image in Figure 14-10.**

   Keep your weight evenly distributed between your legs and arms.

5. **Hold for a count of five again.**

Do two or three repetitions initially and work your way up to about five repetitions. Be sure to make your movements slow and smooth.

Inhale through your nose as you arch your back and exhale through your mouth as you let your back sag.

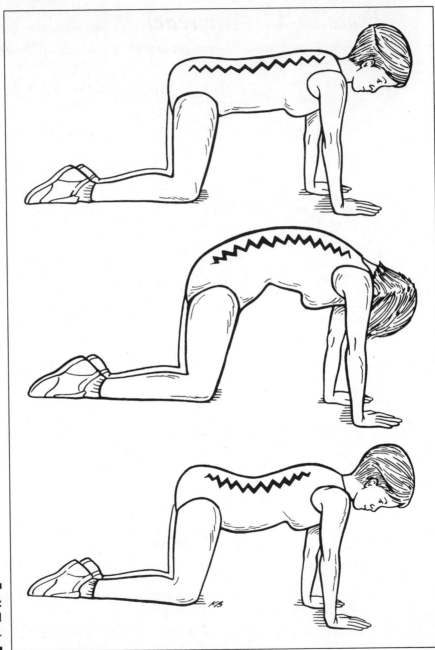

Figure 14-10:
The cat and
camel.

Exercise 11: Arm reach

This exercise is designed to strengthen the muscles of your shoulders and upper back.

1. **Start on your hands and knees with your weight evenly distributed and your neck parallel to the floor.**

2. **Stretch one arm out in front of you being careful not to raise your head (see Figure 14-11).**

   Keep your weight evenly distributed between your knees and the one arm on the floor.

3. **Hold the arm reach for a count of five.**

4. **Return to the starting position.**

5. **Do five repetitions with the same arm.**

6. **Switch to your other arm and repeat Steps 2 through 5.**

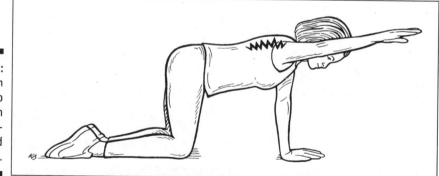

Figure 14-11: Arm reach to strengthen your shoulders and upper back.

Exercise 12: Leg reach

This exercise is designed to strengthen the muscles of your buttocks.

1. **Start on your hands and knees with your weight evenly distributed and your neck parallel to the floor.**

2. **Slowly extend one leg straight out behind you and hold it parallel to the floor, as shown in Figure 14-12.**

   Your foot may be pointed or flexed — whichever is comfortable for you.

As you extend your leg, don't let your back, head, or stomach sag. And make sure no one is behind you when you do this move.

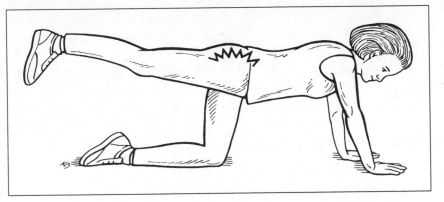

Figure 14-12:
The leg stretch strengthens your buttocks muscles.

3. **Hold this position for a count of five.**

   You may be able to hold this pose for two or three seconds when you start out. This is typical when first practicing this exercise and your endurance will improve as you gain strength and stability through practice.

4. **Return to the starting position and repeat this movement three to five times.**

5. **Switch legs and repeat Steps 2, 3, and 4.**

Exercise 13: Alternate arm and leg reach

If you find this challenging exercise difficult initially, practice Exercises 11 and 12 for a few weeks before adding this one to your routine.

1. **Start on your hands and knees with your weight evenly distributed and your neck parallel to the floor.**

2. **Extend one leg backward, parallel to the floor (as in Exercise 12), and at the same time reach forward with the opposite arm (refer to Exercise 11).**

   Try to make your leg, torso, head, and arm form a straight line parallel to the floor, as shown in Figure 14-13.

3. **Hold this position for a count of three.**

4. **Lower your leg and arm to the starting position.**

5. **Repeat the same movements with your other side.**

Work your way up to five repetitions of this exercise on each side.

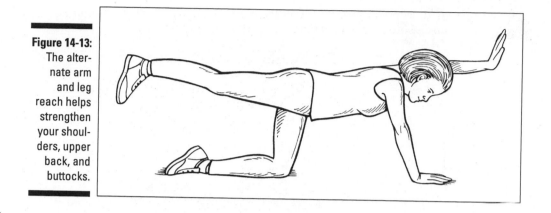

Figure 14-13:
The alternate arm and leg reach helps strengthen your shoulders, upper back, and buttocks.

Exercise 14: Wall slide

Although the name sounds like a new dance step, the wall slide is actually a valuable exercise that strengthens your back, hip, and leg muscles (as you will be able to tell after you start doing it!).

1. **Stand with your back against a wall and your feet shoulder-width apart as shown in the first image in Figure 14-14.**

   Place your hands on your hips or let your arms hang at your sides, whichever is more comfortable. Keep your head level by focusing directly in front of you.

2. **Slide gracefully down the wall into a crouched position with your knees bent to about 90 degrees. (See the second image in Figure 14-14.)**

   If you have trouble going down this far, slide down halfway.

3. **Hold this position for a count of five.**

4. **Slide smoothly up to your starting position.**

Initially, you may be able to complete only two or three repetitions of this exercise. Your goal is to complete five repetitions while holding the crouched position for one minute each time. Work up to this goal gradually.

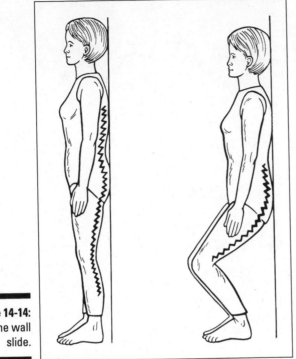

Figure 14-14:
The wall
slide.

Exercise 15: Side stretch

After completing Exercise 14, step away from the wall and remain standing (that sounds like a command out of a Dragnet episode).

This exercise stretches the muscles in your back and sides.

1. **Stretch one arm over your head and bend your upper body to the opposite side in a fluid motion, as shown in Figure 14-15.**

   Put your other hand on your waist, and do not twist your body as you bend.

2. **Hold the stretch for a count of five.**

3. **Return to the starting position with your hands and arms at your sides.**

4. **Repeat this movement five or more times.**

5. **Switch to the other side and repeat Steps 1 through 4.**

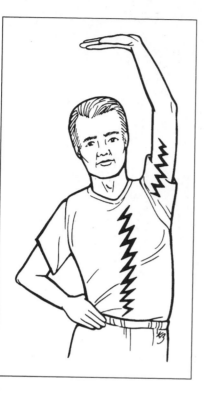

Figure 14-15:
Stretch the
muscles of
your back
and sides
with the side
stretch.

Do this stretch with a flowing movement and avoid jerking.

Exercise 16: Back arch

Your shoulder, back, and hip muscles get attention with the back arch.

1. **Stand up straight with your feet shoulder-width apart and pointing directly forward. Place the palms of your hands on your lower back as shown in Figure 14-16.**

2. **Gently breathe in and out until you feel relaxed.**

3. **Bend your upper body backwards, supporting your back with your hands and keeping your knees straight.**

   Try exhaling as you lean back.

4. **Hold the arch for a count of five.**

5. **Gradually return to your starting position.**

Repeat three to five times.

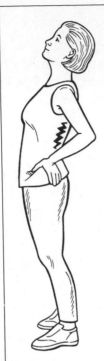

Figure 14-16:
Back arch to
stretch your
shoulder,
back, and
hip muscles.

Cooling down after your exercise program can help you get ready for the rest of your day. Cooling down exercises can be as simple as taking a short walk to keep your muscles loosened up.

Chapter 15

Products for Better Back Health

● ●

● ●

*A*ll postural products have one important function: to support your spine and extremities in a natural, neutral position. This promotes pain relief, recovery, and tolerance to future episodes by lowering the harmful joint stresses that come with poor posture.

For example, when you stand, you assume a posture that keeps your spine in more of a comfortable, neutral position. This neutral position is why most people stand up and walk around to find relief from sitting, sleeping, or reclining in poor postures.

When you're not standing, the furniture you use dictates your posture. Because you probably spend the majority of your time off your feet, proper furniture is an important and effective area to focus on. The posture of your back during rest or activity is a choice and gives you power over your spinal health.

Postural products come in two basic designs:

> ✔ **Products that support from the ground up:** These products include properly designed office chairs, adjustable beds, and recliners, for example. These pieces of furniture are user-friendly because of their adjustability and, by design, provide the greatest benefit. However, these products are typically more expensive than other postural products.

> ✔ **Support-enhancing products that you add to poorly designed furniture:** These products are mainly portable supports used for your lower back and neck. The main advantages of these products are affordability and transportability; they may be your only options when you're away from home or the office.

This chapter covers various products that may be helpful for your back pain problem. These products are grouped by *lifestyle zones,* or those areas where each type of product comes into play. Given the numerous sources of helpful back pain products, we can't list every manufacturer and retailer. However, Appendix B lists a wide variety of Internet sites that you can check out for more information.

Since thousands of back pain products are available, you may wonder how we selected the ones in this chapter. Well, we didn't. We went to the folks at Relax the Back — a U.S. chain of retail stores specializing in products designed to help back pain — and asked them to suggest some of their most popular items.

For Your Home

Home is where you expect to find relief from the day's stresses. Your home environment, however, may actually stress your back to an even greater degree.

Beware of sofas and recliners that you "sink" into. This position rounds out your back and brings your chin into your chest. You trade a couple of minutes of early bliss for pain and tightness that cause you to shift and eventually get up. A good guideline to follow is that you should feel as good, if not better, when you get out of your furniture than when you got in.

Home is where you have great control over the health of your back.

BackSaver Zero-Gravity Stress-Free Recliners

The recliners in the BackSaver Zero-Gravity Stress-Free line are anatomically engineered. The recliners use a NASA-designed reclining position to relieve back pain, reduce muscle tension, and increase circulation, which lowers stress on your heart and promotes healing. This position maintains an optimal angle between your torso and thighs to support the natural spinal curves in a variety of positions, from upright through fully reclined.

Built-in lumbar supports are available that you can either inflate manually or automatically. One automatic unit is the BackCycler CPM. The BackCycler automatically cycles to inflate and deflate the back support, thereby moving the lumbar region to enhance circulation, flexibility, and health. The recliner places cervical support behind your neck rather than your head. This neck support decreases a forward-head position, which rounds out your spine and contributes to back, neck, and arm discomfort. Recliners can be both manual and powered.

BackSaver Rolling Ergo Desk Mate

Working or reading while using a recliner or adjustable bed is comfortable with the BackSaver Rolling Ergo Desk Mate. This height-adjustable work surface has a split-top design. One side stays level for such items as a beverage and pens, while the larger side tilts. Placing your laptop, pad, or book on a tilted surface means that you don't need to bring your head forward and down, or strain your eyes; the materials are closer to you and at a proper height.

Relax the Back Zero-Gravity Massage Lounger

The Relax the Back Zero-Gravity Massage Lounger is a massage chair based on NASA-inspired reclining designs. The chair includes the therapeutic benefits that users get from the BackSaver recliners (which we mention earlier in this chapter), but also features deep-penetrating massage. You can use both manual and programmed settings for combinations of shiatsu, kneading, and rolling massage.

BackSaver Wonder Cushion

The BackSaver Wonder Cushion is a back support that you add to any non-supportive chair or recliner. The cushion's temperature-sensitive WonderFoam conforms to your back's natural contours, improving your posture while reducing painful pressure.

While You Are Sleeping

Sleep is essential to good health and mental alertness. Back pain is the most common nighttime pain, and many back pain sufferers unfortunately wake up feeling unrefreshed.

When you sleep, you have no conscious control over your posture and may irritate your back if your mattress gives poor support. A good mattress will support you properly no matter how many times you move during the night.

Following are a few products that can support you properly as you sleep.

Relax the Back Pressure Relief Mattress

The Pressure Relief Mattress is made of NASA-inspired, temperature-sensitive material that molds to your body's natural contours. The mattress supports you without allowing your spine to "hammock," a position that commonly occurs with overly soft sleep mattress systems. The conforming surface also decreases the amount of tossing and turning you do on an overly firm mattress by up to 80 percent.

The mattress has a progressive design of support from top to bottom, which eliminates the sinking effect you get with traditional body-conforming systems such as air or water. Unlike coil-spring systems, the Pressure Relief Mattress is perfect for an adjustable bed frame (where you can raise or lower parts of the bed).

Adjustable bed frames

Nighttime and morning pain may result with adverse stress from time spent propped up reading or watching TV in a rounded position. Adjustable bed frames allow for an infinite number of therapeutic positions while awake or sleeping. You may prefer to sleep on your stomach, but you may be able to start sleeping on your back by adjusting the bed to slightly elevate your lower legs and chest. This modified back position puts you in the same low-stress body posture as side sleeping the pressure on your shoulder and thigh that causes you to turn. Split sleep systems allow you to adjust each side of the bed according to personal preference. Various designs may include such things as wireless controls, position memory recall, and wavelike massage.

Tempur-Pedic pillows

Foam chip and feather pillows lose their ability to support your head shortly after you lie on them. If you place your hand under your pillow or head while sleeping, you do so to make up for lost support. Sleeping in this position "shrugs" your shoulder up. You round your back, and you stress your back and neck, making pain in the morning more likely.

The Tempur-Pedic line of cervical pillows uses temperature-sensitive material molded to fill the nape of your neck in all sleeping positions, ensuring support for your upper spine in neutral positions that don't promote rounding out the lower spine. A variety of pillow sizes are available to fit a variety of body types, sleeping habits, and sleeping surfaces.

BackSaver Relax 'n' Read Pillow

The BackSaver Relax 'n' Read Pillow is a high-back, fully adjustable bed pillow equipped with back, neck, and arm support that you can use to sit upright in bed. A moveable lumbar support and adjustable headrest allow you the luxury of moving around without constantly manipulating the pillows to find support. You should use this pillow with a small support under your knees to keep your lower back in proper posture. The Relax 'n' Read pillow is a great addition to a non-adjustable sleep system.

BackSaver Zero-Gravity Bed System

The BackSaver Zero-Gravity Bed System consists of two sectional units of back or leg bed wedges. You can use the bed wedges separately for support or together to create a pain-relieving, zero-gravity position. The wedge sectionals convert to different shapes to adapt to your positioning needs.

For Your Office

If you are like many people, you sit at a desk for countless hours every day. With the wrong workstation equipment, you're liable to experience discomfort and even job dissatisfaction. This section suggests office furniture that can help, not hinder, your back.

Relax the Back Signature Series chairs

A proper seating system begins with a versatile chair that adapts to both you and your task. All Signature Series chairs have height-adjustable backs that place the variable-air lumbar support directly behind your belt line to maintain lumbar curvature. This support keeps your body upright with your head held back, a position that effectively lowers disc pressure throughout your spine when compared to slouching. Contour seat pads decrease seated pressure that would normally cause you to shift frequently.

Chair arms are height-adjustable and pivot in or out with a gentle pull or push. The arms provide upper body support when doing computer work or any task in front of you. Having the upper-body weight placed on the inward-turn arm reduces stresses placed on your wrists and may diminish the likelihood of repetitive strain injuries.

All Signature Series chairs feature a "float" mode: The chair provides support as it follows you when you reach forward or behind. Low-back management/task and high-back executive chairs with adjustable neckrests are available. BackCycler gentle motion lumbar support is also available.

Mid-priced management chairs

The therapeutic features in mid-priced chairs are similar to those found in the more expensive chairs we discuss earlier in the chapter. Features that you should expect on any worthwhile chair include an adjustable back, built-in lumbar support, contour or traditional flat seat, height-adjustable arms, and knee tilt.

BackSaver Executive Chairs

This series is crafted in multiple sizes, each shaped and contoured proportionally to support a wide range of body builds. Each chair is fitted with its pivot point just behind the knees so as not to change the seat-to-floor height when leaning back. Your feet stay on the ground when rocking the chair or when the chair is locked in any position. Adjustable lumbar support, adjustable cervical support, and a contoured seat that promotes circulation play an important role in being comfortable for long periods of sitting. BackCycler gentle motion lumbar support is also available.

Portable back and seat supports

An adjustable, portable back and seat support chair insert can be a useful tool in managing back pain. Use this type of insert as a cost-effective way to enhance a nonsupportive chair. The insert's seat provides firm support that doesn't allow the pelvis to roll, thereby reducing slouching. The back portion of the insert provides soft comfort. The BackSaver WonderFoam BackAide by Relax the Back is an example of such an item.

Changeable-height workstations

A changeable-height work surface is an optimum tool against back, shoulder, and neck problems. In some of these devices, you can raise or lower the workstations to any position between two and four feet by using a small foot pedal and a gentle touch. After you set up the work surface with all your equipment, you can lift or lower the station as you change your body position. Set your monitor directly in front, use a wrist rest with the mouse, and use a headset to work smart.

Ergonomic footrests

An ergonomic footrest, which can lower the occurrence of back problems, is an often overlooked component to a proper workstation. Most footrest products tilt to keep the feet at a 90 degree angle, thereby enhancing blood circulation. But more important, placing the feet on the footrest assures you that you aren't sliding forward. This type of product allows you to sit without crossing your legs to lock yourself in place, which causes "rounding" of the lower back and decreases the benefit of your chair.

While You Travel

You shouldn't have to worry about possible back pain when you travel — for business or for pleasure. As a back pain sufferer, you may see travel as being far way from the security of your practitioners and home. However, with a bit of foresight, the thought of travel can become more secure for you.

Self-inflating back rests

Self-inflating back rests (by Relax the Back and others) assume a tailored fit between any seat back and the small of your spine. The support maintains your body upright, keeps seated disc pressure to a minimum, and allows you to sit longer without discomfort. The pillow folds or rolls to a compact size — small enough to fit in a purse or flight bag. Use this pillow in a car or plane — even at the theater or a restaurant.

Sacro-Ease Commuter Supports

Sacro-Ease Commuter Supports are portable back and seat supports custom-shaped to fit you at the time of purchase. The seat provides hip and lumbar support and has additional support pads that you can lower or raise. These supports are suitable for long-term placement (in car seats or kitchen chairs) but light enough to use anywhere. You can choose between standard and deluxe models.

Tempur-Pedic Transit Pillow

The chameleon of travel pillows, you can use the Tempur-Pedic Transit Pillow in one configuration for lower back or neck support while sitting in a car, train, or plane. You can then unroll the pillow to form a sleeping pillow when you get to your hotel. Temperature-sensitive material molds to your body's natural contours in whatever situation you use it.

While You Stay Healthy and Fit

Exercise is the cornerstone of your body's health, and education is the cornerstone of a safe exercise program. If you're smart when beginning your exercise program, you're less likely to suffer setbacks.

Always check with your doctor before initiating any home therapy or exercise program.

Bodytech Golf Belt

The Bodytech Golf Belt is a back support that has six times the compressive force of traditional back belts. Developed within the medical community, this belt splints the back while providing abdominal compression. Use just one hand on the patented pulley system to adjust compressive force. You can wear the washable belt, designed initially to accommodate the changing positions of a golf swing, under or over your clothes.

Swiss ball

The Swiss ball is versatile, therapeutic, and affordable. Used for spinal rehabilitation first in Germany and Sweden, these balls have been recommended for the last 15 years in the United States.

A library of literature is available for their use — their only limitation is your imagination. Sizes are available for different body types and exercise routines. Ask your doctor about specific exercises for you.

Part V

Resuming Normal Activity and Preventing Future Injury: Work, Play, and Sex

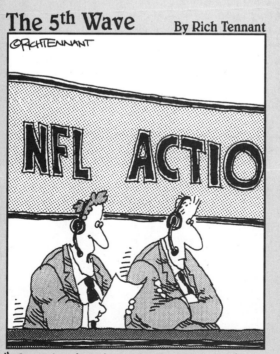

The 5th Wave   By Rich Tennant

"That back injury's come back to haunt number 78. He doesn't have nearly the snap in his end zone that he used to have."

In this part . . .

*B*ack pain permeates every area of your life, including that intimate, behind-closed-doors part. Sooner or later, though, you will be able to return to *all* your normal activities. Doing so, however, can be harder than you think if you fear re-injury or feel like you must go to great lengths to protect your back. That's where this part comes in. We tell you how to keep your back healthy and work to diminish your fears as you return to work — and play.

Chapter 16

Getting Back to Work

• •

In This Chapter

▶ Returning to a risky occupation

▶ Removing roadblocks to your return to work

▶ Planning your return to work

▶ Staying at work after you return

• •

*I*f your back pain has kept you from your job, returning to work can be scary. You may doubt your ability to do your job, especially if your work is somewhat physical, and you may wonder whether you can spend eight hours at work — not to mention your commute — without resting your back.

On the other hand, returning to work can be very exciting. Work gives you a sense of purpose and makes your life more normal and routine. Shedding the discomfort and unpredictability of pain is a relief in itself.

This chapter talks about the pros and the cons of heading back to the job and helps you develop a successful return-to-work plan.

The Purpose of Work

If you're like the average person, you probably spend at least one third of your day pursuing your chosen vocation. Strictly in terms of time commitment, work is a major part of your life. But even more than just time, work gives you a sense of self-esteem and identity (not to mention a paycheck). Arguably, the type of work you do identifies you in society more than any other factor.

A back pain injury that disables you from work isn't just a physical blow to your body, but also a mental and emotional one. The longer you're disabled from work because of back pain, the more your pain affects you emotionally and within your social circles.

You're not alone!

Back pain disability is approaching epidemic proportions. In the United States alone, an estimated 5.2 million American adults are disabled by low-back pain. Of this 5.2 million, approximately one half (2.6 million) are temporarily disabled, and the other half are permanently disabled.

Low-back pain is the most common cause of disability in the working population under the age of 45. It is also the third most common cause of disability in the working population between ages 45 and 65. Studies show that if you have a low-back pain disability, you may be out of work longer as compared to workers disabled from other injuries.

Studies indicate that if you have been off of work because of back pain disability for about six months, the chances of your ever going back to work are about 75 percent. After 12 months, those chances decline to 50 percent. Amazingly, if you have been disabled from work due to back pain for more than two years, your chances of ever returning to work approach zero. Keep in mind that these statistics are based on large groups of injured workers and may not predict what can happen to you as an individual. But knowing these statistics can help ensure that you don't become a "statistic." See G.B.J Anderson, "The Epidemiology of Spinal Disorders," in *The Adult Spine* edited by J.W. Frymoyer, (New York: Raven Press, 1991).

Even if you've been disabled for quite some time because of a back injury, the tips and suggestions in this chapter can help you get back to some type of work.

Identifying Risky Occupations

In this section, we don't cover specific jobs but rather the *types* of activities that you may perform as part of your job that can be risky. If you're working on improving your back problem, this information can help you avoid a future back pain disability. If you're disabled from your job because of a back injury, this information can help you more successfully design a return-to-work program.

Jobs that require lifting and bending

If your job requires heavy lifting, pulling, or carrying, the repetitive motion and strain can lead to lumbar disc disease. (See Chapter 3.) Many studies show a significant association between lifting, pushing, pulling, and low-back pain and sciatica.

Particularly important is the posture that you adopt during lifting moves. As we discuss in Chapter 13, one of the worst positions is lifting while twisting at the same time. Laboratory experiments show that this type of movement can produce tears in the structures that surround the disc. If you lift and twist improperly at work, you can expect to have a two- to threefold increase in the risk of lumbar disc herniation.

If your job involves heavy labor, a number of factors can determine if you have a back injury: the amount of weight you're lifting, the frequency of lifting, and your lifting technique. Your overall physical fitness also comes into play. For instance, if you exceed your overall physical capacity for lifting on a regular basis, your risk of low-back injury increases as much as four times. We discuss a rough guide to lifting in Chapter 13. Although your maximum lifting load is highly variable depending upon your physical condition, generally, the maximum lifting load is 30 to 35 pounds for women and 50 to 60 pounds for men. If you regularly lift objects that are much heavier than these guidelines, watch out. Consider getting help or using some other technique to avoid lifting, such as using a cart or dolly.

If you have a job that requires heavy lifting, check out Chapter 13 on posture. Using proper posture techniques and staying in good physical condition can help prevent back injury. (A good back brace may also help; see Chapter 23.) If you're already disabled from heavy lifting because of a back injury, you need to decide if you will ever be able to return to that type of work. We discuss important issues related to a return-to-work program later in this chapter.

All shook up: Exposure to vibration

Prolonged exposure to vibration, especially that caused by motor vehicles, creates a significantly higher risk for low-back pain problems, sciatica, and disc herniation. Laboratory studies have shown that the frequency of vibration that is stressful to your back is similar to the vibration you experience when riding in a car. If you're exposed to vibration during work, then your risk for developing one of these conditions is two to three times that of the general population, according to studies.

Also, you're at greater risk for a back injury if you commute to work more than 20 miles per day or drive a truck as part of your workday. In fact, if you spend more than half your job driving a motor vehicle, you're three times more likely than the average worker to suffer a herniated disc.

A sitting position places additional stress on your back. (For more on this issue, see Chapter 13.) As your spine is exposed to vibration in the sitting position, your spine is exposed to greater stress. Vibration also fatigues the muscles that support your spine.

If your job exposes you to excess vibration and you have not yet suffered a back pain disability, the information we discuss later in this chapter can help prevent one. You can take steps to reduce vibration to your spine by driving a car with a softer ride, trying not to drive over rough terrain, using proper posture as we discuss in Chapter 13, and using a seat cushion and/or back brace that provides proper support. If you're on disability from a job that exposes you to vibration, you need to take special steps to safely return to that type of work. For more about returning to work, see "Returning to Work" later in this chapter.

Sitting down on the job

If your job requires a great deal of sitting, you have an increased risk for a back injury. Sedentary occupations in general aren't good for your back because sitting puts great pressure on the disc between your vertebrae.

Commuting

Chances are you commute in some manner to work. Commuting by car, bus, train, or subway causes you to be in a sitting position while your spine is subjected to vibration. The following tips can help you as you commute.

- **Watch your position:** Using the healthy posture information we describe in Chapter 13, be sure that your sitting position is upright with your pelvis tucked back. Move your seat up so that you can easily reach the pedals and do not have to stretch your lower extremities. Reclining the backrest about 5–15 degrees can also be helpful.

- **Do some easy commuter stretches:** As you drive, occasionally push your arms straight on the steering wheel to help decompress your lower back and pelvis. You can also periodically arch your lower back forward and away from the back of the seat while doing a slight stretch.

- **Check your seat:** If you're driving in your own car or flying in a plane, check your seat to see whether you need better back support. This can be obtained by such things as using a lumbar roll, repositioning yourself, and repositioning the seat. You can also take weight off your spine by using an arm rest.

- **Avoid keeping your head turned to one side:** While you're driving, avoid keeping your head turned to one side for too long. This can cause muscle tension beginning in your neck and also occurring in your lower back. If you do notice tension from turning your head, look in the opposite direction for a few seconds to help balance yourself out.

- **Stay relaxed:** Being in stop-and-go traffic can be one of the worst situations for tensing up. To combat stress, try playing relaxing music or a book on tape; or take a few deep breaths, exhaling slowly each time (as we discuss in Chapter 12).

- **Take breaks on a long drive:** If you're driving for a long time, take breaks and get out of the car.

Even if you feel that you're sometimes "chained" to your desk, you can use a few techniques to prevent injury: having correct body position, taking frequent breaks, utilizing a back stretching program, and trying to limit your overall sitting time.

Check out Chapter 13 for more details on how sitting places greater stress on your spine, how damage can occur, and what you can do to prevent an injury.

Returning to Work

In this section, we discuss how to design a return-to-work program. Before planning your return to work, you need to try and remove any blockades to your return to work.

Identifying what's blocking you from returning to work

Even though you may be motivated to return to work after a low-back injury, several challenges may get in your way. Here are some of the likely factors that may cause difficulty:

- **Legal intervention:** If legal aspects are involved in your work injury case, this can act as a blockade for return to work. Legal action often creates an adversarial relationship between you and your employer. You may consciously or unconsciously believe that returning to work will hurt your legal case, which ultimately affects your ability to successfully return to work.

- **Job dissatisfaction:** Recent research indicates that how much you like your job (or don't like it) may be one of the most important risk factors for getting a back injury that results in disability. This makes sense: The more you like your job and the more satisfying it is, the more motivated you will be to return to it regardless of back pain.

- **Disability income:** The type and amount of your disability income can also affect your return to work. For instance, if your disability income closely approximates your normal take-home pay, you're likely to be on disability longer after a back injury. This makes sense: If you're not receiving enough income to support yourself while on disability because of a back injury, you're more likely to return to any type of work in order to support your family.

- **Psychological factors:** Psychological factors such as occupational stress, job dissatisfaction, anxiety, and depression are all risk factors for back injury and pain. Also, any of these psychological factors can delay or even prevent your return to work after a back injury.

- **Inappropriate medical care:** Receiving proper medical care for your back problem can delay your return to work. Inappropriate medical care can include such elements as too much bed rest, inactivity, or overmedication.

- **Chronic health problems:** If you have other health problems aside from your back injury, you're less likely to be able to return to work. Your back injury may be "the straw that breaks the camel's back," in terms of your physical ability to perform your job duties.

- **Poor labor market:** If the labor market in your area is particularly bad, this can delay your return to work due to a decrease in the number of options. This is especially the case if you will not be returning to your previous job or career.

- **Limited education/job skills:** If your education is limited and your jobs have always been in heavy physical labor, you may have difficulty returning to work after a significant back injury.

Choosing to return to work

In the past, your general physician — with very little influence from outside agencies — decided whether you returned to work. This isn't the case today. Returning to work most likely requires the coordinated involvement of healthcare providers, governmental officials and programs, providers of rehabilitation services, medical utilization review organizations, lawyers, your employer, and your disability company, among others.

Getting all of these systems and people working together toward successfully returning you to work can be quite a daunting task. Even so, the decision to try and begin the process to return to work ultimately will be yours.

You have many options in your decision to return to work.:

- **Return to work with no restrictions:** Under this option you decide to return to your previous job without any restrictions relative to your back injury. You return on a full-time, full-duty capacity.

- **Return to work with restricted duties:** Under this option, you decide to return to your previous job, but with appropriate medical restrictions for your back injury. You can be restricted from bending, lifting, and twisting. You may also be subject to a weight lifting restriction. In addition, you may begin working on a part-time basis.

When you return to work after a period of prolonged disability, it is always a good idea to return part-time with appropriate medical restrictions. Unfortunately, some employers do not allow this type of return to work. If it is possible in your case, try to return to work on a part-time basis initially. Easing back into your job allows your body to become accustomed to the increased physical demands of returning to work and to gradually increase your work endurance. For example, a part-time schedule may be three hours per day, five days per week or four to five hours per day, three days per week.

✔ **Pursuing vocational rehabilitation:** Under this option, you and your doctor decide that your back injury precludes you from returning to your previous job. For instance, if you were an auto mechanic and performed repetitive bending and lifting throughout your day, a serious back injury may preclude you from ever going back to that occupation. You may choose to pursue vocational rehabilitation to learn a new job within your medical restrictions such as a more sedentary job without bending or lifting.

✔ **Return to work isn't indicated:** Under this option, you and your doctors decide that returning to work isn't an option given your back injury. This situation might exist if you're a 58-year-old truck driver who has sustained a significant back injury resulting in multiple spine surgeries with partial loss of nerve function and a chronic back pain problem (see Chapter 3). Given your age, the type of back injury and resulting medical restrictions, and any of the other variables discussed previously, it may not be realistic nor even appropriate for you to try and return to any type of work. Therefore, permanent disability and retirement would be recommended.

Preparing to Return to Work

A *return-to-work program* includes anything you and your doctor can do to increase the chances that you can successfully return to work and stay there. Some of these things are done prior to returning to work, while others are done in the early phases of your return to work.

Physical reconditioning

Part of preparing to return to work should include physically reconditioning your body to be able to complete your job tasks. If you have been on disability for any length of time because of a back injury, chances are that your body has become physically deconditioned. *Deconditioning* can result in a loss of muscle strength and endurance, decreased aerobic capacity and mobility, or inability to coordinate your movements properly. Physical reconditioning prepares your body to do your work activities. We have found that if you return to work prior to your body being physically ready, you increase the chances of experiencing another back injury and more disability. The better shape you're in, the more likely you can successfully return to work.

A physical reconditioning program should be designed by your doctor and may include many of the exercises and treatments that we discuss in Chapters 7 and 14.

Part of your ability to do your job over an eight-hour day and a 40-hour workweek is the aerobic efficiency of your body. If you've been on disability for any period of time because of a back injury, your aerobic conditioning has likely diminished. Thus, part of your physical reconditioning should include aerobic exercise. Your doctor should guide this activity.

Education

Your most important defense against a re-injury is being a knowledgeable worker. You need to understand what your capabilities are, how to work safely, and when you must refrain from an activity at work that might cause re-injury. Being knowledgeable in the following areas is extremely important for a successful return to work:

- **Body mechanics:** *Body mechanics* involve how you position and move your body, especially related to your back. (These issues are also discussed in Chapter 13.) Using proper and safe body mechanics helps decrease any stress on your lower back and prevent re-injury.

- **Pacing:** When you pace yourself, you take regular breaks throughout your workday in order to prevent a buildup of stress on your spine. For example, if your job requires extended sitting, you should take regular breaks to stand up, walk around, and do some stretching exercises. If your job requires bending and lifting, then you take regular breaks from that activity.

- **Setting limits:** When you return to work, be sure to set appropriate limits based on your physical capabilities to protect your spine. You may limit the amount of bending, lifting, and twisting you're doing. You may also limit the amount of repetitive spinal movements done at one time.

Sometimes setting limits can be difficult when your supervisor is requesting you to complete a certain task "as quickly as possible." It is at these times that you must be assertive and protect your back and prevent re-injury. Trying to save a few minutes by doing a task quickly isn't worth risking another episode of disability.

Preparing for flare-ups

You can usually expect flare-ups in your back pain after you do return to work due to the increased physical demands on your body. If you plan on flare-ups, you won't be surprised or overly concerned if they do occur. Using some of the suggestions in Chapters 7 and 14 can help you successfully get through the flare-up phase. Returning to part-time work with restrictions can also help prevent a serious flare-up or setback.

If your flare-up seems to go beyond something temporary, be sure and discuss it with your doctor. A common pattern we see in patients that return to work is "three steps forward one step back." By this we mean that your work abilities and back pain will improve, followed by a slight regression. Don't be concerned if you notice this pattern; it's fairly common.

Returning to the Office

If you work in an office, your spine is exposed to stress placed on your spine due to sitting for long periods of time as well as bending over certain office equipment. If you work in this type of environment, you should certainly pay attention to the good posture rules we discuss in Chapter 13. In addition, you can try the following ideas:

- **Avoid keeping your head down:** When sitting at your desk or computer terminal, or when standing over the copy machine, avoid the head-down position for an extended period of time. Pointing your head down places your neck and back in an unhealthy position.

- **Reposition yourself frequently:** Reposition yourself to a healthy position frequently. We discuss healthy sitting positions in Chapter 13 and suggest such maneuvers as pushing your pelvis back in your chair, not crossing your legs excessively, and using a chair that supports your spine.

- **Stretching at your desk:** In addition to the stretching exercises discussed in Chapter 14, you can use a couple of good stretching exercises while you're working at your desk. Simply take a short break every once in a while and perform the following stretching exercises.

  - **Pelvic rocking** involves simply taking a deep breath through your nose and stretching your body in the directions indicated by the arrows in Figure 16-1. As can be seen in the figure, you stretch by posturing your body upward and tucking your chin toward your chest. Exhale through your mouth while relaxing after the stretch. Do this exercise about every 30 to 60 minutes of sitting.

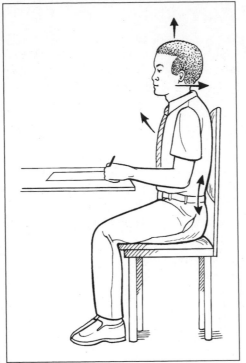

Figure 16-1:
Stretch your upper body in the direction of the arrows.

- **Forward stretch is** useful if your back or neck becomes uncomfortable because of muscle tension from sitting too long. To do this exercise, sit up in a tall, relaxed, upright manner with your hands on your thighs to take the weight off of your spine. Breathe in through your nose as you take this position, stretching yourself tall and in the directions of the arrows shown in first image of Figure 16-2. As you exhale through your mouth, allow your head to gradually release forward. As you allow your head to release forward, you can think of the bones of your spine as the links of a chain. Allow each link to release sequentially, one at a time, from top to bottom. (See the second image in Figure 16-2.) Stop lowering your body either when you feel ready to inhale or you achieve an adequate stretching sensation in your back. (See the third image in Figure 16-2.) At this point, release your body a little bit further as you inhale and then exhale again.

    Continue this breathing pattern, releasing your body a little bit further each time you exhale. You should feel a release of tension in your neck, middle back, and lower back. Ultimately, you can reach the position, as shown in the fourth image in Figure 16-2. Hold this position a few moments before slowly returning to the upright position.

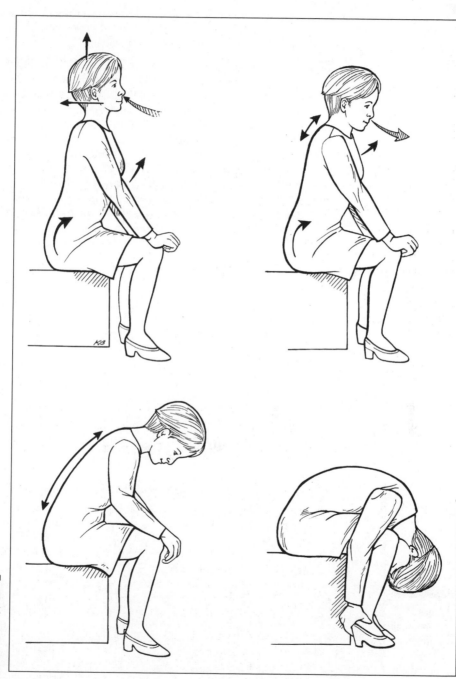

Figure 16-2:
A great
stretch to do
while sitting
in a chair.

Temporary changes in your blood pressure may occur when doing this exercise (that may cause dizziness), so we don't recommend that you immediately stand up afterwards.

- **Spine release rotation** is another good exercise to do while sitting at your desk. After doing the forward stretch that we describe previously, bring one arm to the outside of the opposite knee and turn so that you can reach your other arm over the back of your chair. See the first image in Figure 16-3. Gently turn your head, shoulders, and spine as far as you comfortably can in this same direction. Do this while keeping your knees straight ahead. You should feel a comfortable and gentle stretch of your back. Don't worry if you notice little "clicking" sounds coming from your spine — these are normal. Each time you exhale, you can allow your arms to twist your back a little further, as you feel comfortable. After you inhale and exhale between one and three times, unwind slowly to the front position. Repeat the process in the opposite direction. See the second image in Figure 16-3.

This is a gentle stretch and should not be done to the point of causing pain or discomfort.

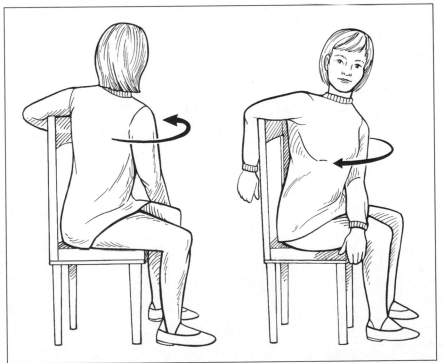

Figure 16-3:
A rotational stretch that you can do in a chair.

Chapter 17

Safely Returning to Your Favorite Sports: The Weekend Warrior

• •

In This Chapter

▶ Reaping the benefits of sporting activities

▶ Enjoying sports — even with back pain

▶ Being smart about your sporting activities

▶ Participating in specific sports with back pain

• •

*E*xercise is good for your back. One of the best ways to get exercise is through sports. Sporting activities provide several positive benefits:

✔ Sporting activities provide you with recreation and enjoyment.

✔ Sports are good for your overall general physical health.

✔ Sports are good for your mental condition. They can help improve your concentration, your sleep, as well as decrease negative emotions such as depression, anxiety, and anger.

✔ Most sporting activities have a social component, which can help as a distraction from your back pain in addition to getting important social support.

✔ Sporting activities increase the chances that you actually get regular exercise because meeting a friend for a sporting activity makes you accountable to be there. Solitary exercise programs are certainly good for your body and general health, but for many people they lack the excitement and sociability of sports.

Unfortunately, we find that sporting activities are among the first things to go after you suffer from a back pain problem. You may feel afraid of re-injury or that your spine can't take the pressure of sporting involvement. Stopping the sporting activities (and usually exercise in general) can lead to the *deconditioning syndrome* as we discuss in Chapter 3 with its associated depression, sleep disruption, muscle weakness, and more back pain.

In this chapter we review methods to help you return to sporting activities even with an ongoing back pain problem. We also review some of the more common sports relative to your back pain.

Getting Involved in Sports Safely

You can do many things to increase the safety of getting involved in sports and decrease the risk of injury to your back. Of course, some sporting activities carry more risk of injury to your back than others. Certainly, the positive benefits associated with being involved in sports far outweigh the risks of injury.

In this section, we discuss how to get involved safely in sporting activities.

Warming up and cooling down

Getting involved in sports includes: the warm up, the warm-up stretch, the cool down, and the cool-down stretch.

The warm up

Whether or not you have a problem with back pain, your body needs to warm up before engaging in any sporting activity. The logic behind warming up is that you prepare your body for the increased physical stress it is about to experience.

When you warm up, your heart rate increases, as does your circulation. This allows your muscles to react quickly without straining.

You can do a warm up in a variety of ways: walking, easy cycling on a stationary bike, or spending some time on a treadmill. Warming up for five to ten minutes is an excellent precursor to participation in sports.

Set an easy, unhurried pace during your warm up. At the end of your warm-up session, your heart rate should be elevated somewhat and you should be perspiring very slightly.

The warm up stretch

After you warm up, you're ready to begin stretching (you can find some good stretching exercises in Chapter 14). Warming up is crucial to being able to stretch your muscles to their limits without strain. If you try to stretch out prior to warming up, you risk injuring your muscles just from the stretching activity.

The focus of your stretching program depends on the type of sport you are about to engage in. Concentrate your stretching program on the parts of your body that will be under the most stress while you're playing. For instance, before playing a racquet sport, focus on stretching the muscles of your arms, legs, shoulders, and lower back.

To be sure that you stretch in a healthy and safe manner, follow these guidelines:

- ✔ **No bouncing:** You may be tempted to bounce as you stretch in order to increase your range of motion, but bouncing may injure your muscles. Instead, simply stretch a particular muscle group to the end of its range and hold the position. You should sense a muscle "pulling" while stretching, but never pain or tearing.

- ✔ **Go slowly:** Do your stretching exercises slowly and gradually, always exhaling as you stretch. Hold each stretch for 20 seconds minimum to 60 seconds maximum.

The cool down

After you finish your activity, remember to cool down. The cool down is probably the most neglected area of safe sporting. The rationale behind cooling down after the sport is to return your body gradually to its usual resting state. Cooling down allows your heart rate, circulatory system, muscle tension, and respiration to return to normal slowly and naturally. Examples of good cool-down activities including light walking, slow biking, or gentle swimming.

The cool down stretch

When you engage in strenuous activity, your muscles contract and lactic acid may build up in your muscles and cause muscle pain if not given a chance to dissipate. When you do your cool-down stretch, contracted muscles return to normal, and lactic acid is carried away. The cool-down stretch also helps prevent muscle pain later on.

Competition: Putting your sport in perspective

Depending on your personality, the competitive aspect of a sporting activity may be an important issue in keeping your back safe from injury. If you are a highly competitive person, you may be more likely to sustain a back injury or cause a flare-up in your back pain during a sporting activity.

The movements often resulting in back injuries or pain flare-ups are those in which you go for the miraculous and heroic "big play" of the game. For example, a tennis ball may be outside of your normal range of motion, but you decide to "go for it" rather than letting it go and conceding the point.

Participating in sports safely when you have a back problem necessitates that you let these kinds of shots go. Think in terms of reserving your energy for other shots throughout the game. You'll end up doing better overall and decrease the risk to your back.

Another risk factor with sporting activities is playing when you are physically and/or mentally fatigued. Unfortunately, the weekend athlete follows this exact pattern. If you are working and thinking hard Monday through Friday, you may be physically and mentally tired on Saturday morning. So pay particular attention to warming-up and cooling-down techniques when participating in a weekend game.

Knowing the risks

Understanding the potential pitfalls of a particular sport can be very helpful. Basically, four types of movements or postures can exacerbate your back pain problem. Even though you use these positions throughout the course of your normal day, they become risky when you perform them excessively or repetitively. These movements and postures are:

- **Flexion:** *Flexion* is simply bending forward from a standing position. Flexion puts additional stress on the discs of the lumbar region of your spine.

  Think about how many times during the course of a racquetball or tennis game you have a choice of either bending from the waist (flexion) to pick up the ball or properly bending your knees. The effects of repeated flexion can be *cumulative*; in other words, the stress of bending over 40 or 50 times to pick up the ball during the course of a game can add up to an irritation of your disc problem.

- **Extension:** *Extension* is the opposite of flexion. Extension is a medical term for arching or bending backwards. Extension movements put stress on the facet joints of your lower back because when you arch backwards, the facet joints in your lower back are brought closer together. As with flexion, the results of repeated extension can be cumulative. For example, your tennis serve involves repeated hyperextension as you throw the ball up and arch your back as part of the serve. You may not notice the effects of a single serve, but 30 to 40 serves can result in an increase in back pain.

- **Rotation:** *Rotation* and twisting motions are key movements in a number of sports. Imagine an invisible line passing vertically through the center of your body, from your head to your buttocks. Now imagine that your body (especially from your neck to your hips) is rotating or twisting around that imaginary line; this is "rotation." Twisting places increased stress on the discs of your lower spine. Although twisting movements are involved in many sports, from ballet to basketball and beyond, you can usually develop techniques to keep this type of movement to a minimum.

Cumulative versus acute effects

The effects of a movement can be either cumulative or acute. *Cumulative* means that repeating a particular motion increases its effect. Examples of cumulative effect or injury include such things as the hyperextension of a tennis serve, a wrist or forearm injury due to the bowling motion, or a low-back problem exacerbated by the repeated twisting motion of a golf swing.

An *acute effect* or injury is something that occurs after a single event — a quick movement outside of your normal range of motion without warming up — which causes a muscle strain. An acute injury may be caused by reaching for a tennis shot that is just outside your normal range, trying a skating move that causes you to fall on your rear-end and lower back, or attempting to lift a barbell weight that is beyond your physical capabilities.

✔ **Lifting:** Any type of lifting can place increased stress on your spine especially if you use a flexion movement, which we describe previously in this section. Two important components of proper lifting techniques include keeping the object you're lifting as close to your body as possible and bending your knees while using your thigh muscles to bear as much of the weight as possible. Some sports involve more lifting than others, and you can't always follow proper lifting rules when you're playing. Bowling, for instance, requires you to lift a rather heavy ball and swing it away from your body

Follow proper lifting techniques as best you can and be sure to do warm up and cool down exercises.

Playing Sports with Back Pain

In this section, we review a number of commonly enjoyed sporting activities. We discuss these sports moving from the ones that have the least risk for back problems to those that have the greatest risk. Table 17-1 shows how we divide up common sporting activities by risk.

Assessing the risk for any particular sport is highly subjective and influenced by a number of factors beyond the actual sport itself. Of course, the intensity with which you participate in a particular sport helps determine how hazardous the sport is: There's a big difference between shooting a few baskets and engaging in a full court, competitive basketball game.

Table 17-1		Risk Levels for Back Problems Associated with Common Sports		
Low	*Low to Medium*	*Medium*	*Medium to High*	*High*
Bicycling	Baseball	Basketball	Golf/Bowling	Football
Swimming	Jogging	Racquet sports	Skating	Gymnastics
Dance/ Aerobics	Skiing	Weight lifting	Horseback riding	Skydiving

Low-risk sports

Bicycling, swimming, low-impact aerobics, and dancing pose the least risk for injury to your back.

Bicycling

Whether you cycle indoors on a stationary bike or outdoors on the open road, biking is generally considered a low-risk sport relative to your back pain problem. In fact, if you jogged prior to a back injury and are finding it difficult to resume that activity, cycling can be a good substitute.

Cycling provides you with excellent leg exercise, cardiovascular stimulation, and the experience of being outdoors without the repeated jarring associated with jogging or running. The only way you may irritate your back on a bicycle is by riding on a high seat and using low handlebars so that you hyperflex your lumbar spine and place stress on the parts of your spine (like the discs; see Chapter 2). Remedy this position by adjusting your seat height downward so that your knee is slightly bent when at full extension on the lower pedal. Of course, mountain biking is rougher on your back than the smooth terrain of road work.

If you experience sciatica pain while riding, take breaks more frequently.

Five to ten minutes on a stationary bike can be an excellent way to warm up prior to stretching and engaging in other sports.

Swimming

In general, swimming is a very safe exercise and can be excellent therapy for a back pain problem. Swimming works virtually all of your muscles in addition to providing cardiovascular conditioning. Also, being in the water protects your spine because the buoyant properties of water help provide support and force you to move slowly and smoothly.

The type of stroke you use can increase the physical stress on your back. Generally, strokes done on your stomach (such as the breast stroke and the crawl) are more stressful because they may place you in a position of hyperextension with your back arched. The butterfly stroke is the most irritating to your back because it requires flexing and extending. Your best bets, and the most beneficial, are the back stroke and side stroke. Experiment with different styles to see which is most comfortable for you.

As with any exercise program, warming up and stretching is important prior to beginning to swim.

Dancing and aerobics

The physical intensity of dancing — we group all forms of dancing and aerobics together in this section — varies depending on whether you do demanding dances such as ballet, the Twist, and break dancing, or practice more sedate styles such as waltzing and ballroom dancing. The same is true for aerobics: High-impact routines are more stressful than low-impact ones.

You can pretty much figure out which type of dancing is high risk and which is low. Slow, ballroom dancing is in the very low-risk category. But, even with this type of dancing, you need to avoid dipping if you have a facet problem, and don't tango if hyperextension causes you more back pain. Higher risk dances include the more physically demanding such as the various types of swing dancing. (For you rockers, slam dancing is very high risk and we don't recommend it if you have a back problem!)

The following guidelines can help make dancing and aerobics safe and rewarding, even with a back pain problem:

- ✔ Maintain a good general conditioning exercise program.
- ✔ Pace yourself while dancing, doing aerobics, or practicing your routines.
- ✔ Avoid any movements that obviously aggravate your back pain.
- ✔ As with any other sport, remember to warm up and stretch prior to engaging in dance or aerobics.

Low- to medium-risk sports

Participating in the following activities carries some risks to your back, but with attention and care, you can enjoy these sports.

Baseball

Baseball, purported to be America's favorite sport, is usually not a problem in terms of your back pain. The pace of the game is rather slow with lengthy periods of inactivity. Running during the game is usually brief and for short distances. Therefore, the weekend athlete need not be in particularly good shape because the physical demands are minimal.

Even so, certain positions and parts of the game can be risky for your back:

- ✔ Pitcher is the riskiest position to play because you can hyperextend your back during each pitch. If you must pitch, try to develop a smooth technique and avoid any extreme arching of your back.

- ✔ Batting, with its twisting motion, can be stressful to your lower back, and may exacerbate your pain. Concentrate on keeping your swing smooth, and absorb some of the twisting motion with your hips and knees rather than with your lower spine. Also, don't use a bat that is too heavy for you.

- ✔ Staying warmed up during the game can be difficult due to the long periods of inactivity. Try to warm up and stretch before the game as well as during the slow periods. You don't want to strain a cold muscle reaching for a fly ball.

As with others sports, you can decrease your chances of back injury and pain simply by keeping the competitive aspects of the game in perspective. Doing so keeps you from diving for the big catch or running over another player while sliding into home plate.

Jogging and running

The intensity of jogging or running ranges from speed walking to sprinting. The bumping and jarring as your feet hit the road transmits directly to your spine and can aggravate a lower back problem. Luckily, you can do several things to minimize the impact of these forces:

- ✔ **Warm up and stretch:** Be sure to warm up and stretch before you start, and cool down and stretch when you finish.

- ✔ **Begin gradually:** If you're a beginning jogger, start slowly. Start out at slower speeds and go shorter distances, until you build up your endurance and get in shape.

- ✔ **Wear good shoes:** One of the most important ways to decrease the impact of road vibration to your spine is to invest in a good pair of shoes. Appropriate shoes provide excellent support for your feet as well as absorb some of the jarring shocks to your knees, legs, and lower back. A good guideline is to change your shoes every 150 miles or six months, whichever comes first.

✔ **Run on soft, smooth, flat surfaces:** Running on a grass field or gravel track is much easier on your spine than running on concrete or asphalt. Running on a flat surface causes the least amount of stress to your spine. Running uphill puts your lower spine into a position of flexion because you bend forward. Running downhill also puts extra stress on your spine because you are in a posture of extension in which you arch backwards.

Pursuing jogging or running given your back pain problem is ultimately your decision. By using the preceding guidelines, you can certainly safely enjoy some level of jogging while keeping your symptoms under control and avoiding reinjury.

Skiing

You may be surprised that we even mention skiing as a possible sport for people who have back pain problems. Actually, skiing is not a bad exercise for your back, and falling while skiing rarely causes back injuries. (In this section, we primarily focus on downhill skiing although similar issues apply to cross-country skiing.)

The common skiing stance — hips and knees flexed with body weight forward — actually helps protect your lower back. The primary risk of exacerbating your back pain due to skiing is falling or the repeated twisting motion while skiing down the mountain as the top of your body faces one direction and your lower body goes another.

The following pointers can help you make skiing a safe activity even with back pain:

✔ **Warm up and stretch:** Proper warming up and stretching is particularly important before skiing. Not only is the outside temperature likely to be cold, but your body may also be subjected to unexpected movements as you negotiate moguls that seem to come out of nowhere.

✔ **Strengthen your leg muscles:** Your pre-ski season strengthening program should pay particular attention to developing your *quadriceps muscles* (the ones running from your hips to the front of your knees). These muscles are critical shock absorbers for your entire body when you're skiing and can absorb much of the jarring that would normally impact your spine — if they're strong enough.

✔ **Avoid twisting:** Avoid twisting your shoulders and hips in opposite directions. Keep your shoulders and hips as parallel as possible to lessen the stress on your lower back.

✔ **Don't ski when you're fatigued:** Most ski accidents occur at the end of the day when skiers are tired and not concentrating on safe techniques. Therefore, you're more likely to avoid a back injury if you stop skiing at the first sign of fatigue.

✔ **Start gradually and lower your sights:** Whether you're just learning to ski or are returning to it after a back pain episode, start gradually and proceed slowly. If you're an advanced skier, start back on the intermediate slopes. You need to put your ego aside while building up to your normal level of expertise.

✔ **Watch the ski conditions:** When you ski, avoid bumps and moguls, choose well-groomed ski runs, avoid deep powder, and watch out for icy conditions that make for a hard fall. (Also, avoid skiing off of 20-foot cliffs while doing flips.)

Medium-risk sports

By taking the proper precautions, you can enjoy basketball, racquet sports, and weight-lifting.

Basketball

Experts don't completely agree about the degree of risk to your back when you play basketball. As with any activity, the way you play the game helps determine how risky it is. If you casually shoot baskets, you're at low risk for hurting your back. Conversely, if you play a full-court, highly competitive game as part of a league, your risk for injury is greater.

Basketball movements associated with back injuries include a variety of things such as twisting, extension, flexion, and running. Keep all these risk factors under control by paying attention to how you approach the game: As with any other sport, warm up and stretch prior to playing and be sure to play within your range of physical ability, expertise, and safety relative to your back problem. You may need to adjust your level of competitiveness relative to the type of back pain problem you suffer from.

Racquet sports

We group *racquet sports* together to include tennis, racquet ball, squash, and badminton. The primary risks in all of these come from the twisting you do throughout a game and from the same shots: the serve, an overhead smash, the backhand, and the lunging shot to make a save.

Follow these guidelines to avoid back pain problems:

✔ **Adjust your style:** If you have a back pain problem, adjust your serve, overhead shots, and backhand. Consider taking lessons from a tennis professional who can help you focus on adjusting your style to avoid hyperextension and excessive twisting.

✔ **Stay in shape:** Stay in shape and in good overall conditioning, part of which involves allowing for an adequate warm-up time prior to playing. Racquet sports tend to be quite social, so you may be tempted to omit proper warm up exercises. Doing so can increase your risk for exacerbation of a back pain problem.

✔ **Stay warm:** If you play outdoors in chilly weather, be sure to dress warmly.

✔ **Don't lunge:** The temptation to "go for it" and get that tough shot depends on your level of competitiveness, but lunging for a shot is probably the most frequent cause of a back injury. Don't do it. Rather, let the shot go and make up points later in the game. You'll do better overall while protecting your back.

✔ **Try doubles:** If you suffer from a severe back pain problem or are returning to a racquet sport after a back injury, consider starting out playing doubles. Doubles is easier on the back simply because you are less likely to move beyond your normal range of motion.

✔ **Wear good shoes:** Wearing good, supportive footwear when playing racquet sports helps decrease the jarring motion on your spine in addition to providing beneficial support for your feet.

✔ **Consider a back brace:** If you have a chronic back pain problem or you are returning from a back injury, consider wearing a back brace while playing a racquet sport. A brace can provide support and protection for your back while you get in shape. We discuss braces in Chapters 7 and 23.

✔ **Consider your type of racquet:** Many different types of racquets are available. Consider purchasing a racquet that absorbs the most shock when contacting the ball and provides the greatest reach. Your tennis professional can make recommendations for you.

Weight lifting

Weight lifting is a medium-risk sport for back injury. Weight lifting exerts immense stress on your lumbar spine. Studies show that evidence of spine damage runs as high as 40 percent among young weight lifters (much higher than the general population).

Of course, the amount of stress placed on your spine is greatly dependent on the type and intensity of weight lifting that you do. Because weight lifting is the cause of so many back injuries, see your doctor immediately if you have an increase in back pain as a result of this activity.

Some tips for making weight lifting safer include:

✔ **Develop your technique:** As with any other sport, you can lift weights in a safer way or a more dangerous way. Be sure to develop your technique and train adequately to be safe. Start weight lifting under the guidance of a qualified trainer. Also, don't try to increase your weight too rapidly or beyond the capabilities of your body.

- ✔ **Watch your movements:** The series of movements in typical lifting can be a stressful combination for your back: You flex your back when you pick up a barbell from the ground, stand erect as you bring it to your chest, and then hyperextend as you raise the weight over your head.

- ✔ **Do weight lifting that spares your back:** In working with a trainer, you can develop a weight lifting routine that essentially spares your back. Focus on doing routines that don't require placing excessive stress on your spine.

- ✔ **Use a weight-lifting belt:** A weight-lifting belt helps stabilize your lower spine and protects the muscles of your abdomen. The belts help diminish strain on that entire area of your body. Weight lifting belts are sold at most sporting goods stores.

- ✔ **Stay within your means:** Be sure to stay within your abilities relative to the amount of weight you are lifting. One way to protect your back is to lift lighter weights and increase the number of repetitions. Again, working with a qualified trainer can help you develop a safer routine.

Medium- to high-risk sports

Medium- to high-risk sports require more careful attention and using safer techniques because of the increased risk to your back. Even so, by taking appropriate precautions, you can still enjoy bowling, golf, and skating.

Bowling

Depending on which expert you talk to, bowling is rated anywhere from a low- to a high-risk sport. We believe that the threat to your back depends mostly on your technique and classify bowling as a medium- to high-risk sport.

Two aspects of bowling can cause problems for your back. One is the twisting motion when you throw the ball — your shoulders and upper torso twist in one direction while your hips and legs twist the opposite way. And, before you throw your strike, you flex your back and hold a heavy ball at arm's length, a position and motion (especially given the weight of the ball) that can irritate your spine, especially the discs and facet joints.

The following guidelines can help you bowl without causing more problems for your back:

- ✔ **Develop a good technique:** One of the best ways to avoid back problems when bowling is to develop a good technique. If you have chronic back pain and plan to bowl regularly, get an evaluation occasionally from a bowling professional to ensure that your technique is safe for your back.

✔ **Use an appropriately sized ball:** Don't use a ball that is too heavy for you and be sure that the ball fits your fingers well. Make sure that you can manage the weight of the ball while releasing it smoothly and easily from your hand.

✔ **Do strengthening exercises:** If you are a regular bowler with a back pain problem, doing strengthening and stretching exercises consistently is extremely important to prevent re-injury or acute flare-ups. If you rarely bowl, take it very easy when you do bowl. The occasional bowler who is not conditioned and whose technique is not particularly good is probably the most at risk for a back problem.

✔ **Consider a corset:** Consider wearing a lumbar corset while you bowl, especially after an acute flare-up of a chronic back problem. Of course, don't rely on the corset to the exclusion of stretching, strengthening, and conditioning. See Chapter 23 for more information.

Golf

Back problems are the bane of golfers. The twisting motion of the golf swing causes fairly significant stress on the discs and facet joints — especially if you have a tendency to arch your back extensively through the swing and try to shift your hips "through the ball" as you hit. Most regular golfers are truly in love with the sport and are reluctant to let a back pain problem hold them back. The following guidelines can help:

✔ **Be sure to warm up:** Given the highly social component of golf and the fact that it doesn't seem like a strenuous exercise, proper warm up is probably most neglected in this sport. But, in addition to sand and water hazards, golf includes back hazards, which makes warming up and stretching out important before you play.

✔ **Develop a safe swing:** As you know if you spend any time at a golf course, golfers' swings vary. Certain types of movements in a swing — such as severely arching your back as you hit the ball — can cause extra stress on your back. Consider having a golf professional help you develop a swing that causes the least amount of stress on your back.

✔ **Take care after long absences:** Many golfers don't get in much golfing time during the winter months. Come springtime, you may want to run out to the driving range and hit buckets of balls in order to get back into the game as quickly as possible. After a season of inactivity, you may be vulnerable to a back problem because your body isn't properly prepared to re-enter the sport. Pay attention to proper conditioning exercises as you ease back into play.

✔ **Respect your driver and long irons:** Your back is probably most at risk when you use your driver and long irons and you're likely to utilize a full golf swing with maximum effort, putting more stress on your back. When hitting with these clubs, pay particular attention to swinging smoothly and easily. Try deciding mentally to hit the ball 10 or 20 yards shorter than usual. You may actually end up hitting the ball farther and more accurately.

> ## Don't forget the cool down after golf
>
> How many times do you finish playing 18 holes feeling great only to wake up the following day with every muscle aching — especially your back? One likely cause is going straight from the course into an air-conditioned car and sitting in one position all the way home. You need to cool down after playing any sport, including golf.
>
> After a round of golf, your body is generally limber and warm. If you jump into a car and drive home, your body cools down too rapidly without having a chance to recover from the physical demands of the game.
>
> Use one or more of these tips to cool down after a round:
>
> ✔ Go out to the range and hit a few short iron shots.
>
> ✔ Take some time to do some gentle stretching including your neck, lower back, and legs. (Chapter 14 sets forth some exercises.)
>
> ✔ Take a warm shower.
>
> Don't go immediately from bending over a one-putt on the 18th green to slumping over an ice-cold drink in the air-conditioned "19th Hole."

✔ **Stay warm if you use a golf cart:** Riding in a golf cart essentially lets your body cool down between each golf shot. Be aware of this tendency and try to walk at least a little between shots. Also, dress warmly on cool days.

✔ **Wear soft-spiked shoes:** Many golf courses now require you to wear soft-spiked golf shoes. Wearing this type of shoe may actually help reduce the impact to your back at the end of your swing. These shoes give you some traction but they do not make your stance nearly as solid as regular golf shoes.

Horseback riding

The risk associated with horseback riding involves the vertical impact or bumpy "up-and-down" motion in the saddle that jars your spine. Also, horseback riding involves primarily the sitting position which puts a greater load on your spine.

If you're recovering from a back injury, you should probably stop horseback riding until your pain has been minimal (or gone) for several months and you have had a chance to recondition your body.

If you use good riding techniques, riding should not cause a problem for your back. For instance, you should rarely be hitting the saddle with any significant impact while riding. Similar to skiing, your legs should act as shock absorbers and minimize any impact to your spine. As with any sport, you should stay within your level of expertise and start out gradually if you are either a beginner or are returning to the sport after a back pain flare-up.

Skating

Skating includes ice skating, roller skating, and in-line skating. Skating is generally a medium- to high-risk sport if you have back pain as long as you stay away from stunts and very long strides. Skating is a good form of general exercise and involves smooth, fluid movements, which are just the type of moves you want to make to prevent back strain.

Three skating activities can aggravate your back condition. You can take steps to manage these problems and enjoy skating while keeping your back problem under good control.

- ✔ **The basic skating position** puts your spine in a slightly bent forward position which can be irritating to your lower back. Take it easy when skating and stay as upright as possible.

- ✔ **The spinning motion** associated with ice skating is perilously close to the twisting motion you should avoid.

- ✔ **Landing after a jump** in either ice skating or in-line skating (including an unplanned fall) is not healthy for your back. If you have a back problem, consider leaving jumps out of your skating routine.

High-risk sports

If you have a back problem, watch out for the sports we describe in this section. These sports are high risk for starting and exacerbating back pain problems. For some of them (football and gymnastics), it is difficult to do anything to make the sport more "back friendly." If involvement in the following sports continually flares your back problem, you may want to consider some other activity.

Football

Football is considered a high-risk sport whether or not you have a back pain problem.

Full contact or tackle football involves excessive twisting, hyperextension, and weight-bearing. It causes stress to your discs, facet joints, muscles, and ligaments. Also, if you are tackling, your back is likely flexed more than 45 degrees, and if you are being tackled, you are likely to land with your spine hyperextended or rotated.

Touch football is less of a menace but still has the potential to cause problems for your back, especially when you and your teammates are weekend athletes who may not be in particularly good shape or condition.

Our recommendation is that if you have a back problem, don't consider playing football. If you must play, an appropriate strengthening, stretching, and conditioning program is essential. You should also warm up adequately prior to playing. Ask your doctor about wearing some type of back brace while playing.

Don't play if your back is in an acute flare-up. If you have a significant flare-up after playing be sure to have your doctor check it to determine whether you sustained some type of significant back injury.

Gymnastics

Gymnastics is considered a high-risk sport even if you don't have a back pain condition. Some of the variety of back stressors include:

- ✔ Wear and tear to the facet joints from severe hyperextension of the spine
- ✔ Strained spinal ligaments from dramatic flexion postures
- ✔ Traumatic displacement of a vertebra from fracture due either to falling or cumulative effects of certain positions

The bottom line is that your body is not designed to extend to the degree required for many gymnastics postures, nor is it designed to change quickly from a position of full flexion to one of full extension.

This sport is most dangerous to youngsters and teenagers, the group with which it is most popular. For instance, a study of young Bulgarian gymnasts showed that 50 percent developed spinal problems. If you or your child engages in this sport, you must pay attention to proper warm up and stretching exercises. Also, be sure not to push your child to do the movements too quickly. Be absolutely rigorous in using spotters to protect yourself or your child.

Because the risk of back injury is so great in this sport, if you or your child have prolonged, severe, and unimproved backaches, seek appropriate medical evaluation and treatment.

Chapter 18

Sex and Back Pain: Getting "Back" in the Saddle

*A*ny ongoing back pain problem can seriously affect your ability to enjoy a sexual relationship. Whether the back pain is your own or your partner's, an injured back can lead to anything from an occasional disruption of sex due to a muscle spasm, to not having sex for a year or more.

Many of our patients list sexual problems as one of their primary concerns related to their back pain. They often point out that no previous doctor has ever asked them about this aspect of their lives. To help an injured back, remember that pain of any type can indeed disrupt your sexual interactions, but, worse, it can disrupt your entire relationship.

Understanding Back Pain's Vicious Cycle

Frustration, anger, guilt, fear, and depression can all accompany a serious back problem. These emotions, along with the physical aspect of having back pain, can virtually wipe out any type of sexual relationship. Back pain can diminish your physical ability to have enjoyable sex, as well as decrease your sex drive.

Back pain is invisible, which can cause even more problems in a couple's physical relationship. If you're the person in the relationship who's coping with back pain, you may begin to feel inadequate and experience self-critical thoughts like, "Why would anybody want to be with me?; I'm unappealing; I'm an invalid." (See Chapter 12 for more information on negative thoughts.) As you accept these negative thoughts, you're more likely to withdraw from any type of sexual interaction.

If you're experiencing back pain, you may begin to engage in spectatoring which can result in performance anxiety. *Spectatoring* consists of mentally watching, evaluating, and criticizing your every sexual move as it occurs. Engaging in spectatoring can lead to *performance anxiety* — you become so anxious that sex is no longer enjoyable and actually becomes something you avoid.

If your spouse or partner is dealing with back pain, your thoughts and emotions can also affect your physical relationship. For instance, you may be afraid that you may further injure your partner during any type of sexual interaction. As a result, you don't initiate sex. If you withdraw from physical interaction, your partner may misinterpret these signals as having something to do with a lack of attraction on your part.

Thus, as intimacy dissolves, a vicious cycle perpetuates: As a couple, you and your partner end up moving away from each other physically and emotionally, communicating less, and eventually feeling even more isolated.

The good news is that even though back pain may limit your ability to perform physically, it does not have to limit your overall sexual relationship, which includes mental, emotional, and intimacy aspects not dependent on the physical relationship. Couples can have a very fulfilling sexual relationship even with the back pain problem. To restore your sexual relationship, you have to do the following:

- ✔ Communicate
- ✔ Focus on sensuality and romance
- ✔ Understand intimacy
- ✔ Discover comfortable positions
- ✔ Put in the effort to make it all work

Don't Be Shy: Communicate

The most important aspect of any relationship is good communication. When communication is effective, you feel understood and satisfied. But, when communication breaks down, you feel embarrassed, unappreciated, misunderstood, defensive, and hostile. All these emotional reactions, either positive or negative, are amplified when the issue is sex.

Many people, however, have difficulty communicating openly about sex usually due to the attitude their parents left them with from childhood or cultural pressures that such talk is taboo. ("Nice children don't talk like that.") When couples cannot openly communicate about their sexual relationship, they create fertile ground for the vicious cycle of sex-related problems.

Following are important helpful hints for effective communication, especially when dealing with sex:

- **Practice listening carefully to one another:** If you're like most people, during a conversation with someone, you are all too commonly thinking about what *you* are going to say next, rather than focusing fully on hearing the other person. Effective communication involves learning to listen attentively to the other person's message. And, when you really do listen, you can often gain a full understanding of your partner's thoughts and feelings about an issue. To be sure you are understanding your partner, you can use an *active listening* approach in which you paraphrase what you think your partner said in order to check for accuracy. To engage in active listening, when your partner is finished speaking, say, "So what you are saying is . . ." paraphrase what you heard, and conclude with, "Is that accurate?"

- **Watch your body language:** When you communicate, be sure that your body language matches your message. Your body language gives you away every time. Research has shown that more than half of what you communicate is done through body language, not words! You may tell your partner that you really enjoy the love-making, but if you're averting your eyes or sighing at the same time, your body language communicates your true message.

- **Avoid threatening and judgmental behavior:** Non-threatening and non-judgmental communication opens the door to meaningful discussion without causing arguments. When the topic is sex, communication that involves no threats or put-downs becomes even more important. The worst possible way to deal with a sexual problem is to criticize each other, which only fosters defensiveness and hostility.

- **Respect one another's conversational styles:** Investigations (also known as research) show that different communication styles are often responsible for triggering misunderstandings. Women and men tend to have different communication styles. For instance, women tend to ask more personal questions, while also sharing feelings and experiences. On the other hand, men are more likely to interrupt and dominate a conversation while discussing problems with the sole intent and focus on finding a solution. Other variables, aside from gender, also determine your conversational style. These include such things as family background, culture, occupation, and education. Be sure to be aware of your partner's style of communication and be respectful of differences.

✔ **Set aside time for communication:** You and your partner absolutely must set aside time to communicate about problems and issues — especially sex. Waiting for the subject to "just come up" at some point is like having a ticking bomb resting over your relationship. Try to choose a time for conversation when you and your partner won't be pressured, rushed, or interrupted.

✔ **Do not discuss sex problems in the bedroom:** Discussing or mentioning sexual problems while you're being intimate is a sure-fire way to light the fuse on that bomb we just mentioned. Always discuss sexual issues outside the bedroom in a non-threatening atmosphere.

✔ **Phrase your comments carefully:** Thinking before speaking is especially important when you're discussing sex or considering bringing it up. Be careful to phrase issues or concerns in a way that does not hurt the other person's feelings. Remember, too, that some things are best left unsaid — the invention that retracts the spoken word is not on the market yet.

✔ **Compliment each other frequently:** Research shows that a very high frequency of negative statements toward one another — relative to the number of positive statements — characterizes troubled relationships. When discussing issues with your partner — including your sexual relationship — compliment the positive and phrase areas of concern in a non-negative way.

✔ **Make your requests specific:** If you want to communicate an issue, be specific. In being specific, remember to do the following:

- Focus on the behavior rather than the person: For instance, it is not useful to make global personality statements such as "You are a lazy !@#%*&." Rather, a statement like, "It seems to me that you have not been taking the trash out as often as you used to. Is that accurate?" The second statement addresses the actual behavior and invites discussion towards finding a solution.

- Use "I" statements rather than "You" statements: For instance, notice the difference in how the following statements feel, "You didn't buy ice cream at the store because you think I'm fat!" versus "When I ask you to buy ice cream at the store and you don't, I feel like you think I'm fat." The first is accusatory and likely to make the other person defensive. The second "I" statement communicates the issue but is much softer and invites useful discussion.

✔ **Write a letter:** If you feel shy about sexual communication, you may want to write your thoughts, feelings, and concerns in the form of a letter to your partner. Letter writing helps you organize your thoughts and be sure that you are presenting them in a non-threatening manner (be sure that the letter has a good number of compliments). Writing letters to one another about sexual issues can be an excellent way to overcome the shyness that often comes with communicating about these issues. You may find that asking your partner to respond with a letter is helpful in getting the communication going.

✔ **Go through this chapter with your mate:** You can use this chapter in several ways, all of which are effective. You can read it together and talk about each section as you go, or you can read each section separately and then discuss it. The most important part is to discuss the information in each section, and to practice good communication skills as you do.

Check to make sure your comments are heard accurately. Ask your partner to paraphrase and summarize what you said or to explain the point you are trying to make. You can then correct any misunderstandings.

Getting in the Mood

A wise person once said, "If there was more courting in marriages, less marriages would end up in court." When back pain is an aspect of a couple's sexual relationship, romance and sensuality are more important than ever.

Even when back pain is not an issue, the romance and excitement of sex can yield more pleasure than the actual physical activity itself. However, contrary to what the movies lead us to believe, romance and excitement do not descend from the clouds with a lush symphony playing in the background. In the real world, communication and planning are usually necessary for romance to occur. Back pain doesn't have to interfere with romance and sensuality in your relationship. Following are a few tips for setting the stage for romance:

✔ **Plan a "back friendly" date:** Planning a date or a series of dates is a good way to build romance. However, people with back pain sometimes forget that they can still have fun, too. (Yes, it's true and good for you!) If you are concerned about going on a date with your back problem, take steps to plan a sensual and romantic interlude that won't stress your back. Perhaps you could plan a romantic dinner, a night time swim, a soothing whirlpool session, or a night in a hotel (you can even stay down the street, as long as the kids are at home). You can add the spontaneity later. Simply planning time together can create sexual excitement, as you anticipate the approaching date.

✔ **Create a romantic atmosphere:** A romantic setting (whatever it is) fosters intimacy that can start many hours — even days — before you and your partner become physically intimate. Pay attention to all your senses as you plan and try to incorporate as many relaxing elements as possible: passionate music, soft lighting, delicate incense or potpourri, a delicious dinner, and satin sheets or pajamas.

> ✔ **Foster emotional intimacy:** Emotional intimacy can begin long before you have sexual contact. Try sending flowers, tucking seductive notes in your partner's lunch, briefcase, or pockets, leaving phone messages, and so on. The possibilities for emotional intimacy are limited only by your imagination. Emotional intimacy builds the anticipation of your physical encounter, helps you focus on the relationship rather than the back pain, and enhances the sensuality of the whole experience.

Getting Physical

Emotional and physical intimacy are intertwined and linked by such things as touching, holding hands, hugging, certain glances, using pet names, and love talk, among other things. After you build up the sensuality, romance, anticipation, and emotional intimacy of your relationship, chances are that you'll start "getting physical." Try creating some physical intimacy by doing the following:

- ✔ Massaging your partner (with or without oils)
- ✔ Soaking in a hot tub or taking a bath
- ✔ Kissing
- ✔ Holding hands
- ✔ Hugging

Physical intimacy may also include activities that help you manage your back pain more effectively during sex. For instance, many individuals with back pain obtain relief from such things as massage, hot packs, or taking a hot bath. You can incorporate all of these pain-relieving activities into your intimate activities.

If back pain has had a very significant impact on your sexual relationship, you should begin slowly in terms of building sexual activity back into the relationship. Open communication is important and may include such detailed items as planning how you will engage in pre-sexual activities and discussing physical positions that are most comfortable given the back pain problem.

Sex is often exciting (are we masters of understatement or what?), and that excitement can lead to greater physical activity, especially as you approach orgasm. Given this heightened level of physical exertion and focus, you may not notice much back pain at the time. Even so, keeping the level of physical activity under some control can be important, especially if you're one of the many people prone to acute back pain flare-up *after* sex.

Back Friendly Sexual Positions, or "Getting Down to It"

This section outlines sexual positions that are generally most comfortable for someone with a back pain problem. You and your partner should experiment with these positions to find those that work best for you. As you experiment with the love-making positions that we describe in this section, remember to take things slowly and communicate openly.

If your back pain is severe, take a more passive role in love-making initially. You can be more passive by paying particular attention to non-intercourse sexual activity (to be discussed in the following section). Also, you may want to talk with your partner about needing to be more passive at first until you work up to being able to tolerate greater activity. Discussing this issue openly will help you feel more comfortable about being passive and your partner will understand that you are not simply being selfish.

Getting started: Doing it without doing it

Not all sexual encounters involve actual genital intercourse. Many people with back pain may be more comfortable if they start out by not making intercourse the goal of physical interaction.

If you have back pain, you may find that lying on your back on a firm surface and placing your legs on pillows is a comfortable position. You may also gain comfort by rolling or folding a small hand towel under your lower back, giving it a slight arch, and providing additional support for your back. This position is fairly passive for the person with back pain, but you can still do a lot from it.

Your search for a firm surface can double as a way to create a romantic atmosphere — try out the family room floor, the dining room table, or any other place that suits your fancy.

Outercourse

Pain — or the fear of pain — is one of the primary obstacles to sexual pleasure and orgasm, so proceed slowly and patiently. The goal is to avoid any type of frustration or significant increase in pain. Genital intercourse is sometimes too painful to attempt and should not be your initial goal. While recovering from a flare-up, or adjusting to the changed condition of your back, you can limit love-making to other forms of sexual interaction, all done from a relaxed position.

Outercourse (a term we borrowed from *Sex For Dummies* by Dr. Ruth K. Westheimer) is a modern term for what used to be called "heavy petting." You can be involved in sexual stimulation even from a relaxed position. Either partner can provide manual and/or oral stimulation. In fact, you can provide sexual stimulation in a variety of ways. You and your partner can have fun exploring these possibilities.

The missionary position

The *missionary position* is basically the male superior position. No, we are not referring to any power hierarchy based on gender: Simply put, the man is on top and the woman is on the bottom. Variations on the missionary position can be useful, depending on the type of back pain you are experiencing.

The missionary position can be fairly comfortable for a woman with back pain:

- ✔ Lie on your back with your legs bent, which allows you to maintain some curve in your spine. The degree your spine curves is relative to how close you bring your knees to your chest. If this traditional missionary position is not comfortable, try placing a towel or small pillow under your lower back to help keep it somewhat arched. You can then adjust how much you bend your legs.

- ✔ Another variation on the traditional missionary position is to lie on your stomach. You can then adjust your position to provide the most comfort for your back by placing a pillow under your chest or stomach, or propping yourself up on your elbows.

- ✔ You can modify the missionary position if you have one-sided back pain problems. Lie on your back with one knee bent up and the other leg lying flat.

A man with back pain can benefit from the missionary position in the following ways:

- ✔ A modified missionary position can be particularly useful for one-sided back pain. Place a pillow or two underneath your partner to raise her buttocks. You can then lay between her legs with one of your legs bent into a deep kneeling position, keeping your other leg straight behind you. Which leg you bend and which leg you keep straight depends on which side you have back pain.

- ✔ Another variation on the conventional missionary position (you probably had no idea how versatile this position can be!) is typically done if you find the standard missionary position too painful to tolerate. Have your partner lie on her back with one or two pillows underneath her back and buttocks. This position raises her enough to allow you to draw both knees into a kneeling position between her legs. You can then enter her in this position with minimal stress on your back.

The female superior position

The female superior position is simply woman on top. This position can be useful for both men and women with back pain.

For the man with back pain:

- ✔ In the female superior position you can keep your back comfortable and non-stressed by straightening your knees or bending them more upwards, depending on what is most comfortable.

- ✔ You can also adjust your position by using towels and pillows for support. This passive position allows you to protect your back while you enjoy having intercourse.

- ✔ Your partner's movements can range from very gentle to more physically active. Keep her informed of your comfort level, so she can adjust her movements in order to keep your pain at a minimum.

For the woman with back pain:

- ✔ This position allows you virtually complete control over physical movement. You can control the depth of penetration and speed of thrust, depending on your back pain.

- ✔ You can lay your chest down on your partner's, which may be more comfortable if rounding out your back reduces pain.

- ✔ A variation on the standard female superior position is to face away from your partner. Try this variation to see whether it provides you with more comfort for your back. Besides, it can add some creative variety to your experience.

Doggie style

Doggie style is the slang term for the position in which the man enters the woman from behind, the way most animals do. The woman is usually "on all fours" (on her hands and knees) while the man kneels behind her. This position can be great for controlling back pain but may be a little hard on the man's knees if the surface isn't soft (of course, he can always go for the knee pads).

For the woman with back pain:

- ✔ This position allows you to adjust the posture of your lower back, controlling your comfort level.

- ✔ You can position yourself either with your torso more upright (by resting on pillows or the corner of the bed) or on your hands and knees on the bed.

For the man with back pain:

- ✔ This position can be comfortable for you since it allows you to keep your lower back rounded out.

- ✔ You can control the aggressiveness of your movements very effectively from this position in order to keep your back pain at a minimum.

Side by side

Three side-by-side positions can be useful in managing a back pain problem during sex: spooning, the T-bone, and the scissors position.

Spooning

Spooning is essentially a variation of the doggie style, but done sideways. In this position, the man still enters the woman from behind, but the woman lies on her side, not her knees. Many couples find this position more physically relaxing than the traditional doggie style.

- ✔ For the man with back pain, the spooning position lets you control the position of your back during intercourse by how you place your body next to your partner. You can bend your back either slightly forward or backwards depending on what is most comfortable.

- ✔ As a woman with back pain you can control the position of your back either by bending slightly forward to bring your chest down toward your knees or by arching your back backwards and leaning towards your partner.

The T-bone

Either the man or the woman with back pain can use this position — we just made the name up, in case you're wondering. In this position, the woman lies on her back and the man lies beside her on his side, facing her. She bends both of her legs upward enough to allow him to bring his legs underneath hers. She then places her legs down over his. This position allows you and your partner to touch other body areas and have direct face-to-face communication.

For the woman with back pain:

- ✔ You are in a very relaxed and comfortable position for your back.

- ✔ You can control the position of your back by how you position your legs.

- ✔ You can improve your comfort if necessary by placing a small towel or pillow under your lower back.

For the man with back pain:

- ✔ You control the position of your back during intercourse by how you place yourself next to your partner. You can lean forward, closer to her, or move backwards away from her depending on what is most comfortable.

- ✔ You also control the aggressiveness of your movements while being in a position in which your entire body is supported by the bed (or lawn, or carpeting, or whatever).

The scissors

This position is known as "the scissors" even though you may look more like a pretzel when you try it. In this position, the woman lies on her back while the man lies next to her on his side. The woman bends the leg closest to her partner and he brings his top leg forward and places it under her bent leg. She then lowers her upper leg and rests it on top of his. Each partner has one leg bent and the other leg straight. (Huh?! Keep re-reading that one until it makes sense.) He can then enter her from the side.

This position can be quite comfortable if either person, or even both partners, have general back pain or one-sided back pain. This position is a very relaxed one for both participants and allows for face-to-face communication and touching.

Putting It All Together

Approach the information in this chapter — we know that it seems overwhelming at first — in a fun and adventurous manner. We like to use the acronym GREAT SEX to summarize our advice for getting your relationship together — even with back pain.

- ✔ **Give it a try:** You must begin by simply giving "it" a try. "It" may be anything in this chapter. Start out with whatever seems easiest for you and your partner, then progress to other areas. It is important to make communication one of the first "its" to practice. An easy way to get started is to go through this chapter as a couple.

- ✔ **Romance and sensuality:** Don't forget, romance and sensuality are primary components of a good sexual relationship.

- ✔ **Express and communicate:** Expressing yourself and communicating in an open and non-threatening manner are important elements of a good relationship, especially when it comes to sex and back pain.

- ✔ **Accentuate intimacy:** Especially when dealing with a back pain problem, remember to accentuate emotional and physical intimacy.

✔ **Time:** Make time and plan ahead for your romance, love-making atmosphere, and sexual encounters. Don't count on spontaneity, and make sure that your sexual relationship happens.

✔ **Slow:** Go slowly when trying out the different things we discuss in this chapter and in the other resources we offer. Proceed at a pace that keeps pain at a minimum and avoids any type of frustration, hostility, or defensiveness.

✔ **Explore variability:** As you work on your relationship (emotional and physical) be sure to explore variations. Be creative and have fun!

✔ **Xcellent:** Yes, we know "excellent" doesn't really begin with "X" but finding a word that fit this acronym and started with an "X" was somewhat challenging. Anyway, we hope that after you and your partner work with this chapter a little, you develop an excellent physical and emotional relationship regardless of back pain.

Additional resources

You may find the following resources useful for more detailed information about sex and back pain.

Sex and Back Pain. L. Hebert. Greenville, ME: Impacc USA, 1994, 24 pages; 800-762-7720.

This booklet offers very straightforward and explicit love-making positions for the back pain sufferer and includes illustrations that help the reader avoid any misunderstanding in developing safe and comfortable positions.

The Townsend Institute, P.O. Box 8855, Chapel Hill, NC, 27515; 800-888-1900.

This company provides a variety of materials designed to enhance a couple's sexual relationship.

Sex Smart: How Your Childhood Shaped Your Sexual Life and What to do About It., A. Zoldbrod, Oakland, CA: New Harbinger Publications, 274 pages; 800-748-6273; www.newharbinger.com.

This book explores how your childhood family environment shaped your sexual attitudes and behavior. Self-tests and exercises help you understand your own sexual issues and develop strategies for counteracting problem areas.

Part VI
The Part of Tens

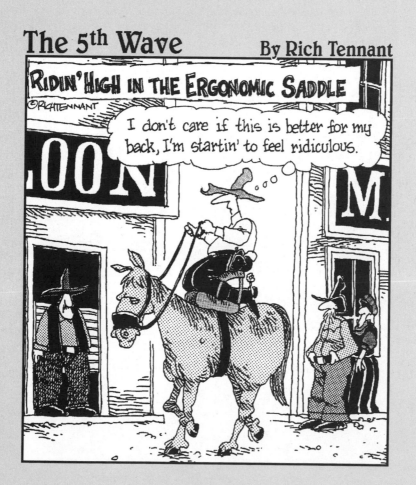

The 5th Wave   By Rich Tennant

RIDIN' HIGH IN THE ERGONOMIC SADDLE

©RICHTENNANT

I don't care if this is better for my back, I'm startin' to feel ridiculous.

In this part . . .

This part of the book is really fun. All ...*For Dummies* books include a Part of Tens, which features a few chapters that give you ten or so tips, ideas, or suggestions. These quick chapters condense information into little sound bites that you can read on the run. Think of them as Top Ten lists with substance.

Chapter 19

Ten Most Common Questions about Back Pain

*R*emember the old saying, "The only silly question is the one you don't ask" from your grammar school days? As you deal with the medical community, you may feel like you should already know the answers to your questions — so much so that asking your doctor can be intimidating. In this chapter, we answer the ten most common questions we get about back pain from our patients. Hopefully, the answer to at least one of your own "silly" questions is here.

Can I Manage My Herniated Disc without Surgery?

You can almost always manage your herniated disc successfully without surgery. Only a very small percentage of patients actually require surgery for a herniated disc (see Chapter 3). Many research studies show that patients with a herniated disc can recover nicely with nonsurgical, conservative management. In one study, 92 percent of patients with documented disc herniations recovered without surgery. (See J.A. Saal, et al. "The Natural History of Lumbar Intervertebral Disc Extrusions Treated Non-operatively," Spine 15 (1990): 8–20.) Many of these patients had large herniated discs that were compressing nerve roots. In another study, patients with disc herniations were treated either surgically or nonsurgically. After five years, the researchers found no difference in the groups. (See H. Weber, "Lumbar Disc Herniation: A Controlled, Prospective Study with Ten Years of Observation," Spine 8 (1983): 131–140.) In our own research, recently presented at the 1999 meeting of the American Academy of Orthopedic Surgery, we followed a large number of patients with massive lumbar disc herniations who received conservative treatment. On average, the MRI follow-up evaluation after six months showed disc herniation size reduced by 62 percent. (See Chapter 23 for more on this study.)

We often see symptoms of a herniated disc with nerve compression (back pain, buttock pain, and sciatica) resolve spontaneously as the disc shrinks. Your body has a natural ability to heal and reabsorb disc herniations and return to a normal state.

Surgery may be appropriate for your disc herniation in some cases. If your neurological symptoms, such as weakness in your legs, decreased sensation, and bowel and/or bladder problems, are getting progressively worse, your doctor may recommend surgery to prevent permanent neurological damage. If you experience these symptoms, consult a spine specialist who is aware of nonsurgical treatment options. We discuss these issues further in Chapters 3 and 7.

What Kind of Doctor Should I See for My Back Pain?

As we discuss in Chapter 4, many types of healthcare professionals treat back problems. You may find all the options quite confusing as you decide whom to seek treatment from. Much of your decision depends upon your symptoms and your history of back pain problems. For instance, if you have a long history of a recurrent back pain problem, you probably already have a doctor who knows your case and with whom you consult when you have flare-ups.

For simple acute back pain problems in which you experience no significant associated symptoms (such as bowel or bladder problems, debilitating pain down one or both legs, or severe throbbing pain that awakens you at night), you can see your family physician, chiropractor, or a physical therapist.

Certainly, your family physician can give you a physical evaluation. He can also probably rule out any serious problems, provide medications such as anti-inflammatories and painkillers, and recommend any appropriate limitations to your activity, although most family doctors do not provide specific instruction on back exercises.

Your chiropractor can also provide initial treatment of your back problem (see Chapter 10). Chiropractors cannot prescribe medications but may be more likely to provide exercise guidelines — although they don't always. Of course, if you see a chiropractor, you need to be open to his method of treatment.

Make sure that any doctor that you choose monitors you closely and focuses on gradually increasing your activities through strengthening and stretching. If your doctor primarily prescribes medications and recommends prolonged rest, you may want to consider consulting another doctor — research shows that this approach is likely to be ineffective and may actually make you worse.

If your back pain goes on for more than four to six weeks, you don't seem to be improving, and your activity level continues to be quite restricted, then you need to see a spine specialist. Spine specialists come in all shapes, sizes, and types. Typically, the type of physician who specializes in spinal problems includes orthopedic surgeons, neurosurgeons, physiatrists, neurologists, and osteopaths. Of these, you want a specialist who focuses on nonsurgical, conservative treatment of back pain. Statistically, physiatrists fit this role (see Chapter 4 for more information). If you're interested in alternative medicine treatments, then you may also want to find a spine specialist who is comfortable working with practitioners of this type.

If you have a more complex back pain problem — symptoms that don't resolve after several months or severe symptoms like those we discuss in the preceding paragraph — then you may be better off searching for a center that specializes solely in spinal problems. Spine centers usually offer a multi-disciplinary approach including physicians, surgeons, physical therapists, pain psychologists, and chiropractors, among others. The different specialists evaluate and treat all aspects of your spine problem simultaneously (see Chapter 7). You can find a spine center by asking your family physician, checking with your local hospital, calling your local university medical center, or reviewing the resources in Appendix B.

Use your family doctor, friends, or the resources in Appendix B to find a doctor to see initially (after four to six weeks of pain) or for complex cases. Unfortunately, in today's era of managed care, your insurance plan guidelines may heavily influence your choices.

Why Do I Still Have Pain When My Imaging Scans Are Normal?

Many known and well-understood structural reasons for back pain may be applicable to your specific problem. However, in a large percent of all back pain cases, doctors find no specific, identifiable structural diagnosis (see Chapter 3). One reason your scans may be normal while you still have discomfort is that your back pain may come from sources that current imaging technology can't identify. In fact, high-tech instruments may never be able to identify things like pain from inflammation, sprain or strain in the muscles or ligaments, and back pain due to unconscious mental stress.

Imaging studies are not the last word on diagnosing back pain. The results can be difficult to interpret because people with no back pain can have abnormal MRIs while people with back pain often have normal MRIs (see Chapter 6 for more information). As we point out in Chapter 3, imaging studies and high-tech assessments are only one part of a good back pain evaluation.

The prognosis for a full recovery is extremely good even if your doctors never find the exact cause of your back pain. Treatments often work whether you know the exact cause of pain or not.

What About Alternative Treatments for My Back Pain?

People are pursuing alternative treatments for a variety of medical problems (including back pain) in record numbers. As you may know, a great many alternative treatments are available for back pain. (We review many of these in Chapters 9 through 12.) Some of the more common alternative treatments for back pain include acupuncture, chiropractic, yoga, meditation, magnets, herbal therapies, and bodywork. Whether or not you pursue these types of treatments is really an individual decision, but you can approach these treatments in a safe manner.

Alternative treatment can nicely complement traditional treatment for your back pain problem. Prior to pursuing any alternative treatments, have a good evaluation by a physician to ensure that your back pain doesn't stem from a serious problem that requires medical attention.

If you are getting only alternative medicine treatments for your back pain, continue to have periodic physician evaluations. Look very carefully into any alternative medicine treatment, regardless of whom provides the referral. To make sure that the alternative treatment you're receiving is safe, obtain answers to the following questions:

- Does this treatment involve any risk?

- How commonly is this treatment used for back pain?

- How long has this treatment been around?

- In what percentage of cases is this treatment successful for back pain?

- What are the potential side effects of this treatment?

- Can better or more proven treatments accomplish the same goal?

- How much, or how many sessions, of this treatment should I expect to undergo before I see results?

- How do you determine when and whether this treatment has been successful for my back pain?

Is My Diagnosis as Terrible as It Sounds?

As we mention in Chapter 3, doctors may use a number of scary sounding spinal diagnoses even though the reality of the condition may be nothing serious at all. Two such examples are *disc protrusion or bulge* and *degenerative disc disease*. Many diagnoses were not at all common prior to the advent of sophisticated imaging studies such as MRI and CT scan. Unfortunately, practitioners often over-interpret these imaging studies as being abnormal rather than as simply a part of normal wear-and-tear changes in the spine as you age.

Disc bulges generally aren't a cause for concern and, in fact, are present in a high percentage of the population who don't have any back pain or symptoms. Similarly, so-called arthritis of the spine and degenerative changes are most often not associated with any back symptoms. Spinal degeneration actually starts when you are about 20 years of age and continues throughout your lifetime. In the vast majority of cases, you should think of this condition as similar to other aging processes, such as your hair turning gray.

When Should I Consider Surgery for My Back Pain Problem?

Surgery is medically necessary to correct only a few spinal problems. These conditions include severe nerve compression in the lower spine, spinal tumors, and some spinal infections. In all other situations, having surgery is your choice. Making that decision can be very difficult. The guidelines we discuss in Chapter 8 and summarize in the following list can help you make a good decision:

- ✔ Consider surgery only after appropriate, conservative treatment in most cases.

- ✔ Make sure that your surgeon has a very good idea of what's causing your pain and that surgery can correct the problem.

- ✔ Be sure that your *objective findings* — such as the physical examination and imaging studies — closely match your *subjective findings* — such as your complaints about the symptoms.

- ✔ Don't agree to exploratory surgery. Your surgeon should have a pretty good idea of what he or she is going to surgically correct.

- ✔ Eliminate psychological or emotional factors — depression, anxiety, or a great deal of stress — that would get in the way of a good surgical response.

✔ Make sure that you have no other issues that may ruin your response to surgery, such as drug abuse or other medical problems.

✔ Get a second surgical opinion that is in agreement with the surgery recommendation before proceeding.

✔ Consider surgery only if your back pain is interfering with your quality of life to an unacceptable point.

Can Stress and Emotions Cause My Back Pain?

Thoughts and emotions are part of any back pain problem. Take this issue seriously if you believe — or your doctor suggests — that stress is making your back pain worse. Your brain evaluates all pain impulses and either amplifies or minimizes them. Your thoughts and emotions (and the resulting stress you experience) have great power over the way you perceive pain: Stress and emotions can worsen any pain impulses coming from your back.

Stress and emotions can actually cause your back pain. Although the exact mechanism is not clear, doctors think that unconscious stress causes muscle tightness in your lower back. The resulting pain is similar to having a tension or stress headache in your back. In this situation, your back pain originates entirely from emotional stress, and traditional medical treatments are not likely to be effective until you address the emotional stress. For more information about stress-related back pain, see Chapters 3 and 23.

How Can Pain Only in My Legs Be Related to My Back?

Think of a telephone line extending from the operating terminal to your home. If the line just outside the terminal has a problem, you experience static on your telephone even though you may be several miles away. Spinal nerves travel into your buttocks, down your legs, and all the way to your toes (see Chapter 2). If anything irritates those nerves, you can experience pain along the nerve. Thus, irritation of certain nerves in the lower spine can cause pain as far down as your feet and toes even if you don't experience any back pain, buttock pain, or upper leg pain.

What Does a Good Medical Evaluation Consist of for Back Pain?

Before high-tech tests come into the picture, your medical evaluation should certainly consist of a thorough history and physical examination. The history and physical examination can usually categorize most back pain problems, including such things as determining whether you have a sprain or strain, disc problem, or some other condition (see Chapter 6).

Your physical examination should include specialized tests such as raising each of your legs while you are lying flat on your back to test disc problems (straight leg raise), checking sensations in your lower extremities (legs, ankles, and feet), checking your muscle strength (especially in your lower body), checking your reflexes, having you walk on the balls of your feet and then your heels, and looking at your gait (how you walk).

Beyond the history and physical examination, your doctor may take an X ray of your spine. *Note:* X rays are generally not routine on your first visit to the doctor for back pain. You can usually expect an X ray if your back pain started with some type of traumatic event such as a car accident or a fall. In this case, your doctor looks for some type of fracture in your vertebra.

Your doctor may request blood and urine tests if he wants to assess other medical problems that may relate to your pain.

Reserve tests such as MRIs and CT scans for later on in your treatment, should they become necessary. These tests can help confirm a diagnosis such as a herniated disc, and they can also help your doctor determine whether invasive conservative treatment such as nerve-block injections may be helpful. Allow other diagnostic tests such as a *myelogram* (an imaging study done with you in different positions — such as bending forward and backward — after a dye is injected into your spine) or a *discogram* (a painful test to pinpoint a problem area in your spine) only if you are considering spine surgery.

Should I Continue Exercising If Doing So Worsens My Pain?

The answer to this question really depends on your situation. First of all, if at any time your activities or exercise program are making your back pain worse, you should consult with your doctor. Given that understanding, we can offer general guidelines to answer this question.

In the acute or initial stages of your back pain problem, let pain be your guide. We recommend two days of relative bed rest — up to five days only if necessary — after acute onset of your back pain; then a gradual increase in your activities (see Chapter 5). As you increase your activities and add an exercise program at this stage, stop or reduce it if your pain worsens. Letting pain be your guide also applies to other spinal conditions that require a certain healing time such as a spinal fracture or recovery from a fusion surgery.

If a chronic back pain condition causes *deconditioning* (you become physically weak from not using your muscles), you can expect to experience an increase in pain with your exercise program. This increase in pain is similar to the aches and pains you experience after a good workout at the gym, because you are using muscles that you haven't used for a while. In this case, you're experiencing "good pain" because the pain indicates that you're getting stronger.

Even if you're receiving physical rehabilitation, you should still consult your physician if exercise causes your back pain to worsen. Your physician will make sure that the pain is part of the rehabilitation process and that you have no other problems or re-injuries.

Chapter 20

Ten Steps to a Healthy Back

• •

• •

*P*revention is one of best ways to treat back pain. And one of the best ways to prevent back pain is to incorporate simple steps to keep your back healthy. The common sense methods in this chapter are not only good for your back but also for your overall health.

Stay in Shape

One of the best ways to keep your back healthy is to stay physically fit. You need to get regular, aerobic exercise. Some good overall conditioning activities that can be safe for your back include brisk walking, swimming, certain types of aerobics (low impact or in the water), and the recumbent stationary bike (in which you sit in a more reclined position with your back supported while you pedal). If you want to play sports, we recommend that you partake in an athletic activity that provides you with exercise and enjoyment. If you enjoy the activity, you are much more likely to follow through with it on a regular basis. Regular aerobic exercise is good for your mental health, too, because it relieves stress.

Do Your Back Exercises

Starting a home exercise program for your back can be a great way to keep your back healthy. A good home exercise program (we provide one in Chapter 14) keeps your back and abdominal muscles in good shape. This type of back program in conjunction with a cardiovascular or aerobic exercise program is an excellent combination.

Maintain Your Proper Body Weight

Being overweight can increase stress on all of your body's structures, including your back. A beer belly, in particular, increases the stress on your lower back, setting you up for a back injury. Therefore, part of maintaining a healthy back — not to mention heart — involves trying to maintain your proper body weight through a healthy diet. Before you start a weight-loss program, check with your doctor. Avoid the temptation to *crash diet* — starving yourself to get the weight off fast — which can be dangerous to your health and doesn't work over the long term. To get help in setting up an effective weight-loss program, you can consult a nutritionist or get involved with an organization such as Weight Watchers or Overeaters Anonymous (check your telephone directory for local numbers). As always, before starting any diet or exercise program, consult your physician.

Watch Out for High-Risk Sports

We discuss a variety of different sports and back pain in Chapter 17. Some sports are higher risk for back injuries than others. Aside from physically aggressive sports such as football, sports that require a lot of twisting can be risky, too. For instance, racquetball forces you to bend at the waist, twist, and hit the ball. This action can be stressful to your spine, especially if you don't warm up and stretch properly. Golf is another very twisty sport that can be hard on your back. Again, properly warming up and stretching are important.

If you play sports that require much twisting, bending, or impact, take special care to have a thorough warm-up routine. In many of these sports (especially golf and racquet sports), you can learn techniques to minimize your risk for back injury through lessons with a professional.

Foster a Positive Attitude

Some research studies show that job dissatisfaction and other emotional variables can increase your risk for a back injury with extended disability. Maintaining a positive attitude toward your job and home life can certainly help prevent a back pain problem. And, the converse is true, too: If you experience a back pain problem, having a positive attitude in your work and home environments helps you recover more quickly. If you feel that you can't maintain a positive attitude in these situations, talk with family and friends about options for solving the problems. Professional counseling can be helpful in this regard.

Lift and Move Properly

As we discuss in Chapter 13, lifting objects and moving them properly is an important part of protecting your back. When lifting an object, never bend over at the waist. Instead, bend at the knees, pull, and hold the object close to you, and lift from that position. Always look up before you lift to help put you in a proper lifting position.

Of course, you should also use common sense when it comes to trying to lift anything that is simply too heavy for you. Always stop and ask yourself whether lifting a too-heavy object is worth the chance of an acute back attack. Then, if you think that the object may be too heavy for your back, either use a dolly or get some help.

Don't Lift and Twist

Lifting an object and twisting at the same time is risky — you may very well cause yourself a back injury. Turn your entire body rather than twisting your back while lifting a heavy object. Also, instead of tossing something heavy, walk it to its destination. Always stretch and warm-up prior to any lifting or twisting activity (such as playing sports). See Chapter 13 for more information about twisting and posture.

Don't Stand or Sit for Long Periods

If you are in a situation where you must stand for a long period of time, try changing positions frequently and propping one foot up on a stool. Leaning against something occasionally, such as a wall or column, can also be helpful. If you can predict when you may have to stand for a long time, plan to stretch, bend, or walk prior to your standing stint, or incorporate those activities into your regular breaks. Good, supportive shoes are always helpful when you must stand for long periods (see Chapter 13), as is a surface that absorbs some shock such as a rubber mat or grass, if you have that option.

Long periods of sitting can also be quite stressful on your back because sitting puts a great deal of pressure on your spine. Driving is even worse because the road vibrations transmit to your spine. If you have to sit or drive for long periods, try to take a break at least once an hour to stretch, loosen up, and walk around.

Use a Good Chair

If you must sit for long periods of time, using a chair specially designed to put your back in the most proper and healthy position can be very helpful (see Chapter 15). Many companies design ergonomically correct chairs for those whose jobs require sitting, and some of these resources are listed in Appendix B. If you don't have — or can't get — a special chair, roll up a towel and place it behind your back for support while you sit. Propping your feet on a low foot stool or large book — a telephone book works great — can also be helpful.

Avoid Carrying Heavy Luggage

To keep your back healthy, avoid carrying heavy luggage when you travel. This advice is especially important for people who travel regularly as part of their job. Carrying heavy luggage by using a shoulder strap can be awkward and quite stressful on your back. Also, you are very likely to lift and twist heavy luggage as part of your traveling experience.

Your best bet is to get a pull cart or luggage with wheels for long walks through airports and parking lots. If no cart is available and your suitcases don't have wheels, try to balance the weight of the load on each side of your body and take frequent rest-breaks (see Chapter 13).

Chapter 21

Ten Reasons to See a Doctor for Back Pain

*W*e very much believe that you can do a tremendous amount to manage your back pain at home, on your own. In fact, we spend a good deal of time in Chapter 5 (and elsewhere throughout the book) explaining many self-care treatments. However, your doctor really does need to treat certain symptoms. This chapter lists ten occasions when you should go straight to the doctor, without passing Go or collecting $200.

You're Weak in the Legs (or Feet)

If you begin to experience weakness in one or both of your legs and/or feet, see a physician who specializes in spinal problems quickly (within 24 hours) or go to the emergency room. With *foot drop,* your foot becomes so weak that you have trouble pulling your toes up toward your head, causing your foot to "drop" and drag when you walk. Nerve compression in your spine may be the culprit (see the next section for more information).

You Can't Control Your Bowels or Bladder

If you experience a loss of bowel or bladder control, see a physician who specializes in spinal problems within 24 hours, or go to the emergency room. Also head straight for your doctor if you have any of the following:

- ✔ Loss of feeling during a bowel movement
- ✔ Inability to start or control your bowel movements
- ✔ Inability to start or control urination
- ✔ Loss of feeling to your groin or anal area
- ✔ Inability to get an erection (if you are male, of course)

Cauda equina syndrome (see Chapter 8) may cause the preceding symptoms. The cauda equina syndrome involves a compression or "pressing" on important nerves in your lower spine. These nerves supply function to your bowels and bladder, as well as sensation to your groin and anal areas. This condition usually requires quick, surgical treatment because permanent damage can occur if the nerves are compressed for too long.

Your Back Pain Gives You a Rude Awakening

If you have a back pain problem, pain may awaken you from sleep at night every once in a while. But, in some cases, *rest pain* — back pain that consistently awakens you from sleep at night — can indicate a spinal infection or tumor, although both are quite rare. A bone scan or MRI can help diagnose these conditions (see Chapter 6). People with weakened immune systems may be at greater risk.

The constant throbbing or aching pain that occurs with a tumor or spinal infection may be quite severe throughout the day, worsen with rest, and be markedly different from the type of back pain that occasionally awakens you at night. Although a tumor or spinal infection is not quite the medical emergency that a cauda equina is, see a specialist quickly if you notice rest pain symptoms (see Chapter 8).

You Have New Symptoms or Excruciating Pain

See a spinal specialist as soon as possible — or go to the emergency room — any time you have pain so excruciating that you feel unbearable. "Unbearable" is really an individual determination, but is usually defined as pain that makes you go to the ER or doctor because you just can't stand it. (What a nice circular definition: The pain is unbearable if you need to go to the ER and you should go to the ER if the pain is unbearable.)

The choice between specialist or emergency room depends upon when you experience the excruciating pain (weekday or weekend), whether you have a back specialist doctor, and how soon you can see your specialist.

✔ If your pain kicks in on the weekend when your family doctor is not in the office, or if you don't have a spine specialist, then go to the ER.

✔ If you have a back pain doctor or you have been seeing your family doctor, try to contact him or her first to get guidelines on what to do. If you are unsuccessful, go to the ER.

A physician should always check any significant increase in pain to an unbearable level.

You should also call your doctor if you begin to experience any new symptoms, including the type of symptoms we discuss earlier in this chapter and in Chapter 8, such as bowel or bladder problems, foot drop or weakness, as well as radiating pain, numbness or tingling, or shooting pains in your legs.

You Undergo a Serious Trauma

If your back pain starts with a serious trauma — like a bad fall — or is worsened by some type of accident, you should call your doctor. If your pain is unbearable, and your doctor's office is closed, you may have to go to the ER, but try to contact your doctor or back pain specialist first.

Although most back pain does not require an imaging study such as an X ray or CAT scan, in the case of trauma your doctor may need to use one of these tests to check for a possible vertebral fracture. Only your doctor can determine whether some type of vertebral fracture has occurred.

A vertebral fracture is generally not a serious problem (see Chapter 3) and usually just requires limited rest, time to heal, and appropriate treatment (such as wearing a brace, appropriate activity restrictions, and/or medicines). Once the fracture heals, your back should return to functioning normally and painlessly. A small percentage of spinal fractures are unstable and require surgery to repair.

You Want to Pursue Alternative Treatments

As we discuss in Chapter 9, we prefer the term *complementary medicine,* even though alternative medicine is a more popular term. We believe that the most powerful treatment approach is to combine both traditional and complementary medicine in an appropriate manner (see Part III).

Your physician should usually evaluate you if you decide to pursue complementary medicine treatment for your back pain (see Chapters 9 and 22 for tips on how to work with your doctor relative to complementary treatment approaches). A medical evaluation ensures that your back pain isn't due to a serious or dangerous condition. After your medical evaluation rules out any significant problems, you can pursue your complementary medicine treatments without worry.

Many alternative treatments face no federal regulations, nor does any government agency oversee them. As your complementary medicine treatment proceeds, plan to see your physician periodically to ensure that the treatment you're receiving is being provided in a safe manner.

You Need More than Chicken Soup

You can use a number of home remedies to treat your back pain, including such things as limited bed rest, ice and heat, over-the-counter anti-inflammatory medicines, and mild exercise. (See Chapter 5 for more information.) When these approaches aren't working adequately, see your doctor (if you haven't already). Your doctor can prescribe other treatments such as physical therapy, different medicines, spinal injections, and so on. (Chapter 7 has more on medical treatment for back pain.)

You're Not Seeing Improvement

Conservative treatments for your back pain include home remedies or more formal medical treatment, such as physical therapy. Back pain doctors commonly prescribe a four- to six-week course of physical therapy and then follow up with you when you finish.

Physical therapy treatment can initially aggravate your back pain due to the increase in activity. But, after a few weeks you should begin to feel some relief from your symptoms. If you don't notice improvement, see your doctor before you end the physical therapy. If the physical therapy doesn't seem to be either helping or hurting, consult your doctor. He or she may suggest changing the physical therapy approach or adding other treatments (such as medicine, nerve blocks, or complementary approaches; see Chapter 7) to help make the physical therapy more effective.

Your Medications Aren't Working

See your doctor in either of these medicine-related situations:

✔ **You experience any side effects to either prescription or over-the-counter medications:** Your doctor may want to alter your dosage or switch you to another medication (see Chapter 7).

Herbs are medicines, too. Always tell your doctor whether you are combining herbal and prescription medicines. If you begin to experience side effects, your physician may need to evaluate any drug interactions.

✔ **You are using drugs to self-medicate your back pain:** Self-medicating in this sense includes such things as using more medication than is prescribed for you, using alcohol to treat your back pain, using someone else's medication, or using other substances or drugs (such as marijuana or opiates) to manage your pain.

Your Doctor Recommends Surgery

Consider the following when choosing to have spine surgery: whether your symptoms warrant surgery, whether your symptoms match your test findings, whether conservative treatment has failed, and whether or not you judge your quality of life to be unacceptable. (See Chapter 8 for more information.)

If your doctor recommends spine surgery, always get a second opinion. Spine surgery is often a significant, irreversible, and invasive medical procedure that you should not undergo lightly. A second opinion gives you the opportunity to hear what another trained specialist thinks about your back pain condition, to determine whether other nonsurgical treatments may be helpful, and to decide whether spine surgery may be effective.

Chapter 22

Ten Tips for Working Successfully with Your Doctor

· ·

In This Chapter

▶ Practicing assertive communication

▶ Planning your interview and doctor visit in advance

▶ Preparing your medical fact sheet

▶ Maintaining a positive attitude

▶ Engaging in a dialogue with your doctor

▶ Understanding the course of treatment

▶ Taking a friend

▶ Directing your questions to the appropriate person

▶ Exploring other sources of information

· ·

Surveys show that most people generally are satisfied with the care they get from their doctors. Unfortunately, good care doesn't always translate into good communication. A recent American Medical Association survey shows that only 42 percent of patients feel that doctors usually explain things well and only 31 percent believe that physicians spend enough time with their patients.

Patients commonly make the following complaints about their doctors:

✔ My doctor doesn't spend enough time with me.

✔ My doctor isn't friendly.

✔ My doctor doesn't answer questions openly.

✔ My doctor doesn't explain problems understandably.

✔ My doctor doesn't treat me with respect.

Doctors, as busy professionals, are sometimes lacking in the active communication department. That's where you come in. The ability to work with your doctor and other treatment providers effectively is a critical part of enhancing your response to treatment. The tips in this chapter show you how to communicate with your doctor while preserving the quality of the overall relationship. By following these techniques, you and your doctor can work together to create the best possible treatment program for you.

Identifying Your Communication Style

Your personal communication style can have a great impact on the doctor-patient relationship. Research shows that people tend to use one of four different types of communication. You may notice that you tend to use one style of communication in one type of situation and a completely different style in other interactions. See M. McKay, et al., *Messages: The Communication Skills Book, 2nd Edition* (Oakland, CA: New Harbinger Publications, 1995).

- **Non-assertive or submissive:** *Non-assertive behavior* is giving in to another person's preferences while discounting your own rights and needs. If you're chronically non-assertive, you may often feel the need to please others around you, and you may be afraid that people won't like you if you actually express desires. At the same time, you may feel guilty or resentful that your rights are being "violated," when, in truth, no one knows how you feel. People around you may not even realize that you are being non-assertive or submissive because you never express your needs.

- **Aggressive:** *Aggressive behavior* involves expressing your wants and desires in a way that is hostile or attacks. Aggressive people are typically insensitive to the rights and feelings of others around them and use coercion and intimidation to get what they want. People who are the targets of aggressive communication respond in one of two ways: Either they leave the situation or they become defensive and fight back.

Being aggressive when seeking treatment for your back pain can be disastrous. An aggressive attitude toward your doctor, nurses, and social support network can cause them to withdraw from you or counterattack in a similarly aggressive manner.

- **Passive-aggressive:** *Passive-aggressive behavior* is a means of expressing anger in a passive manner. Passive-aggressive people are likely to express hostile urges or anger in a sullen, disgruntled attitude and actions that obstruct the wishes of others. Passive-aggressive behavior is designed to frustrate others by such things as postponing decisions, constantly raising objections, or taking ineffective action. Expressing anger in a passive-aggressive way is a very ineffective means of communication, which usually leaves your needs unmet and others around you frustrated.

- **Assertive:** *Assertive communication* allows you to express how you feel or what you want while respecting the rights of others. Assertive communication is simple and direct without attacking, manipulating, or discounting those around you.

Becoming an Assertive Communicator

You can teach yourself to communicate in an assertive fashion. The following bulleted list provides guidelines for making assertive requests with your doctor:

- ✔ **Use assertive nonverbal behavior:** Your body language goes above and beyond your verbal expression. Assertive behavior includes such things as establishing eye contact with your doctor, keeping your head up, standing straight, maintaining an *open posture* (facing your doctor with your head up and arms uncrossed), and staying calm.

- ✔ **Keep your request simple:** An assertive request is simple, direct, and straightforward. Ask for only one thing at a time, because a multitude of requests can be quite confusing for your doctor. Easy-to-understand sentences, such as "I would like more information about my treatment program," or "I would like more information about how to obtain a second opinion," are effective and assertive communications.

- ✔ **Be specific:** Before you see your doctor, determine your wants, needs, and feelings so that you can express them in a specific fashion. Avoid vague requests like, "I would like to get more help from your office staff regarding your recommendations," which your doctor may not interpret correctly. Instead, opt for the more effective, "I would appreciate your office staff's help with getting insurance approval, setting up my appointment for the MRI, and getting me information about pain control."

- ✔ **Use "I" statements:** People have a tendency to tell others what they want them to do by using "You-statements" such as, "You need to help me out more." To the person listening, these statements may feel threatening, which puts the receiver on the defensive. Instead, use "I" statements, which frame your request in terms of your own needs. "I would like to better understand my treatment plan" elicits a totally different response than, "You're not giving me enough information about my treatment."

- ✔ **Avoid the temptation to address personality flaws; concentrate on behaviors instead:** You may be tempted to say, "I know that as a doctor, you're very impatient, but can you explain this test to me again?" Your doctor will respond to your needs much more favorably if you instead say, "I would like you to explain this test to me again so that I better understand my treatment."

- ✔ **Don't apologize for your request:** If you tend to be a non-assertive communicator, you may have trouble believing yourself that your request deserves a response. This feeling surfaces in your statements: "I'm really sorry to ask, but could you, if possible, explain the test results again?" With an apologetic approach, your actual request is often ignored. Instead, go with a more assertive, "I would appreciate it if you would explain the test results again."

✔ **Don't make demands:** Assertive communication involves either making a request of another person or setting a limit by saying, "No." In either case, always communicate in a way that respects the rights and dignity of the other person.

Planning Your Interview and Doctor Visit in Advance

Before you see your doctor, think about what you want to get out of this particular visit and then make a list of your questions and concerns in a simple and straightforward format. Be realistic about the number of questions you can ask on any given visit. Although you may feel as if you should be able to spend as much time with your doctor as you like (and ask as many questions as you want), this simply cannot happen. Your doctor needs to balance the time available for all patients throughout the day.

As you look over your list of concerns and questions, you should be able to summarize them into about five main questions, which will allow adequate time for discussion. Writing the questions down on a piece of paper and bringing them with you helps ensure that you get the information you require. Depending on the situation, you may want to fax your questions to the doctor's office prior to your visit so that your doctor can review the questions before he or she meets with you.

Communicating your goals at the outset can help the visit go smoothly. For instance, you may start out your visit by telling your doctor that you have five questions or concerns that you would like to address with her.

Preparing Your Medical Fact Sheet

Writing up a *medical fact sheet* — a written summary of your important medical information — can help you get the best possible treatment while avoiding any dangerous or harmful mistakes. Some doctors send you a fact sheet to fill out before your initial visit. You should check to make sure that the doctor's fact sheet contains at least the following information (and add the information if it is not addressed). Otherwise, you need to do your own fact sheet. Your sheet (or sheets) should be concise and neat and include at least the following information:

✔ Your name, address, phone numbers, emergency contacts, and any special problems or disabilities

✔ Current medical conditions with brief explanations

✔ Previous treatments and your response

✔ Previous tests (such as an MRI) and the results

✔ Past medical conditions with brief explanations and dates

✔ Surgical history with dates and outcomes

✔ Current medications with dosages and side effects

✔ Allergic reactions to medications

✔ Other physicians and specialists involved in your medical care (name, address, phone number, and conditions being treated)

After you prepare your medical fact sheet, take a copy to each of your health-care professionals. By providing this information, you help them to facilitate coordination of your treatments and do a better job overall.

Checking Your Attitude

Your attitude about your doctor visit can affect the outcome greatly. For instance, if you are angry because you're in pain or don't like doctors, you are likely to be aggressive. Although some doctors are more understanding than others about your pain and the irritability that goes with it, most doctors meet aggressiveness with either defensiveness or counter-aggressiveness. Either situation does not lead to a pleasant and productive visit.

Another way to keep your cool is to bring along something to do while you are waiting in the doctor's waiting room. Your attitude can go from pleasant to sour when you're left sitting in the waiting room with magazines from the early 1960s. Take an interesting piece of reading material — like this book, maybe? — or some other hobby (crochet, knitting, a video game, or your big screen TV, for example) to keep yourself pleasantly occupied.

A common perception is that doctors do not value their patients' time, but demand that patients honor theirs. Although some doctors certainly have such an attitude, most will keep their patients waiting only when uncontrollable circumstances arise (such as an urgent phone call related to patient care, an emergency patient visit, or a surgery that goes on longer than expected). Unfortunately, in the business of *doctoring*, these unforeseen problems causing delays happen more frequently than in other lines of work.

Allowing the Doctor to Ask Questions First

Your doctor needs to gather a great deal of information in a relatively short period of time, so let him or her ask questions first. After that, you can ask for any information not covered or that is unclear. Even though waiting to tell your doctor information that you think is important can be difficult, resist the urge to go into the visit with a prepared monologue because you may end up giving the doctor information that is not relevant to your diagnosis and treatment. Your doctor will usually open with questions about how you're doing and what symptoms you're experiencing. Answering these opening questions is your opportunity to tell your doctor what is going on. The doctor has to gather certain information in order to formulate a treatment plan and assess your progress (that's what you're paying for). After he or she obtains that information, you can express your specific questions and concerns.

If you're concerned that you will run out of time before you can ask your questions, simply alert the doctor at the beginning of the appointment by saying something like, "I have several questions for you, so would you please save enough time for me to ask them before we finish with the appointment?"

Making Sure That You Understand the Conclusions

Summarize any conclusions you and your doctor have come to at the end of the visit. If you're uncertain about any instructions or guidelines, address these before you leave. You may want to take notes during the office visit, but avoid getting so focused on recording every detail that you don't pay attention to what you doctor is saying. If you don't understand a recommendation (especially one related to medicines), be sure to ask for clarification.

Bringing a Friend

Bringing a friend or family member is an effective way to get the most out of your doctor visit — especially if you're facing an important medical decision or gathering information from a specialist.

Dr. T. Ferguson concludes that bringing another person with you can help in many ways. See T. Ferguson, "Working with your doctor" in *Mind-Body Medicine: How to Use Your Mind for Better Health,* edited by D. Goleman and J. Gurin (Yonkers, NY: Consumer Reports Books, 1993).

> ✔ Your friend's presence has a calming and relaxing effect, allowing you to focus better.
>
> ✔ You're less likely to feel intimidated with someone else along.
>
> ✔ Your companion can bring up questions or concerns and help you recall the discussion with the doctor. If you and your friend do not agree on what was heard, then you can raise these questions with your doctor on the next visit.
>
> ✔ Your friend can act as a reality check on how the visit with the doctor went.

Using the suggestions we present in this chapter, you may want to develop an overall strategy for your doctor's visit with your friend or family member beforehand.

Directing Your Questions to the Appropriate Person

Many doctors have a physician's assistant or nurse who works closely with him or her. This person can frequently be one of your best sources of additional information about your back pain problem. Your doctor can help you determine who in the office can gather information. Also, think ahead about who may be the best person to ask a specific question. For instance, appointment and insurance questions usually go to the administrative personnel, so you don't have to use your appointment time to discuss those issues with your doctor.

Exploring Other Sources of Information

You may be able to get further information about your back pain problem from resources other than your doctor. For instance, your doctor may mention a certain diagnosis or treatment approach but not go into much detail due to time constraints. You may be able to find more information by reading books about the problem or procedure, searching the Internet, and joining self-help groups. The resources in Appendix B can be a good place to start searching out more information.

Carefully scrutinize the source and content of the information you obtain, especially from the Internet. (Information on the Internet is completely unregulated and often invalid.) Countless patients have been unduly frightened by information they found about their diagnosis and/or treatment plan. Generally, medical information from a Web site associated with a university or the U.S. government is more reliable than sites representing commercial ventures. Appendix B has several good Web sites for collecting more medical information.

Chapter 23

Ten Hot Topics in Back Pain

*R*esearchers and healthcare professionals are constantly developing new evaluation and treatment methods for back pain problems. Emerging technology and testing methods allow for quicker and more accurate diagnoses. As with any evolving field, there are a number of hot topics in back pain evaluation and treatment.

This chapter covers ten of the hottest topics in the back pain world today. Some of these developments are already in use while others are just in the testing stages; even so, they are all exciting.

A Revolutionary New Medicine: Celebrex

Nonsteroidal anti-inflammatory drugs (NSAIDs) such as aspirin, ibuprofen, and naproxen (in addition to many prescription NSAIDs) are among the most commonly used pain medicines in the world. In fact, it's estimated that more than 100 million people worldwide take NSAIDs on a regular basis for a vast array of medical conditions in which pain and inflammation are part of the problem, including arthritis and back pain. NSAIDs can be quite effective, but they can cause serious side effects such as stomach and intestinal upset, bleeding ulcers, and kidney problems.

Studies show that if you take NSAIDs for a long period of time, you have a one-in-five chance of developing an ulcer. Also, it's estimated that there are 80,000 cases of bleeding ulcers and 6,000 deaths in the United States each year due to NSAID use.

For many years, scientists have been searching for an alternative type of anti-inflammatory medication that does not have these serious side effects. The search is now over with the release of a new medicine by Searle Pharmaceuticals: Celebrex. The Food and Drug Administration recently approved Celebrex, the first medicine in a new class of drugs known as *COX-2 inhibitors*. The important feature of these new medicines is that they provide an anti-inflammatory benefit without the side effects of wrecking your stomach and intestines.

Currently, Celebrex is approved for use only in rheumatoid and osteoarthritis, although it is anticipated that the medicine will be approved for more general pain relief, such as for back problems, in the near future. You should ask your doctor about the COX-2 inhibitors; they are available by prescription only.

Back Pain and the Unconscious Mind

Mind-body medicine is among the least understood areas in Western medicine today, although much of the future war against back pain may be battled on this front.

One diagnosis that takes into account mind-body issues in back pain is *tension myositis syndrome* (TMS). John Sarno initially coined the term TMS in his first book, *Mind Over Back Pain,* back in 1981. He described the *psychosomatic* (in other words, mind affecting your body) process in which your back pain is the result of repressed emotions, most commonly anger or rage. TMS is not dangerous and is reversible. To treat TMS pain successfully, you need to recognize it as a mind-body problem and see it as a distraction from underlying emotions. You don't necessarily need to identify the specific emotion or unconscious cause to get better. (This explains how thousands of patients around the United States have gotten over their back pain simply by reading Dr. Sarno's book and diagnosing themselves.)

Self-diagnosis can be dangerous. In rare cases, something serious like a tumor or infection can be causing the pain. If you self-diagnose TMS and don't get better, see a doctor familiar with TMS to confirm the diagnosis.

According to Dr. Sarno, even though you may receive a structural diagnosis such as a disc herniation, degenerative disc disease, osteoarthritis, or scoliosis, TMS may actually be the culprit. If that is the case, the structural problems may be irrelevant. Many people without back pain show various structural problems on X rays and MRIs. TMS is actually quite common, and we successfully treat people with this condition every day. You are likely to improve just by recognizing repressed anger or rage as the source of your pain.

At first, you may have difficulty accepting that structural findings shown on imaging tests (such as an X ray) may have absolutely nothing to do with your pain, especially when your doctor reinforces structural diagnosis. Unfortunately, only a handful of physicians across the country are skilled in diagnosing and treating TMS.

TMS is a hot topic because Dr. Sarno recently released a new book, *The Mind-Body Prescription.* His entire theory remains controversial among most medical professionals, but we are strong advocates of his work and believe it applies to a significant number of back pain sufferers. Dr. Sarno has made a dramatic impact with the public through his popular books. Andrew Weil's best-selling book, *Spontaneous Healing,* references the entire subject of back pain to Dr. Sarno's work with TMS.

The Cybertech Back Brace

Although back braces of various designs and styles have been around for years, something new is on the horizon: the *Cybertech orthosis.* This back brace (or *lumbar orthosis,* as it is called) offers a level of comfort, support, and stability unparalleled in comparative products. In fact, Dr. Stephen Hochschuler, a spine surgeon who is Chairman of the Texas Back Institute, feels that the Cybertech brace is the most user-friendly support available. With an ingenious yet simple pulley system, the brace can reach compressive forces previously unobtainable except in large, bulky, extremely expensive, custom-made back braces.

The Cybertech brace is easy to take on and off, as well as adjust for tightness. By increasing the pressure in your abdominal area as the brace tightens, the stress on your spinal structures is reduced. This reduction, in turn, reduces the likelihood of injury to your spine while also supporting an already injured area. Thereby, you have a decreased chance of re-injuring yourself or worsening your back pain. While offering support and stability, the Cybertech brace also enables you to move around and function better overall during an episode of back pain and spasm. The supportive pressure of the Cybertech brace on your muscles and nerves can reduce pain by altering the signal sent up the nerves to the spinal cord where pain is carried.

You may have heard that back braces cause muscle weakness and atrophy. Part of this general belief is a myth, because it depends upon how you use the back brace. Lumbar braces can be worn daily without causing muscle weakness or atrophy as long as you continue to exercise your back muscles. We typically prescribe a Cybertech brace in conjunction with a back exercise program. The Cybertech brace can also help support your back area during such activities as prolonged sitting or driving. The Cybertech brace is now being used for spinal fractures and after spinal surgery.

MR Neurography: Taking a Picture of Your Nerves

In the field of spinal problems and back pain, a good medical history and physical examination can often reveal to your doctor much information about what may be causing your symptoms. When the problem is still not obvious, you may need medical imaging studies such as X rays, CAT scans, and MRI scans. As we describe in Chapter 6, imaging studies may also be called for in other spinal problems, such as when a tumor is suspected or a surgery is being considered.

As one of the innovators of a new type of imaging study, Dr. Aaron Filler of the UCLA School of Medicine states that your doctor can now obtain detailed pictures of your nerves through the use of MR Neurography.

MR Neurography fine-tunes MRI technology to give an excellent picture of your nerves. Prior to this innovation, this level of image detail was simply not possible with a regular MRI. The results of MR Neurography are amazing, given the size of a nerve and the complexity of the details. For example, if you have a pinched nerve, an MR Neurogram can actually show the dent in your nerve. The procedure for getting an MR Neurogram is the same as for an MRI. Refer to Chapter 6 for more information on MRIs.

Your doctor must ultimately decide whether MR Neurography can be helpful in identifying what is causing your pain.

Unfortunately, MR Neurography is so new that your doctor may not have even heard of it! Only a small fraction of the MRI scanners in the United States are of high enough quality to be able to produce the MR Neurogram image. In addition, most radiologists have not been trained in the area of reading and interpreting this type of scan. You're most likely to find MR Neurography available at a university medical school, or check out Appendix B in this book for facilities with Neurogram capability.

If you're going to have spine surgery, a Neurogram prior to your operation is not usually necessary. Most of the time, the routine imaging of your lumbar or cervical spine is very accurate. As such, your surgeon will be very sure of what is wrong and what needs to be done about it surgically. However, if the images don't quite add up and your doctor is uncertain about where your pain might be coming from, consider asking about Neurography. Dr. Brad Jabour, Chief of Neuroradiology at the Medical Imaging Center of Southern California, states that MR Neurography will have expanding clinical applications in the next five to ten years.

Preparing Psychologically for Your Spine Surgery

Psychological preparation for your spine surgery is easy to do, safe, side effect free, and cost-effective. Over the past thirty years, more than 200 research studies with thousands of patients investigating psychological preparation for surgery have found the following beneficial effects.

A surgery preparation program is straightforward, and you can do most or all of the preparation on your own. You can expect the following benefits from psychological preparation for surgery:

- Decreased distress before and after your surgery
- Less need for pain medications
- Fewer postoperative complications
- Quicker return to health
- Increased satisfaction with your overall surgery experience

Even though these techniques have overwhelming scientific support for their effectiveness and are widely available, you do not find them used much in surgical practice. The reasons for this are many, but probably the primary explanation is that surgery has traditionally been viewed in mechanical terms, attending to the parts of your body that need to be "fixed" without taking *you,* as an entire person, into account.

Technological advances related to spine surgery, as well as the managed care movement, have prompted a strong trend toward shorter hospital stays and more outpatient surgeries. As a result, your doctor, surgeon, nurse, and other healthcare professionals have much less contact with you during the entire surgical process than they would have a decade ago. This lack of contact makes it much more difficult for your doctors to adequately prepare you for the procedure as well as monitor, guide, and reassure you during the postoperative phase.

To get the most out of your medical care, you must take more responsibility and play a more active role in your treatment. A psychological preparation for surgery program can help you accomplish this goal.

Following are some important components of a psychological preparation for surgery program:

- **Collecting information about your surgery:** The first step in a preparation for surgery program is for you to find out as much as possible about your surgery. This involves gathering and deciphering medical information and asking questions in order to ensure that you really understand what is going on and what will happen.

- **Getting adequate pain control:** Almost all surgical procedures cause mild to severe postoperative pain and, if you are like most patients, this pain may be one of your greatest worries. Adequate postoperative pain control is essential to the overall success of your surgery. Postoperative pain that is not well controlled can impair your healing and recovery as well as have a demoralizing effect on you and your family. Even though your surgeon may downplay the issue of postoperative pain control, it is important for you to play an active role in establishing your pain control plan with your physician prior to surgery.

- **Cognitive techniques:** *Cognitive-behavioral techniques* is a fancy term for approaches that change the way you think (see Chapter 12 for more details). These exercises can help you prepare for your surgery by decreasing your preoperative anxiety and fear and by giving you coping skills to help decrease distress and pain after surgery.

- **Relaxation techniques:** Stress causes harmful effects on your body, including elevated blood pressure, elevated heart rate, increased muscle tension, rapid and shallow breathing, release of stress hormones, reduced blood flow to certain areas of the body, diminished immune system function, and slowed tissue-healing time. Relaxation techniques can effectively block this stress and help you reduce pain, control nausea, enhance immune system function, and improve your breathing. You can use many methods to achieve the relaxation response, including breathing techniques, progressive muscle relaxation, visualizing a peaceful scene, and meditation, among others. These methods are fully reviewed in Chapter 12, and further information is available in Appendix B.

- **Spiritual issues:** Even though most Americans feel that spiritual issues are important, many doctors are reluctant to discuss them. Thus you as a patient may be reluctant to bring up these issues. Recent research indicates that spirituality can make a positive contribution to your physical health and may help with your surgery.

- **Developing assertiveness skills:** The process of surgery and postoperative recovery can bring up many stressful situations in which assertiveness skills are required for you to get good care. You may need to be assertive in a variety of situations such as work, home, and medical settings.

Preparing for your surgery can yield many positive benefits with a minimal amount of time investment. Even with all the research documenting its effectiveness, psychological preparation for surgery is not yet part of mainstream medicine. Therefore, you probably need to pursue it on your own and educate your doctors and surgeons about what you are doing.

Spinal Endoscopy

Spinal endoscopy is a new high-tech procedure that can be used to help diagnose and treat your chronic lower back and leg pain.

As described by Dr. Mary Jo Ford of Beverly Hills, California, spinal endoscopy is a surgical procedure in which a special viewing instrument (called a *flexible fiber-optic endoscope*) and a very small tube (called a *catheter*) are used to allow your physician to look inside and treat certain parts of your spine, including tissues and nerves. This procedure is considered minimally invasive and is done on an outpatient basis. Compared to traditional spinal surgery, spinal endoscopy has the advantages of being less invasive, offering faster recovery time, and being cost-effective.

If you undergo a spinal endoscopy, you are awake, lying on your stomach, and sedated with special medicines. Local anesthetic is injected to numb any pain you may feel as the doctor inserts the instrument in your back just above your buttocks. The endoscope and catheter are inserted through a small hole into the area inside the spinal column but outside the spinal cord itself. Your doctor uses an X ray to guide the endoscope, and the image appears on a video monitor.

In using the spinal endoscopy procedure, your physician looks on the video monitor for abnormalities in the tissues, inflammation, and adhesions. Although patients are sometimes completely sedated for the procedure, it is very helpful if you are alert and able to communicate with your doctor while it is going on. Your doctor carefully brings the endoscope near suspected problem areas in your spine to see whether it causes your usual symptoms to start occurring or become worse. This procedure helps your doctor confirm that the trouble spots are being accurately pinpointed for treatment.

The entire procedure takes about 30 minutes. You're discharged when you are fully recovered from the procedure and anesthesia (about an hour). You should be given detailed discharge instructions, and schedule a follow-up evaluation with your physician. Plan on having someone drive you home and on resting for the remainder of the day.

Spinal endoscopy is certainly not for everyone. The procedure may be appropriate for you if you suffer from chronic back pain and/or pain that goes into your buttocks and legs. The spinal endoscopy procedure is considered for you only if you have not responded to other conservative therapies that do not require surgery (as described in Chapter 7), such as physical therapy, medications, and so on. Also, if you suffer from other diseases or have psychological problems, you may not be a good candidate. Your doctor or a physician who specializes in this type of procedure can determine whether you are a candidate.

The risks associated with spinal endoscopy are minimal. You can expect some discomfort at the site where the endoscope and catheter were inserted. You may experience temporary symptoms such as an increase in your back or leg pain or a headache. Very rare risks include infection or nerve injury, and these complications usually completely resolve with time if they do happen to occur. Keep in mind that you may not be able to assess the results of the spinal endoscopy for several weeks.

Preemptive Analgesia

As described by Dr. John Reeves in his book, *Preparing for Surgery,* preemptive analgesia has been the focus of a great deal of exciting research recently. It is certainly something you should investigate if you are going to have a spine surgery, although your surgeon and anesthesiologist may not be entirely familiar with it. The research in this area is very promising and generally shows that preemptive analgesia patients usually have less postoperative pain and require less postoperative pain medications.

Preemptive analgesia is based upon the concept that pain messages from tissue damage can actually cause permanent changes in your nervous system that make you hypersensitive to pain. In these cases, you continue to experience a pain signal coming from the area of tissue damage long after the site has healed. It's almost as if your nervous system were sending a false pain signal. One example of when these "false pain signals" can occur is the tissue damage caused by a surgery itself. In this situation, you continue to experience the pain signal (that started with the surgery) long after you have healed postoperatively.

The goal of preemptive analgesia is to prevent the pain message from reaching your spinal cord so that lasting changes in your nervous system do not occur.

As such, preemptive analgesia requires taking action before your surgery and/or during the surgery itself. This action can include such things as:

✔ Giving you opioid medications, nonsteroidal anti-inflammatory drugs (NSAIDs), or other pain-relieving medications before the surgery

✔ Injecting local anesthetics into the area of your surgery (during the surgery)

✔ Injecting local anesthetics around the nerves responsible for transmitting the pain message to the spinal cord (either before or during your surgery)

✔ Injecting your spine with a local anesthetic in order to block nerve impulses

Preemptive analgesia may be addressed before your surgery, during it, or both. The medication you may be given prior to surgery depends on a number of factors that your doctor addresses. For instance, in spine surgery you may not be able to take any anti-inflammatory medicine just prior to surgery, and you must use some other preemptive analgesia medications.

Preemptive analgesia is a relatively new finding and is not yet widely used. If you are facing spine surgery, be sure to discuss this option with your surgeon or anesthesiologist. Preemptive analgesia is especially important to consider if you have already been experiencing significant pain prior to your surgery. Scientific evidence suggests that if you have spine-related pain for some time prior to surgery (especially nerve-related pain), it can be prevented from worsening postoperatively through preemptive analgesia methods.

Treating Massive Disc Herniations without Surgery

In the past, spine surgeons may have recommended spine surgery for a large disc herniation rather than trying a conservative, non-surgical approach. Surgeons suggested surgery because they were fearful of what problems a massive disc herniation might cause if not surgically corrected.

In a recent study in our center, we looked at what would happen when patients who had "massive" disc herniations (from 7 mm to 17 mm) were treated with conservative treatment and time. By common surgical decision-making standards, these patients often would have been considered appropriate surgical candidates due to the size and symptoms of their herniations.

The patients were given an initial MRI that confirmed the presence and size of the herniation. Patients were then given a conservative treatment, which included limited bed rest, physical therapy, medication, epidural steroid injections, and healing time. All patients underwent a follow-up MRI at a minimum of six months later.

Dramatically, our study showed that the disc herniations had decreased in size an average of 62 percent! This study shows that having a large disc herniation does not automatically mean you need surgery. In appropriate cases, even if you have a disc herniation the size of a bus (well, maybe a VW beetle), conservative treatment can be effective.

This study does not indicate that spine surgery for a herniated disc is not a successful treatment. In properly selected patients, as we discuss in Chapter 8, surgery is very successful. Rather, the study outlines a non-surgical treatment option that you may discuss with your doctor if you have a large disc herniation.

Advances in Spine Surgery

Dr. Theodore Goldstein of Cedars-Sinai Medical Center in Los Angeles, describes an especially exciting new development that may revolutionize disc surgery. The procedure is called *IDET* (intradiscal electrothermal annuloplasty), and some researchers believe that it may eventually replace most fusion surgeries. (As we discuss in Chapter 8, *fusion* surgery is a costly operation in which two adjacent vertebrae are "fused" together.)

IDET takes about 15 minutes and is done under local anesthetic. (A fusion involves general anesthesia, several days of hospitalization, and months of post-operative recovery time.)

In order to understand how IDET works, think of the disc between two vertebrae as a car tire made of tightly woven bands of ligaments and filled with a gel-like toothpaste (see Chapter 2 for more information). When the disc is in good shape, it forms a tight seal on the vertebra and provides a cushion. For a variety of reasons (such as injury or aging), the ligaments that encase the disc can wear, tear, and loosen, allowing veins and nerves to get inside the disc (where they are not supposed to be). The invading nerves then get pinched by the vertebra causing significant pain.

You can think of IDET as trying to "repair the tire" (disc) rather than throwing it out. (We're really "wearing out" the tire analogy at this point, aren't we?) IDET uses a Spine-Cath (developed by Drs. Jeffrey and Joel Saal of Stanford University), which is a 6-inch needle and a fine catheter with a heating element on the end. The catheter is inserted through the needle and into the problem disc. It is then heated to 194 degrees for 14 to 17 minutes. The heat kills the nerves that have invaded the disc and tightens the surrounding ligaments creating a new seal (sorta like "patching the tire").

The technique is still under research, with only about 700 patients having been treated with the procedure. The early results are good with 80 percent of patients reporting reduced pain, increased mobility, and decreased need for pain medicine.

Advances in Implantable Pain Therapies

As we describe in Chapter 7, implantable pain therapies are the most invasive of the conservative treatments. As explained by Dr. Joshua Prager of the UCLA School of Medicine, implantable pain therapies consist of two different types: spinal cord stimulation (SCS) and intraspinal drug infusion therapy.

Both of these procedures involve minor surgery to place the devices in your body. These devices have no curative properties but are designed to provide relief of your symptoms. These treatments should be considered only when all other treatments for your pain have been tried and found not to be beneficial.

Advances in spinal cord stimulation technology

As we cover in Chapter 7, spinal cord stimulation involves surgically placing a set of electrodes in the epidural space of your spine. These electrodes send a mild electrical signal to the spinal cord that prevents the pain signals from getting all the way to your brain. In essence, the SCS blocks the pain signal to help give you some relief.

Until recently, SCS was shown to be effective mainly for back pain that radiates down the leg, as opposed to pain in the back itself (see Chapter 7). Research in Europe now demonstrates that electrodes spaced closer together produce a greater effect for the spinal cord stimulation. With a switch to more closely spaced electrodes, called *dual lead systems,* SCS may be effective for both back and leg pain.

As of now, this type of dual lead electrode equipment requires more sophisticated electronics than is currently available from totally implanted systems. Thus, lower back pain must be treated with devices that have an external power source (outside your body) that "drives" a receiver inside your body by an antenna. (The units that treat just leg pain are totally contained inside your body and do not require the external unit.)

Being able to treat back pain with dual lead stimulation is exciting, but the drawback of an externally driven system deters some people. In Europe, a new system has been released that is internally powered and can run sophisticated internal dual lead systems. This technology should be available throughout the world in the near future so that SCS may replace the need for intraspinal drug administration systems in some patients with low-back pain only.

New medications for intraspinal drug infusion systems

The Food and Drug Administration (FDA) currently approves only two medications for use with intraspinal drug infusion systems. Only one of these two medications, morphine, is approved to treat pain with the use of a pumping device.

Pain physicians, many of whom are anesthesiologists, have begun widespread use of other medications in pumps to treat back pain. Local anesthetics are FDA-approved for spinal use as part of spinal anesthesia but not for use with intraspinal drug infusion systems (even though the medication is directed into the identical space in your spine). Local anesthetics mixed with morphine in the pump can lower your morphine requirement and improve your pain relief. Using medications in this way is called *off label use,* meaning the medication is not yet FDA-approved for that use. Off label use of a medication is legal and is the prerogative of your physician *as long as there is a rationale and it is safe.*

Off label use of other medications is rapidly improving the effectiveness of treatment with intraspinal drug infusion systems. Other medications in the morphine family have different characteristics, and you may respond better to one of these medicines rather than morphine.

- ✔ **Clonidine,** a drug developed to treat high blood pressure, is now being used in the pump to treat pain without having to use an opioid. Using a drug like this one eliminates possible opioid side effects such as dizziness, constipation, and nausea.

- ✔ **Ziconotide,** a drug in final-phase testing for use in intraspinal drug infusion systems, was originally derived from the venom of the only fish-eating snail in the world. The dosage of this medication is in micrograms (billionths of a gram). This promising medication has a very special action on nerve tissue that may help with pain relief.

The use of these types of medications with intraspinal drug infusion systems (beyond morphine) provides greater potential use of this treatment approach if you have a complex back pain problem that has not responded adequately to other conventional therapies.

Appendix A

Glossary

● ●

*T*his glossary defines many of the most important — and often most confusing — terms that you encounter reading this book or working with your back pain practitioner. Cross-referenced terms are in ***bold italics.***

Acetaminophen: The pain-relieving or analgesic substance in Tylenol. A non-narcotic pain reliever that does not have anti-inflammatory properties. Less irritating to the stomach and intestinal tract than anti-inflammatory medicines.

Acupoints: Acupuncture points throughout the body that correspond to specific organs. Acupoints are found along the ***meridians.***

Acupuncture: An ancient Chinese medicine approach in which small needles that pierce the skin are placed at specific body locations (acupoints) to cause healing or other benefits (for example, pain relief).

Acute back pain: Back pain that has rapid onset, severe symptoms, and short duration. In contrast to chronic back pain, acute back pain is sometimes defined as continuing for less than three months.

Analgesic: A pain-relieving substance.

Anesthetic: Any substance that causes a loss of sensation or feeling, especially pain.

Ankylosing spondylitis: A progressive inflammatory disease of the spine that is more common in men.

Annulus fibrosis: The tough fibrous outer portion of the intervertebral disc.

Anterior: Toward the front or forward part of the body or an organ.

Anti-anxiety medications: Medications used for the relief of anxiety. They are also termed *anxiolytics.*

Anti-depressants: Medications that provide relief from depression. In much lower doses, they can also provide pain relief and help with sleep.

Anti-inflammatory: A substance that decreases the inflammatory response of tissues as well as reduces swelling and pain. Medication examples include Motrin, Naprosyn, and aspirin.

Arachnoiditis: An inflammatory condition of spinal *arachnoid* (connective tissue around the spinal cord). *Arachnoid* literally means *like a cobweb,* which describes how the structure looks on imaging studies.

Arthritis: Inflammation and irritation of the joints that often includes swelling and pain.

Biofeedback: A treatment approach in which a physical response or symptom, such as muscle tension, heart rate, sweat gland activity, or blood pressure, is electronically measured and fed back to you so you can learn to bring it under voluntary control.

Bodywork: A term referring to therapies such as massage, deep tissue manipulation, movement awareness, and energy balancing.

Bone scan: A scan or *X ray* taken after a radioactive dye is injected and allowed to concentrate in the skeleton. The primary use of a bone scan is to diagnose a fracture, infection, tumor, or *arthritis* of the bones. Any area of increased concentration of the dye is significant.

Bulging disc: An intravertebral disc that sticks out only slightly from its normal space without breaking through the annulus fibrosis. It may or may not cause any symptoms. See also *protrusion,* and *sequestration,* and contrast with *extrusion.*

Bursitis: Inflammation of the *bursa* (a saclike cavity filled with lubricating fluid and located within a joint).

Cervical spine: The seven vertebrae that comprise the neck area of the spine.

Chemonycleosis: A treatment in which a chemical is injected into the disc in order to dissolve the part of it that is thought to cause symptoms. Because of possible severe side effects, this treatment is no longer used in the United States.

Chi: See *Qi.*

Chiropractic: A treatment approach that focuses on the relationship of the spinal column, muscles, and skeleton. Spinal *manipulation* and many other treatment techniques are utilized. A chiropractic practitioner receives a D.C. degree (doctor of chiropractic; chiropractor).

Chronic back pain: Pain that persists for a long time (usually more than three months). Also defined as pain beyond the point of tissue healing. Commonly termed *chronic benign back pain*.

Coccydynia: Pain in the *coccyx* or tailbone area.

Coccyx: The small bone at the end of the sacrum; the tailbone.

Cognitive/cognition: A thought; related to thinking.

Conservative treatment: Treatment for your back pain that is non-surgical and does not cause irreversible changes.

CT or CAT scan: A computerized *X ray* recording of sections or slices of your body; literally means Computerized (Axial) Tomography.

Deconditioning syndrome: Generally refers to the negative consequences of resting your body too much due to back pain. Also termed *disuse syndrome*.

Degeneration: A gradual tissue change resulting in lower or less active function. Commonly used to describe aging changes in the disc. Also known as *deterioration*.

Degenerative disc disease: A condition in which disc degeneration, usually at several spinal levels, causes pain.

Disc (intervertebral): Discs are cartilage tissue that are 80 percent water and sit between the vertebrae. A disc has two main parts: the outer ring *(annulus fibrosis)* and the inner ring *(nucleus pulposus)*. Discs separate the spinal vertebrae and act as shock absorbers.

Disc degeneration: A progressive process during which discs lose water and shrink in size. Disc degeneration may or may not cause symptoms and commonly occurs as part of the normal aging process. This term is inaccurately used interchangeably with *degenerative disc disease.*

Disc narrowing: Occurs when a *disc* degenerates to the point of reducing the distance between two adjoining vertebrae.

Discectomy: The surgical removal of all or part of a *disc* (usually in the case of a *herniated disc*).

Discography: A test in which radioactive dye is injected into a disc to see whether the injection of the dye causes the patient to experience his or her usual pain, thereby confirming the disc as a source of pain. Also termed *discogram.*

Dura: The tough, protective, outermost membrane surrounding the spinal cord and brain.

Electrodiagnostic studies: Any test of nerve function in which electricity is used. Nerve conduction studies and electromyography (EMG) are the most common.

Endorphins: Opiates produced in your brain that act as natural painkillers.

Enzyme: Complex proteins that are produced by living cells and catalyze specific biochemical reactions.

Epidural injection: Injection of an anesthetic or other substance into the *epidural space.*

Epidural space: The area that is just outside the *dura* in the spinal canal.

Ergonomics: The study of how you use your body in situations such as work, sports, and other settings. It is the interaction between the body and environment.

Exercise physiologist: A practitioner who has advanced training in proper exercise approaches.

Extension: Bending the spine backward.

Extrusion: A displacement of a portion of the disc through the annulus into the spinal canal. Contrast with *bulging disc, protrusion,* and *sequestration.*

Facet joints: Paired joints that connect the *posterior* (toward the back) aspects of the *vertebrae.*

Failed back surgery syndrome: A chronic back pain syndrome that develops after one or more unsuccessful spine surgeries.

Fascia: A fibrous membrane covering, supporting, and separating muscles. It unites skin with the underlying tissue.

Fibromyalgia: A clinical syndrome defined by specific points of muscle tenderness as well as sleep disturbance, diffuse pain, and fatigue.

Foramen: A natural passage or opening in a bone or membrane; often an opening that a nerve passes through.

Functional restoration program: A multidisciplinary treatment program emphasizing gradually increasing physical function and abilities. See also *work hardening program* and *pain clinic.*

Fusion: The process of "melting" together. A spinal fusion is an operation in which bone grafts are placed in-between two or more *vertebrae* with the goal of having them grow together. A spinal fusion reduces the mobility or movement in that part of the spine.

Gate control theory of pain: The theory which postulates that spinal nerve gates can open (allowing more pain message to reach the brain) and close (allowing less pain message to reach the brain) due to a variety of factors. These gates cause the perception of more or less pain in your brain.

Hemilaminectomy: The surgical removal of a *lamina* on only one side.

Herbal therapy: An ancient treatment approach that includes pills or liquids loaded with plant extracts used for treating illness.

Herniated disc: The extrusion or herniation of the nucleus of a *disc* through the *annulus fibrosis* (outer ring). If the herniated disc material irritates or compresses a nerve, it can cause symptoms such as pain, weakness, or numbness down the leg.

Hydrotherapy: Any therapy or treatment that uses water.

Hypnotherapy: Treatment to induce a trance-like state to foster healing; supposedly bypasses the conscious mind which may be impeding progress or causing illness.

Hypochondriasis: An irrational fear of presumed illness and a preoccupation with the body.

Idiopathic back pain: Back pain that does not have a well-known or identifiable cause. Investigations indicate that most back pain is idiopathic even though practitioners give some type of diagnosis.

Imaging studies: A general term referring to tests such as *CT scan, Magnetic Resonance Imaging (MRI),* and *X ray* that give an image of a body part or structure.

Impotence: The loss of a male's ability to maintain an erection to the point of ejaculation.

Invasive treatment: Any procedure that includes penetrating the skin. This type is differentiated from noninvasive, conservative treatment.

Kinesiologist: A practitioner trained in the anatomy and mechanics of movement.

Kinesophobia: The irrational fear of movement. It is often part of the development of the disuse syndrome and *chronic back pain.*

Lamina: The part of the *vertebra* just behind the spinal canal.

Laminectomy: A surgery to remove part of the *lamina.* It is usually done to relieve pressure on the spinal cord and nerves coming from it.

Laminotomy: The surgical creation of an opening in the *lamina.*

Lesion: An injury, wound, or single infected area in skin disease.

Ligament: A band of fibrous tissue that connects bones or cartilage; supports and strengthens joints.

Lumbar spine: The five *vertebrae* that make up the lower back area of the spine.

Lumbar stenosis: A narrowing (stenosis) of the spinal canal in the *lumbar* naturally small canal or spondylosis.

Lumbosacral sprain/strain: An ambiguous term for injury to the muscles, ligaments, or tendons of the back.

Magnetic Resonance Imaging (MRI): A commonly used imaging technique that uses a strong magnetic field rather than *X ray* and reveals anatomical structures in great detail.

Magnetic therapy: The use of magnetic fields to treat various disorders, including back pain.

Manipulation: The use of pressure or force by a practitioner (chiropractor, osteopath, physical therapist, and so on) to cause movement of the bones of the spine. The cracking noises that are often heard are the result of gases released from the joints. Also termed *adjustment* or *joint mobilization.*

Meridian: In Eastern tradition, the major energy pathways throughout the body along which *Qi* runs.

Modality: Most commonly refers to the *passive modalities* in which you are the passive receiver of a physical therapy treatment (like massage, hot pack, cold pack, ultrasound, and so on).

Muscle spasm: An involuntary contraction or tightening of muscles which results in pain.

Musculoskeletal system: Pertains to the muscles and skeleton.

Myelography (or CT-myelogram): Used for better viewing of structures, a myelogram is an *X ray* and *CT scan* done after the injection of a contrast or radioactive dye into the spinal canal. The side effects (most notably severe headache) of this procedure have been dramatically decreased with the creation of water-soluble dyes. This test should only be done when surgery is being considered.

Myositis: Inflammation of the muscles.

Nerve root: The part of the nerve that exits the spinal canal, goes through the *foramen,* and extends just beyond the *vertebrae.* Several nerve roots come together to form larger nerves such as the sciatic nerve.

Neurological: Pertaining to the study of nervous system diseases.

Neurologist: A physician who has advanced training in problems of the nervous system. Neurologists use nonsurgical treatment approaches.

Neuromuscular: Pertains to both the nerves and the muscles.

Neurosurgeon: A medical doctor who specializes in surgically treating nervous system problems.

Neurotransmitters: Substances that transmit nerve impulses to the brain.

Nucleus pulposus: The inner part or center of the *disc.*

Objective: In medicine, a symptom or condition that is perceptible to others besides the patient — the opposite of *subjective* findings. For example, *x-ray* results are objective findings and pain complaints are subjective.

Opiates: Any medication that contains opium or any of its derivatives; narcotic.

Organic: Explainable by physical causes or related to being physical. In outdated medical jargon, pain was defined as organic or functional (refers to a psychological or emotional basis). Currently, this distinction is not useful and should not be used.

Orthopedist: A physician who has been specially trained in problems of the skeletal system. The training emphasizes surgical treatments.

Osteopath: A doctor who has been trained in a system of manipulative treatment and other techniques. These doctors have a D.O. degree (Doctor of Osteopathy) and can practice similar to physicians that are trained in a traditional medical school.

Osteoporosis: A weakening of the bones as they lose some of their density.

Pain clinic: A multidisciplinary center that uses a variety of specialists to evaluate and treat pain in a highly coordinated and structured fashion. These programs usually emphasize having you take personal responsibility for getting well. See also *functional restoration program* and *work hardening program.*

Pedicle: The bony part of the *vertebrae* that connects it to *posterior* structures. In *fusion* surgeries, it is the site of placement for pedicle screws.

Physiatrist: A medical doctor who has specialized training in problems of the muscles and bones. Physiatrists do not do surgery, and they focus on a rehabilitation approach. This doctor is often recommended as the most appropriate to treat the majority of back pain problems.

Physical therapist: A practitioner trained in rehabilitation. They generally work under a physician's prescription and have an RPT certification (registered physical therapist).

Pinched nerve: A non-medical, layman's term for compression of a nerve.

Podiatrist: A practitioner who has training in the evaluation and treatment of problems of the feet.

Posterior: Situated toward the back.

Protrusion: A distinct bulge in the *annulus fibrosis* due to displaced *disc* material. See also *bulging disc, sequestration,* and contrast with *extrusion.*

Pseudoarthrosis: A condition in which a *fusion* was attempted but inadequate healing of the bone grafts in-between the *vertebrae* resulted in incomplete union.

Psychiatrist: A physician who specializes in the practice of psychiatry. Psychiatrists often focus on medication management. They should have further training in order to manage back pain problems.

Psychological: Having to do with emotions, mental processes, thoughts, and human behaviors.

Psychologist: A practitioner trained in the evaluation and treatment of problems related to mental processes, emotions, and behaviors. Psychologists typically hold one of three different types of doctoral degrees (Ph.D., Psy.D., or Ed.D.). They should have specialized training in pain management in order to treat your back pain.

Psychosomatic: A physical condition that results from, or is made worse by, psychological factors (also termed *psycho-physiological*). These conditions are incorrectly thought to be imaginary problems by the layperson. Rather, actual physical changes occur due to nonphysical forces. See *stress-related back pain.*

Qi: In alternative medicine, it is the vital life energy that runs throughout the body (also spelled *chi*).

Range of motion: The physiological range of joint movement in several different directions.

Recurrent acute back pain: Episodes of back pain that are of varying duration and are separated by relatively pain-free periods. It may actually be the most common type of back pain condition.

Rheumatologist: A medical doctor who specializes in arthritic problems.

Ruptured disc: See *herniated disc.*

Sacroiliac (SI) joint: The joint between the sacrum and pelvis. There are two SI joints, one on each side.

Sacrum: A thick triangular bone situated at the lower end of the spinal column, where it joins both hipbones.

Sciatica: Pain in the buttocks and the back of the legs due to irritation of the sciatic nerve or nerve roots.

Scoliosis: An abnormal curve of the spine to the side. It is often very mild and usually doesn't cause symptoms even though it is often inappropriately used as an excuse for *manipulation* treatment to "straighten" the spine. In severe cases, it is treated with bracing or surgery.

Sedative: Medication used primarily to induce sleep. Also referred to as *hypnotics.*

Sequestration: Complete displacement of part of a *disc* into the spinal canal with no connection to the remaining disc (also termed a *free fragment*). Contrast with *bulging disc, protrusion,* and *extrusion.*

Specificity theory of pain: States that there is a one-to-one relationship between pain and the amount of tissue damage. Proposed by Descartes hundreds of years ago, this theory has been shown to be inaccurate.

Spinal canal: The "tube" (through which the spinal cord passes) that is formed by the opening at the back of each vertebra as they are stacked upon one another.

Spinal stenosis: An abnormal narrowing of the spinal canal. Stenosis is classified as *developmental* (genetic origin), *congenital* (from birth), and *acquired* (developed after birth). Acquired stenosis is the most common due to degenerative changes in the spine.

Spinous processes: The bony bumps on the *vertebrae* to which muscles and *ligaments* attach.

Spondylitis: Rarely a cause of back pain, it is inflammation of the *vertebrae* usually due to normal wear-and-tear changes associated with aging.

Spondylolisthesis: The slipping forward of an individual *vertebra* over the one below it.

Spondylosis: Degenerative changes of the spine, including the vertebrae, the *discs* and the *facet joints.*

Sprain: An injury in which some of the fibers of a supporting *ligament* are ruptured.

Strain: To overexercise, overstretch, or overexert a muscle.

Stress-related back pain: Back pain that is thought to be caused and maintained primarily by emotional and psychological issues. See *tension myositis syndrome.*

Subjective: Medical findings that are a symptom or condition perceptible only to the patient. Subjective should be contrasted with *objective*. Pain is a subjective symptom.

Tendons: A tough cord or band of dense white fibrous connective tissue that attaches a muscle to some other body part.

Tension myositis syndrome (TMS): A pain syndrome often involving the back and neck muscles, caused by unconscious emotional stress.

Thoracic spine: The 12 vertebrae that comprise the middle part of the back. It's rarely a source of back pain and is the most stable part of the spine due to the attachment of the ribs.

Traction: A treatment in which pressure is applied to the spine in order to pull the *vertebrae* away from one another.

Transcutaneous Nerve Stimulation (TNS): A treatment in which low levels of electricity are applied to areas of pain by electrodes placed on the skin.

Ultrasound: The use of sound waves to generate heat below the surface of the skin for treatment purposes.

Vertebra or **Vertebrae:** A bone of the spine. Each vertebra has three parts: the vertebral body, the transverse process, and the spinous process. (Vertebrae is more than one vertebra.)

Work hardening program: A multidisciplinary treatment approach that emphasizes simulating the demands of the work environment as part of rehabilitation. See also *functional restoration program* and *pain clinic.*

X ray: Electromagnetic radiation. A tissue or organ that is dense (such as bone) absorbs more X rays than surrounding tissue. This difference in density produces a relative transparency or picture on the film.

Appendix B

Resources for Additional Information

··

This appendix lists organizations and Web sites that are a great starting point for collecting as much information as you need. These resources can provide you with more information related to your back pain problem, and they can also help you find information about different types of doctors, practitioners, and centers that deal with back pain and related conditions.

Organizations

The organizations in this section can provide you with more information about back pain. These resources can help you find a specific type of back pain specialist and treatment method. Although it is impossible to be exhaustive with such a list, any one of these organizations can likely provide you with many other resources in their specific area.

Acupressure and acupuncture

Acupressure Institute, 1533 Shattuck Ave., Berkeley, CA 94709; phone 800-442-2232 or 510-845-1059.

American Association of Oriental Medicine (formerly American Association of Acupuncture and Oriental Medicine), 433 Front St., Catasauqua, PA 18032; phone 610-266-1433.

Australian Acupuncture and Chinese Medicine Association Ltd., P.O. Box 5142, West End, Brisbane, Australia 4101; phone 800-025-334 (within Australia) or 617-3846-5866 (outside Australia).

British Medical Acupuncture Society, Newton House, Newton Ln., Whitley, Warrington, Cheshire, U.K. WA4 4JA; phone 44-1925-730727.

Alternative and complementary medicine (general)

Institute for Complementary Medicine, Unit 15, Tavern Quay Commercial Centre, Rope St., London, U.K. SE16 1TX; phone 171-237-5165.

Office of Alternative Medicine (OAM) Information Clearinghouse, National Institutes of Health (NIH), P.O. Box 8218, Silver Spring, MD 20907-8218; phone 301-496-9600 or 888-644-6226.

Biofeedback

Association for Applied Psychophysiology and Biofeedback, 10200 West 44th Ave., Suite 304, Wheat Ridge, CO 80033. Please include a self-addressed, stamped envelope when requesting information by mail.

Center for Applied Psychophysiology, Menninger Clinic, P.O. Box 829, Topeka, KS 66601-0882; phone 785-350-5000 or 800-351-9058.

Thought Technology, Ltd., 2180 Belgrave Ave., Montreal, Quebec H4A 2L8; phone 800-361-3651.

Bodywork

American Oriental Bodywork Therapy Association, Laurel Oak Corporate Center, Suite 408, 1010 Haddonfield-Berlin Rd., Voorhees, NJ 08043; phone 609-782-1616; e-mail aobta@prodigy.net

Associated Bodywork and Massage Professionals, 28677 Buffalo Park Rd., Evergreen, CO 80439; phone 970-282-8086 or 800-458-2267.

Chiropractic

American Chiropractic Association, 1701 Clarendon Blvd., Arlington, VA 22209; phone 703-276-8800.

International Chiropractors Association, 1110 N. Glebe Rd., Suite 1000, Arlington, VA 22201; phone 703-528-5000 or 800-423-4690.

World Chiropractic Alliance, 2950 N. Dobson Rd., Suite 1, Chandler, AZ 85224; phone 800-347-1011.

Consumer information and protection

Consumer Product Safety Commission, Washington, D.C.; phone 301-504-0990.

Council of Better Business Bureaus, Inc. National Headquarters, 4200 Wilson Blvd., Arlington, VA 22203; phone 703-276-0100; Web site www.bbb.org

Drugs, medications, and products

Drug Enforcement Administration, U.S. Department of Justice, 801 1st St. N.W., Washington, D.C. 20001; phone 202-305-8500.

Office of Consumer Affairs (HFE-88), Food and Drug Administration, 5600 Fishers Lane, Room 16-85, Rockville, MD 20857; phone 301-827-4422; Web site www.fda.gov/oca/guide

Homeopathy

British Institute of Homeopathy and Complementary Medicine, 520 Washington Blvd., Suite 423, Marina del Rey, CA 90292; phone 310-306-5408.

National Center for Homeopathy, 1495 St. Joseph Blvd., Gloucester, Ontario, Canada K1C 7K9; phone 613-830-4759.

United Kingdom Homeopathic Medical Association, 6 Livingstone Rd., Gravesend, Kent, U.K. DA12 5DZ; phone 44-1474-560336.

Hypnosis and hypnotherapy

American Society of Clinical Hypnosis, 2200 E. Devon Ave., Suite 291, Des Plaines, IL 60018; phone 847-297-3317.

International Medical and Dental Hypnotherapy Association, 4110 Edgeland, Suite 800, Royal Oak, MI 48073; phone 800-257-5467 (outside Michigan) or 248-549-5594.

London College of Clinical Hypnotherapists, 229a Sussex Gardens, Lancaster Gate, London, U.K. W2 2RL; phone 44-171-402-9037.

Massage therapy

American Massage Therapy Association, 820 Davis St., Suite 100, Evanston, IL 60201-4444; phone 847-864-0123.

Esalen Institute, Hwy 1, Big Sur, CA 93920; phone 831-667-3000; Web site www.io.com/~hambone/web/esalen

Massage Training Institute, 24 Highbury Grove, London, U.K. N5 2EA; phone 44-171-266-5313.

Meditation

Academy for Guided Imagery, P.O. Box 2070 Mill Valley, CA 94942; phone 800-726-2070.

American Holistic Medical Association, 6728 Old McLean Village Dr., McLean, VA 22101; phone 703-556-9728; Web site www.holisticmedicine.org

Center for Spiritual Awareness, P.O. Box 7, Lake Rabun Rd., Lakemont, GA 30552-0007; phone 706-782-4723.

Himalayan Institute of Canada, 371 Berkeley St., Toronto, Ontario, Canada M5A 2X8; phone 416-960-5062.

Himalayan Institute of Great Britain, 70 Claremont Rd., West Ealing, London, U.K., W13 ODG; phone 44-181-991-8090.

Mental health

American Psychiatric Association, 1400 K Street NW, Washington, D.C. 20005; phone 202-682-6000; fax 202-682-6850; Web site www.psych.org

American Psychosomatic Society, 6728 Old McLean Village Drive, McLean, VA 22101; phone 703-559-9222; Web site www.psychosomatic.org

Canadian Psychiatric Association, 237 Argyle Avenue, #200, Ottawa, Ontario K2P 1BP; phone 613-234-2815.

National Mental Health Association, 1021 Prince St., Alexandria, VA 22314-2971; phone 703-684-7722 or 800-969-6642.

Mind-body medicine (general)

American Association for Therapeutic Humor, 222 S. Meramec, Suite 303, St. Louis, MO 63105; phone 314-863-6232.

American Psychological Association, 750 First Street NE, Washington, D.C. 2002-4242; phone 202-366-5700 or 202-336-5500; Web site www.apa.org

Center for the Improvement of Human Functioning, 3100 North Hillside Ave., Wichita, KS 67219-3904; phone 316-682-3100.

Mind-Body Medical Center, Deaconess Hospital, Deaconess Rd., Boston, MA 02215; phone 617-632-9525.

Nutrition

American Dietetic Association, 216 W. Jackson Blvd., Suite 800, Chicago, IL 60606; phone 800-366-1655.

USDA Center for Nutrition Policy and Promotion, 1120 20th St. NW, Suite 200 North, Washington, D.C. 20036; phone 202-418-2312.

Osteopathy

American Academy of Osteopathy, 3500 DePauw Blvd., Suite 1080, Indianapolis, IN 46268; phone 317-879-1881; fax 317-879-0563.

American Osteopathic Association, 142 East Ontario St., Chicago, IL 60611; phone 312-202-8000.

British Osteopathic Association, Langham House East, Mill Street, Bedfordshire, U.K. LU1 2NA; phone 44-158-248-8455.

Pain (general)

American Academy of Pain Medicine, 4700 W. Lake Ave., Glen View, IL 60025; phone 847-375-4731.

American Chronic Pain Association, P.O. Box 850, Rocklin, CA 95677; phone 916-632-0922.

American Pain Society, 4700 W. Lake Avenue, Glenview IL 60025; phone 847-375-4715; Web site www.ampainsoc.org

International Association for the Study of Pain, 909 NE 43rd St., Suite 306, Seattle, WA 98105-6020; phone 206-547-6409; Web site www.halcyon.com/iasp/

National Chronic Pain Outreach Association, 7979 Old Georgetown Road, #100, Bethesda, MD 20814-2429; phone 301-652-4948.

Professional medical societies (see also Surgery)

American Academy of Family Physicians, 8880 Ward Parkway, Kansas City, MO 64114; phone 816-333-9700.

American Academy of Physical Medicine and Rehabilitation, One IBM Plaza, Suite 2500, Chicago, IL 60611-3604; phone 312-464-9700; Web site www.aapmr.org

American Board of Medical Specialties, 1007 Church St., Suite 404, Evanston, IL 60210-5913; phone 847-491-9091; Web site www.abms.org

American Chiropractic Association, 1701 Clarendon Blvd., Arlington, VA 22209; phone 703-276-8800; Web site www.amerchiro.org

American College of Sports Medicine, 401 W. Michigan St., Indianapolis, IN 46202; phone 317-637-9200.

American Medical Association, 515 N. State St., Chicago, IL 60610-4320; phone 312-464-5000 or 800-621-8335.

American Orthopedic Society for Sports Medicine, 6300 North River Rd,. Suite 200, Rosemont, IL 60018; phone 847-292-4900.

American Osteopathic Board of Surgery, 3 Mac Koil Ave., Dayton, OH 45405; phone 937-252-0868 or 800-782-5355; Web site www.aobs.org

Canadian Association of Physical Medicine and Rehabilitation, 774 Echo Dr., 5th Floor, Ottawa, Ontario K1S 5N8; phone 613-730-6245.

Canadian Orthopaedic Association, 1440 Ste-Catherine Street West #421, Montreal, Quebec H3G 1R8; phone 414-874-9003.

Society of Behavioral Medicine, 7611 Elmwood Avenue, Middleton, WI 53562; phone 608-827-7267; Web site www.sbmweb.org

Relaxation techniques

The Mind-Body Medical Institute , 110 Francis St., Suite 1A, Boston, MA 02215; phone 617-632-9525; fax 617-632-7383.

Sleep problems

American Sleep Disorders Association, 6301 Bandel Rd., Suite 101, Rochester, MN 55901; phone 507-287-6006.

Spinal societies

American Back Society, St. Joseph's Professional Center, 2647 E. 14th Street, Suite 401, Oakland, CA 94601; phone 510-536-9929; Web site www. americanbacksoc.org

International Society for the Study of the Lumbar Spine, 2075 Bayview Avenue, Room A401, Toronto, Ontario, M4N 3M5; phone 416-480-4833; Web site www.issls.org

North American Spine Society, 6300 North River Road, Suite 500, Rosemont, IL 60018-4231; phone 847-698-1630; Web site www.spine.org

Substance abuse

Alcoholics Anonymous (AA), consult a phone book for the nearest chapter; Web site www.alcoholics-anonymous.org/index

Narcotics Anonymous (NA), World Service Office, P.O. Box 9999, Van Nuys CA 91409; phone 818-773-9999.

National Institute on Drug Abuse (NIDA), 5600 Fishers Lane, Room 10A-39, Rockville, MD 20851; phone 301-443-6245 or 800-662-4357; Web site www.nida.nih.gov

Surgery

American Academy of Orthopaedic Surgeons, 6300 North River Road, Rosemont, IL 60018; phone 847-823-7186 or 800-346-AAOS; Web site www.aaos.org

American Association of Neurological Surgeons, 22 South Washington Street, Park Ridge, IL 60068; phone 847-692-9500.

American Board of Neurological Surgery, 6550 Fannin St., Suite 2139, Houston, TX 77030-2701; phone 713-790-6015.

American Board of Surgery, 1617 John F. Kennedy Blvd., Suite 860, Philadelphia, PA 19103-1847; phone 215-568-4000.

American College of Surgeons, 633 Saint Clair St., Chicago, IL 60611; phone 312-202-5000; Web site www.facs.org/index

Yoga

American Yoga Association, P.O. Box 19986, Sarasota, FL 34276; phone 941-927-4977; Web site http://m2.aol.com/amyogaassn/index

British Wheel of Yoga, 1 Hamilton Place, Boston Rd., Sleaford, Lincolnshire U.K., NG34 7ES; phone 44-1529-306859.

Sivananda Yoga, 5178 South Lawrence Blvd., Montreal, Quebec, Canada H2T 1R8; phone 514-279-3545.

Internet Resources

This section provides Web site addresses for selected organizations and topics. Browse through the following sites to find doctors and other health-care practitioners, information on treatments, research results, and more.

Achoo Online Health Services: www.achoo.com

Agency for Health Care Policy and Research (AHCPR): www.ahcpr.gov

Alternative Medicine: www.pitt.edu/~cbw/altm.html

Biofeedback Society of Europe: www.bfe.org

CHIRObase: www.chirobase.org

Choosing and working with your primary care doctor: www.coolware.com/health/medical_reporter/choosing.html

Combined Health Information Index: chid.nih.gov

Comprehensive Orthopedics: www.corortho.com

Comprehensive Spine Care: www.spineinstitute.com

Cybertec brace: biocybernetics.net

DocFinder: www.docboard.org

Family medicine related internet resources:
griffin.vcu.edu/~dimlist/index.htm

Finding a doctor: www.lhs-be-well.org

Food & Drug Administration: www.fda.gov

Health hotlines: sis.nlm.nih.gov/hotlines

Health Oasis: www.mayohealth.org/index.htm

Health World Online: www.healthy.net

HSTAT — Health Services/Technology Assessment Text: text.nlm.nih.gov

Johns Hopkins University's IntelliHealth site:
www.intelihealth.com/IH/ihtIH

Medical Matrix: www.medmatrix.org/index.asp

MEDLINE: www.nlm.nih.gov/databases/medline.html

Medscape: www.medscape.com

Medsite: www.medsite.com

Mind and Back Pain: www.tensionmyositis.com

MR-Neurography: www.neurography.com

Multimedia Medical Reference Library: www.med-library.com

National Health Information Center: nhic-nt.health.org

National Institutes of Health: www.nih.gov

National Institutes of Health Office of Alternative Medicine:
altmed.od.nih.gov/oam

National Library of Medicine: www.nlm.nih.gov

New England Journal of Medicine: www.nejm.org

North American Spine Society: www.spine.org

Online medical reference system: www.kumc.edu/service/dykes/ refassist/facts/rankrec.html

Quackwatch: www.quackwatch.com

Reuters Health Information Services: www.reutershealth.com

Sleep information: www.lifedesigntech.com

Surgery Preparation: www.surgeryprep.com

US News Online: America's Best Hospitals: www.usnews.com/usnews/nycu/health/hosptl/tophosp.htm

World Health Organization: www.who.org

Product Resources

Check out these sites for products that can help relieve your back pain.

AHC Products (mattresses, massage loungers, ergonomic seating, adjustable beds, and magnetic therapy): www.ahcproducts.com/back_index.htm

American Back Care Company (ergonomic desk chairs, pillows, and various products): www.americanback.com

Back Be Nimble — Your One Stop Back Shop (products for ergonomic support, videos, books, and massage devices): www.backbenimble.com

Bio Cybernetics International (back braces): biocybernetics.net

Brookstone (various massage and sleep products): www.brookstone.com

Hammacher Schlemmer (various massage tools): www.hammacher.com

Relax the Back (various back pain products): www.relaxtheback.com

Sharper Image (various back pain products): www.sharperimage.com

A Back and Neck Support Store (various back pain products): www.vitalityweb.com/backstore/productindex.html

The Healthy Back Store (ergonomic desk chairs, exercise products, luggage, travel aides, and back savers): www2.healthyback.com/hbs/newstuff.qry

Index

vertebral body, 23
vibration exposure, 245–246
visualization. *See* imagery

• W •

walking. *See also* posture
  breathing and, 208
  head and, 208
  head-forward, 207
  healthy, 208–209
  heel-pounding, 207
  loose, 207
  pelvis and, 208
  posture, checking, 207–208
  shoes, 209
  smoothly, 208–209
  stiff, 207
  stomach-out, 207
  stress, 208
  tension release and, 208
Walking Yourself Healthy, 209
wall slide exercise. *See also*
    back exercise program
  benefits of, 229
  description, 229
  illustrated, 230
warm-up stretch
  defined, 256–257
  golf, 267
  skiing, 263
water therapy
  active, 99
  benefits, 99
  passive, 100
weight lifting, 265–266
whole-person approach, 1
work
  back pain and, 243
  blocking from returning to,
    247–248
  choosing return to,
    248–249
  commuting to, 246
  dissatisfaction, 247
  lifting/bending, 244–245
  office, returning to,
    251–254

preparing to return to,
    249–251
  returning to, 247–249
  risky, 244–247
  sit down, 246–247
  vibration exposure,
    245–246
work hardening program
  characteristics, 96
  defined, 96–97, 332
  quality, checking, 97
  screening evaluation, 97
workbook (surgery), 132

• X •

X rays
  candidates for, 80
  chiropractors and, 157, 158
  defined, 80, 332
  no findings on, 81

• Y •

yoga. *See also* complemen-
    tary medicine
  asanas, 162
  back exercise and, 165–166
  for back pain, 164–167
  daily journal and, 166–167
  defined, 17, 161
  goal for back, 166
  Hatha, 162–164
  instructors, finding,
    165–166
  key for back, 166
  lifestyle changes, 161
  meditation, 162, 164
  pranayama, 162
  resources, 340
  samadhi and, 162, 164
  sleep and, 167
Yoga For Dummies, 161

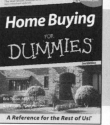
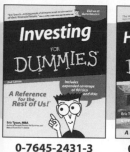
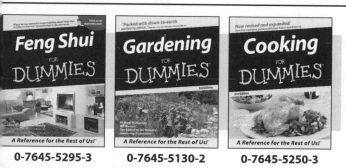
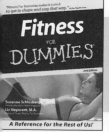
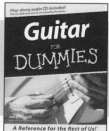
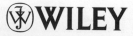

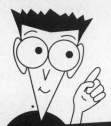

FOR DUMMIES®

A world of resources to help you grow

TRAVEL

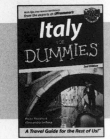

Italy FOR **DUMMIES** 2nd Edition
A Travel Guide for the Rest of Us!
0-7645-5453-0

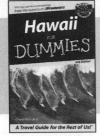

Hawaii FOR **DUMMIES** 2nd Edition
A Travel Guide for the Rest of Us!
0-7645-5438-7

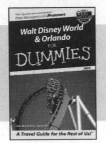

Walt Disney World & Orlando FOR **DUMMIES** 2003
A Travel Guide for the Rest of Us!
0-7645-5444-1

Also available:

America's National Parks For Dummies
(0-7645-6204-5)

Caribbean For Dummies
(0-7645-5445-X)

Cruise Vacations For Dummies 2003
(0-7645-5459-X)

Europe For Dummies
(0-7645-5456-5)

Ireland For Dummies
(0-7645-6199-5)

France For Dummies
(0-7645-6292-4)

Las Vegas For Dummies
(0-7645-5448-4)

London For Dummies
(0-7645-5416-6)

Mexico's Beach Resorts For Dummies
(0-7645-6262-2)

Paris For Dummies
(0-7645-5494-8)

RV Vacations For Dummies
(0-7645-5443-3)

EDUCATION & TEST PREPARATION

Speak Spanish — the fun and easy way!
Spanish FOR **DUMMIES®**
A Reference for the Rest of Us!
Berlitz
Susana Wald
0-7645-5194-9

Algebra FOR **DUMMIES**
Mary Jane Sterling
A Reference for the Rest of Us!
0-7645-5325-9

U.S. History FOR **DUMMIES**
Steve Wiegand
A Reference for the Rest of Us!
0-7645-5249-X

Also available:

The ACT For Dummies
(0-7645-5210-4)

Chemistry For Dummies
(0-7645-5430-1)

English Grammar For Dummies
(0-7645-5322-4)

French For Dummies
(0-7645-5193-0)

GMAT For Dummies
(0-7645-5251-1)

Inglés Para Dummies
(0-7645-5427-1)

Italian For Dummies
(0-7645-5196-5)

Research Papers For Dummies
(0-7645-5426-3)

SAT I For Dummies
(0-7645-5472-7)

U.S. History For Dummies
(0-7645-5249-X)

World History For Dummies
(0-7645-5242-2)

HEALTH, SELF-HELP & SPIRITUALITY

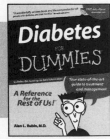

Diabetes FOR **DUMMIES**
A Reference for the Rest of Us!
Alan L. Rubin, M.D.
0-7645-5154-X

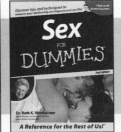

Sex FOR **DUMMIES** 2nd Edition
Dr. Ruth K. Westheimer
A Reference for the Rest of Us!
0-7645-5302-X

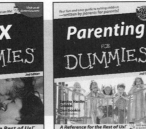

Parenting FOR **DUMMIES** 2nd Edition
Sandra Hardin Gookin Dan Gookin
A Reference for the Rest of Us!
0-7645-5418-2

Also available:

The Bible For Dummies
(0-7645-5296-1)

Controlling Cholesterol For Dummies
(0-7645-5440-9)

Dating For Dummies
(0-7645-5072-1)

Dieting For Dummies
(0-7645-5126-4)

High Blood Pressure For Dummies
(0-7645-5424-7)

Judaism For Dummies
(0-7645-5299-6)

Menopause For Dummies
(0-7645-5458-1)

Nutrition For Dummies
(0-7645-5180-9)

Potty Training For Dummies
(0-7645-5417-4)

Pregnancy For Dummies
(0-7645-5074-8)

Rekindling Romance For Dummies
(0-7645-5303-8)

Religion For Dummies
(0-7645-5264-3)

Available wherever books are sold. Go to www.dummies.com or call 1-877-762-2974 to order direct